Evidence-based Paediatric and Adolescent Diabetes

Edited by

Jeremy Allgrove

Barts and the London NHS Trust
Royal London Hospital
London, UK

Peter G.F. Swift

Leicester Royal Infirmary
Children's Hospital
Leicester, UK

Stephen Greene

University of Dundee
Department of Maternal and Child Health Sciences
Ninewells Hospital
Dundee, UK

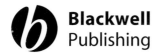

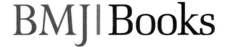

Blackwell Publishing, Inc., 350 Main Street, Malden, Massachusetts 02148-5020, USA
Blackwell Publishing Ltd, 9600 Garsington Road, Oxford OX4 2DQ, UK
Blackwell Publishing Asia Pty Ltd, 550 Swanston Street, Carlton, Victoria 3053, Australia

First published

1   2007

Library of Congress Cataloging-in-Publication Data

Evidence-based paediatric and adolescent diabetes / edited by Jeremy Allgrove, Peter G.F. Swift, Stephen Greene.
     p. ; cm.
   "BMJ books."
   Includes bibliographical references.
   ISBN 978-1-4051-5292-1 (hardback)
1. Diabetes in children.   2. Diabetes in adolescence.   3. Evidence-based medicine.
I. Allgrove, Jeremy.   II. Swift, Peter G. F.   III. Greene, Stephen A.

[DNLM: 1. Diabetes Mellitus.   2. Adolescent.   3. Child.   4. Evidence-Based Medicine.
WK 810 E93 2007]

RJ420.D5.E95 2007
618.3′ 646–dc22

                              2007013626

ISBN: 978-1-4051-5292-1

A catalogue record for this title is available from the British Library

Set in 9.5/12 Minion by Aptara Inc., New Delhi, India
Printed and bound in Singapore by Markono Print Media Pte Ltd

Commissioning Editor: Mary Banks
Editorial Assistant: Victoria Pittman
Development Editor: Simone Dudziak
Production Controller: Rachel Edwards

For further information on Blackwell Publishing, visit our website:
http://www.blackwellpublishing.com

Contents

List of contributors, v

Foreword, ix

Preface, xi

1 Methodology of evidence-based medicine, 1
Jeremy Allgrove

2 Definition, epidemiology and classification of diabetes and structure of the diabetes team, 9
Maria Craig, Sarah J. Glastras & Kim Donaghue

3 Aetiology of type 1 diabetes mellitus – genetics, autoimmunity and trigger factors, 26
Loredana Marcovecchio, David B. Dunger,
Mark Peakman & Keith W. Taylor

4 Type 1 diabetes mellitus – management, 42
Joanne J. Spinks, Julie A. Edge, Krystyna Matyka & Shital Malik

5 Type 1 diabetes mellitus in the very young child, 63
Stuart Brink

6 Adolescence and diabetes: clinical and social science perspectives, 76
Alexandra Greene & Stephen Greene

7 Management of special situations in diabetes, 93
Fergus J. Cameron & Jeremy Allgrove

8 Dietary management: optimising diabetes outcomes, 104
Sheridan Waldron

9 Education in childhood diabetes, 123
Peter G.F. Swift

10 Psychological interventions in childhood diabetes, 141
John W. Gregory & Sue Channon

11 Screening for associated conditions and prevention of complications, 157
Catherine Peters & Jeremy Allgrove

12 Type 2 diabetes mellitus – genetics, diagnosis and management. Polycystic ovarian syndrome, 175
John Porter & Timothy G. Barrett

13 Rare forms of diabetes, 197
Julian Shield, Maciej T. Malecki, Nicola A. Bridges & Jeremy Allgrove

14 Diabetes and information technology, 221
Kenneth J. Robertson

Abbreviations, 228

Index, 232

Contributors

Jeremy Allgrove MB BChir, MA, MD, FRCP, FRCPCH

Consultant in Paediatric Endocrinology and
  Diabetes
Barts and the London NHS Trust
Royal London Hospital
London, UK

Timothy G. Barrett PhD, MB BS, MRCP, MRCPCH, DCH

Professor of Paediatrics
Institute of Child Health
Birmingham, UK

Nicola A. Bridges, DM, MRCP, FRCPCH

Consultant Paediatric Endocrinologist
Chelsea and Westminster Hospital
London, UK

Stuart Brink, MD

Senior Endocrinologist
New England Diabetes and Endocrinology
  Center (NEDEC)
Associate Clinical Professor of Pediatrics
Tufts University School of Medicine
Waltham, USA

Fergus J. Cameron

Associate Professor
Head Diabetes Services
Deputy Director
Department of Endocrinology and Diabetes
Royal Children's Hospital
Parkville, Australia

Sue Channon, BSc D Clin Psych

Consultant Clinical Psychologist
Child Psychology Department
Children's Centre
St David's Hospital Canton
Cardiff, UK

Maria Craig, MB BS, PhD, FRACP, MMed (ClinEpid)

Paediatric Endocrinologist
Institute of Endocrinology and Diabetes
Children's Hospital Westmead
Westmead, Australia

Kim Donaghue, MB BS, PhD, FRACP

Associate Professor
Head of Diabetes Services
The Children's Hospital at Westmead
University of Sydney
Westmead, Australia

David B. Dunger, MD, FRCPCH

Professor of Paediatrics
Department of Paediatrics
Addenbrooke's NHS Trust
Cambridge, UK

Julie A. Edge, MD, FRCPCH

Consultant in Paediatric Diabetes
  and Endocrinology
Department of Paediatrics
John Radcliffe Hospital
Oxford, UK

Sarah J. Glastras, MB BS(Hons), BSc Psychol(Hons)

Junior Medical Officer
Institute of Endocrinology and Diabetes
The Children's Hospital at Westmead
Westmead, Australia

Alexandra Greene

Senior Research Fellow
Health Services Research Centre
University of Aberdeen
Scotland, UK

Stephen Greene, MB BS, FRCP, FRCPCH

Reader in Child and Adolescent Health
Maternal and Child Health Sciences
University of Dundee
Ninewells Hospital
Dundee, UK

John W. Gregory, MB ChB, DCH, MD, FRCP, FRCPCH

Professor of Paediatric Endocrinology
Department of Child Health
Wales College of Medicine
Cardiff University
Cardiff, UK

Maciej T. Malecki, MD, PhD

Senior Lecturer
Department of Metabolic Diseases
Jagiellonian University
Medical College
Krakow, Poland

Shital Malik, MRCPCH, MD, DCH, DNB

Paediatric Specialist Registrar
University Hospital Coventry and
    Warwickshire NHS Trust
Coventry, UK

Loredana Marcovecchio

Research Fellow
University of Cambridge
Department of Paediatrics
Addenbrooke's Hospital
Cambridge, UK

Krystyna Matyka, MRCP, MD

Senior Lecturer in Paediatrics
Clinical Sciences Research Institute
University of Warwick
Coventry, UK

Mark Peakman, BSc, MSc, PhD, MB BS, FRCPath

Professor of Clinical Immunology
Department of Immunology
King's College London
School of Medicine at Guy's
King's College and St Thomas' Hospital
Guy's Hospital
London, UK

Catherine Peters, MD, MRCPCH

SpR Paediatric Endocrinology
Royal London Hospital
London, UK

John Porter, BA (Hons), MB BS

Specialist Registrar
Department of Endocrinology
Birmingham Children's Hospital
Birmingham, UK

Kenneth J. Robertson, MB ChB, FRCP, FRCPCH

Consultant Paediatrician
Royal Hospital for Sick Children
Glasgow, UK

J.P.H. Shield, MD, MRCP, FRCPCH

Reader in Diabetes and Metabolic
    Endocrinology
University of Bristol
Bristol Royal Hospital for Children
Bristol, UK

Joanne J. Spinks, BSc (Hons), BM, MRCPCH

Specialist Registrar Paediatric Diabetes and
    Endocrinology
John Radcliffe Hospital
Oxford, UK

Peter G.F. Swift, MA, FRCPCH, DCH

Consultant Paediatrician
Leicester Royal Infirmary
Children's Hospital
Leicester, UK

Keith W. Taylor, MB, PhD, FRCP
Emeritus Professor
Barts and the London
Queen Mary's School of Medicine and
   Dentistry
London, UK

Sheridan Waldron, PhD
Dietetic Manager
Leicestershire Nutrition and Dietetic
Service
Leicester Royal Infirmary
Leicester, UK

Foreword

There appear to be a number of irrefutable facts about diabetes in childhood: some to do with aetiology and others related to the management of this group of disorders [1]. First, type 1 diabetes mellitus (T1DM) accounts for the vast majority of children and youths with diabetes. T1DM is increasing in incidence worldwide at the rate of 2–5% per year, with immigrant populations relatively quickly assuming the higher incidence in their new countries. Second, there has been a staggering increase in childhood obesity worldwide, bringing with it a significant increase in earlier onset of T2DM, probably not yet of the epidemic proportions in the youth that many have threatened. Third, molecular genetic technologies have helped unravel the mysteries of an increasing number of monogenic types of diabetes, both neonatal and childhood/young adult onset. Finally, the data derived from two sentinel randomised control trials, namely the Diabetes Control and Complications Trial (DCCT) and its extension observation study Epidemiology of Diabetes Interventions and Complications (EDIC) in T1DM, and the United Kingdom Prospective Diabetes Study (UKPDS) in T2DM inform the current approach to the control of hyperglycaemia in order to prevent the onset or slow the progression of diabetes-related complications.

While certain 'facts' may seem irrefutable, what is less robust are the data needed to fill in the details about the why's, when's, what's and how-to's about the cause, course and complications of all types of diabetes. This is where a careful distillation of the available information is required and decisions are made based on the most convincing evidence. The discipline of evidence-based medicine has arisen and rapidly evolved as a means of accomplishing this as accurately and reproducibly as possible in order to provide the state-of-the-art recommendations for diagnosis, treatment and prognosis of the condition under review. There are several caveats that warrant attention here. First, the recommendations can only be as strong as the data that underpin them. Second, there is in the field of diabetes in children and the youth a paucity of data on which to make the highest grade recommendations. This is a fact of life in most areas of paediatric medicine. Finally, the evidence changes, and it may do so quite rapidly with the emergence of new therapeutic agents (e.g. insulin analogues and oral hypoglycaemic agents). Hopefully, this means that as steadily as the evidence accumulates and improves, so does the treatment and outcome of the condition.

A couple of sobering thoughts are in order here. First, a study from the Centers for Disease Control in Atlanta, USA [2], in 2003 reported a loss of almost 20 life years for 10-year-old children diagnosed with diabetes in the year 2000. And Gale from Bristol [3] has pointed out that the majority of children with diabetes worldwide will *not* achieve levels of control commensurate with reasonable protection from microvascular complications. Furthermore, '*the individual and communal legacy of poor glucose control will remain with us for the next thirty years, even if an effective means of preventing new cases of the disease were to be introduced tomorrow.'* Gale concluded that *'the greatest need is for more effective implementation of what is already known'* [3].

In this book, editor Jeremy Allgrove has marshalled the energies and expertise of a highly qualified and accomplished international group of childhood diabetes specialists to sift carefully through the evidence ('what is already known') and make the best possible recommendations for the care of children and the youth with diabetes. The result is an outstanding addition to the literature in this field. This has been a gargantuan, but highly worthwhile, task at a number of levels. First, it helps the reader understand just how strong (or not) the evidence is for recommending one approach over another. Then, it highlights the areas where the evidence is not based on the type of studies needed to provide high-grade recommendations, but in which there is general consensus as to a most sensible approach. In many of these instances, the gold-standard study, a randomised controlled trial, is unlikely to be performed. Finally, it lays bare the issues that remain inadequately addressed such that no definitive recommendations can be made.

Undoubtedly, both the editor and the chapter authors as well as the readers hope that the recommendations will soon be out of date with the emergence of 'newer and better' approaches to diabetes prediction and prevention in both T1DM and T2DM, management that facilitates achievement and maintenance of normoglycaemia without the ever-present threat of hypoglycaemia and prevention or reversal of complications. Until such time as these advances become reality, this volume will stand as a wonderful navigator for health-care professionals involved in the care of children with all types of diabetes. My heartiest congratulations to Dr Allgrove and his contributors for their superb efforts.

Denis Daneman
Past President, ISPAD

References

1 Daneman D. Type 1 diabetes. *Lancet* 2006; **367**: 847–58.
2 Narayan KM, Boyle JP, Thompson TJ *et al.* Lifetime risk for diabetes mellitus in the United States. *JAMA* 2003; **290**: 1884–90.
3 Gale EA. Type 1 diabetes in the young: the harvest of sorrow goes on. *Diabetologia* 2005; **48**: 1435–8.

Preface

This book is intended to be part of a series of evidence based publications on a variety of topics. It is particularly intended as a companion volume to 'Evidence-Based Diabetes' which will deal in a similar manner with the field of adult diabetes. It is not intended to be yet another guideline to the treatment of diabetes as several of these have already been published, but rather to concentrate on the evidence that is available in the paediatric field to support the development of those guidelines. Whilst we have tried to be as comprehensive as possible, there are certain topics that have not yet had a significant impact on paediatric practice and are therefore not covered. These include inhaled insulins, the artificial pancreas and pancreatic cell transplantation. Nevertheless, there are topics covered, not least the chapter on Type 2 Diabetes, which are unlikely to have been included in a similar publication even five years ago but which are of increasing importance today.

It has been an enormous privilege to have been asked to edit this edition of 'Evidence-Based Paediatric and Adolescent Diabetes' and a great pleasure to be able to work with my co-authors, Peter Swift and Stephen Greene, both of them long-standing colleagues and good friends. I wish to thank them and all of our co-authors for their hard work and effort in seeing this book through to its final stages. I also wish to thank the publishers, Blackwell's, for their unstinting support and encouragement in making it possible.

Many thanks also to all of the authors who have contributed to the book and for their efforts in getting manuscripts in on time so that publication can go ahead within the time frame originally envisaged. Finally I wish to thank my wife, Natalie, for her patience and understanding in tolerating my slaving over a hot computer when other attractions beckoned.

When one is responsible for editing a book that is dependent upon evidence, it is, of course, necessary to ensure that the evidence presented is as was originally published, even if the conclusions reached in those papers were dubious. Martin Routh (1755–1854), British academic and President of Magdalen College, Oxford from 1791 until his death in 1854, was once asked by an admiring student, towards the end of his life, to supply a precept which might serve as a guiding principle in a young man's life. 'I think, sir,' he replied, after a moment's thought, 'since you come for the advice of an old man, you will find it a very good practice always to verify your references!' I hope that all of the references quoted here have been verified.

Jeremy Allgrove,
Editor-in-Chief

CHAPTER 1

Methodology of evidence-based medicine

Jeremy Allgrove

When one admits that nothing is certain one must, I think, also admit that some things are much more nearly certain than others.
—Bertrand Russell. 'Am I an Atheist or an Agnostic?' 1947
British author, mathematician and philosopher (1872–1970)

Introduction

Over the past two decades evidence-based medicine has become increasingly important in determining the way in which medicine is practised. The medical profession has always had a reputation for questioning its own practices, as demonstrated by the number of scientific publications that have appeared since medical journals were invented. As a result, considerable advances in health care have been achieved.

Nevertheless, it is not always the case that ideas that have developed are necessarily correct, and dogmatic statements or assumptions that have been made have sometimes turned out to be false when re-examined more rigorously. Although it has been suggested that 'it is curious, even shocking, that the adjective "evidence-based" is needed' [1], it is nevertheless the purpose of evidence-based medicine to limit these false assumptions and incorrect dogma so that patients may be treated in the best possible way with the tools available.

What is evidence-based health care?

The Cochrane library [2] quotes three slightly different definitions of evidence-based health care:
• Evidence-based health care is the conscientious use of current best evidence in making decisions about the care of individual patients or the delivery of health services. Current best evidence is up-to-date information from relevant, valid research about the effects of different forms of health care, the potential for harm from exposure to particular agents, the accuracy of diagnostic tests and the predictive power of prognostic factors [3].
• Evidence-based clinical practice is an approach to decision-making in which the clinician uses the best evidence available, in consultation with the patient, to decide upon the option which suits that patient best [4].
• Evidence-based medicine is the conscientious, explicit and judicious use of current best evidence in making decisions about the care of individual patients. The practice

of evidence-based medicine means integrating individual clinical expertise with the best available external clinical evidence from systematic research [5].

All of these definitions are very similar but differ slightly in emphasis on such matters as patient involvement and reliance on diagnostic tests.

What constitutes proof?

Scientific proof has always depended on probabilities rather than absolute proof and is determined by observation and perception. Both of these are open to misinterpretation and can be refuted by other observations that may be made under different circumstances. Statistical analysis is frequently used to 'verify' observations and it has become usual practice to accept that a probability of something being true with 95% certainty ($p < 0.05$) means that observation is 'true'. By definition, it also means that there is a 5% chance that it will not be true.

In contrast, there is a fundamental difference between a scientific proof and a mathematical proof [6, pp. 21–2]. In the latter, proof is absolute and remains so forever. If proof is not absolute, i.e. if a flaw can be found in the logic, then proof does not exist. A simple example of this is the proof of the well-known formula of Pythagoras:

$$a^2 + b^2 = c^2$$

where a, b and c are the values of the sides of a right-angled triangle, c being the hypotenuse. The proof of this theorem is straightforward [6, pp. 333–4] and it can be shown that the relationship is true under *all* circumstances. Thus, if the values of any two numbers are known, the third can always be calculated.

However, this relationship can be rewritten as:

$$a^x + b^x = c^x$$

where the value of x is any whole number greater than 2. The French mathematician Pierre de Fermat (1601–1665) postulated that there is *no* solution to this equation. This has become known as Fermat's last theorem. He died having claimed that he had found a proof that there is no solution, but the proof was lost and the challenge to rediscover it became the most exciting in the field of mathematics for the next 329 years until finally solved by Andrew Wiles in 1994.

Fermat's last theorem is fiendishly difficult to prove. Initial attempts resulted in proofs that the postulate is true for values of $x = 4$ and $x = 3$. The problem is that even if it is possible to show that for all values between, say, 3 and 1000 the postulate is also true, this does not prove the theorem, as there could still be values greater than 1000 that do satisfy the equation. This is shown by another conjecture, that of the Swiss mathematician Leonhard Euler, which states that there are also no solutions to the equation:

$$x^4 + y^4 + z^4 = \omega^4$$

Initial attempts to solve it proved fruitless and the lack of a counter-example was taken as proof of its truth until a solution* was eventually found in 1988 some two centuries after it was postulated [6]. Therefore, Euler's postulate is absolutely not true in mathematical

---

*$2{,}682{,}440^4 + 15{,}365{,}639^4 + 18{,}796{,}760^4 = 20{,}615{,}673^4$

terms, although in scientific terms it had been taken to be so. Thus, to obtain an absolute proof, it is necessary to go back to first mathematical principles and demonstrate that the conditions apply to *all* numbers.

Scientific proof is not so rigorous and only demands that there is a sufficient body of evidence to suggest very strongly that a fact is 'true'. Medicine is no different in this respect from other scientific disciplines and, particularly because one is dealing with a biological rather than a physical system, is particularly open to variations in response. The most rigorous method available to scientists, in the realm of medicine, for determining the effectiveness of a treatment is the double-blind, placebo-controlled trial, properly conducted under clearly defined conditions with sufficient numbers of patients and with removal of bias. Some treatments have fulfilled these criteria, although others that are regularly used have never been tested under such circumstances. There has, for instance, never been such a trial of the use of insulin in type 1 diabetes mellitus (T1DM). It would, of course, be totally unethical to conduct such a trial now and yet there is little or no doubt that insulin therapy is effective in treating T1DM. The statement 'insulin is an effective treatment of T1DM' is taken to be true. Evidence-based medicine depends upon scientific observation rather than mathematical proof and is always open to some degree of doubt, however small. It is therefore necessary to have some means of gauging how reliable a piece of evidence is in scientific terms.

Grading of evidence

Several methods of grading evidence have been used and different guideline development groups (GDGs) have used different methods of classifying evidence. The classification used by the Scottish Intercollegiate Guideline Network (SIGN) is the most detailed [7]. The 'levels of evidence' are then converted into 'grades of recommendation' (A–D). In addition, they list 'good practice points' (GPPs).

The National Institute for Clinical Excellence (NICE), an independent body set up by the UK Department of Health, uses a similar, though not quite so detailed, classification [8]. It gives grades A–D and GPPs, and also recommendations from NICE technology appraisals.

The American Diabetes Association (ADA) has the simplest classification. This does not describe a level of evidence which is then converted into a grade but assigns a grade directly to a study [9]. The classification is shown in Table 1.1.

All of these grading methods are similar but, since this book is not designed to be another guideline but rather to present the evidence, we have chosen to use the ADA classification which does not include any GPPs, etc. The new International Society for Pediatric and Adolescent Diabetes (ISPAD) guidelines also use the same gradings. Where relevant, gradings have been assigned to references within the text.

Guidelines

Since the beginning of the 1990s there has been a move away from professional consensus towards more rigorous scientific methods, such as systematic reviews and meta-analyses [10]. This has usually been done in the context of creating guidelines, although the quality of these guidelines has varied depending on how rigorously the methodology has been applied. In 2003, Burgers *et al.* published a study, on behalf of the Appraisal of Guidelines,

Table 1.1 ADA evidence grading system for clinical practice recommendations

Level	Description
A	Clear evidence from well-conducted, generalisable, randomised controlled trials that are adequately powered, including: • evidence from a well-conducted multicentre trial • evidence from a meta-analysis that incorporated quality ratings in the analysis • compelling non-experimental evidence, i.e. 'all-or-none' rule developed by Centre for Evidence-Based Medicine at Oxford Supportive evidence from well-conducted randomised controlled trials that are adequately powered, including: • evidence from a well-conducted trial at one or more institutions • evidence from a meta-analysis that incorporated quality ratings in the analysis
B	Supportive evidence from well-conducted cohort studies: • evidence from a well-conducted prospective cohort study or registry • evidence from a well-conducted meta-analysis of cohort studies • supportive evidence from a well-conducted case-control study
C	Supportive evidence from poorly controlled or uncontrolled studies: • evidence from randomised clinical trials with one or more major or three or more minor methodological flaws that could invalidate the results • evidence from observational studies with high potential for bias (such as case series with comparison to historical controls) • evidence from case series or case reports Conflicting evidence with the weight of evidence supporting the recommendation
E	Expert consensus or clinical experience

Note: There is no Grade **D**.

Research and Evaluation for Europe (AGREE) study group [11], in which they described the structures and working methods of 18 national GDGs from 13 different countries worldwide. These did not include guideline development by NICE since this organisation was formed only in 1999 and produced its first report in 2002. They concluded that '*principles of evidence-based medicine dominate current guideline programs*'. As a result, it can be concluded that most of the current guidelines that have been developed are reasonably well evidence based and well referenced.

However, this is not always the case. For instance, the Consensus Guidelines for the Management of Type 1 Diabetes in Children and Adolescents published by ISPAD in 2000 contained no references. It raises the question of how truly evidence-based they were and how much they depended on the views and opinions of the guideline development team. Having said that, they have proved invaluable as a resource. The situation is due to be rectified with the publication of the new ISPAD Clinical Practice Consensus Guidelines 2006/2007, which are heavily referenced. The first two chapters were published in 2006 (**E**) [12, 13], with the rest due to be published in 2007.

Bertrand Russell is quoted as saying [14], '*The fact that an opinion has been widely held is no evidence whatever that it is not utterly absurd; indeed in view of the silliness of the majority of mankind, a widespread belief is more likely to be foolish than sensible*'. Although he was referring to marriage, he could as easily have been referring to clinical guidelines. That is not to say that guidelines should not be followed, but it must be understood that, whilst they are usually well researched, there are often aspects of the guidelines that are based solely on the personal opinions of those drawing them up with little or no hard evidence to support them and there may be individual circumstances where they do not necessarily apply.

There may also be a tendency, in some instances, for recommendations to be 'transferred' from one guideline to another by default. Let us examine, as an example, the statement made in all of the major national and international guidelines for the treatment of diabetic ketoacidosis (DKA) in children that the dose of insulin should be '0.1 unit per kilogram body weight per hour' (E) [8, 15–18]. The British Society for Paediatric Endocrinology and Diabetes (BSPED) guidelines (E) [16] state that '*Modifications (to their previous guideline) have been made in the light of the guidelines produced by the International Society for Pediatric and Adolescent Diabetes (2000) and the recent ESPE/LWPES consensus statement on diabetic ketoacidosis in children and adolescents*', and the NICE guidelines (E) [8] say that '*The current guidelines take account of recently published consensus statements developed by the European Society for Paediatric Endocrinology and the Lawson Wilkins Pediatric Endocrine Society. The guidelines highlight the need for further research to investigate the effectiveness of different concentrations of rehydration fluid, the rate of rehydration and the concentration of insulin infusion in the management of diabetic ketoacidosis*'. The implication of these two statements is that they are merely following previous recommendations and have not re-examined the evidence.

Despite claims to the contrary [15], the evidence for the stated dose of insulin is weak. The Lawson Wilkins Pediatric Endocrine Society/British Society of Paediatric Endocrinology and Diabetes (LWPES/BSPED) guidelines state that '*Physiologic studies indicate that IV insulin at a dose of 0.1 unit/kg per hour, which achieves steady state plasma insulin levels of ~100 to 200 µU/mL within 60 minutes, is effective*'. However, as stated by Edge and Spinks in Chapter 4 of this book, '*there is a body of opinion that a dose of 0.05 units/kg/hour is sufficient to reverse the metabolic abnormalities and overcome any insulin resistance whilst reducing the blood glucose at a steadier rate*', and many units in the UK ignore the national and international guidelines and routinely use this lower dose.

The statement, which is given an **A** grading, is based on a study conducted in six adults with established diabetes who were rendered ketotic by the administration of two doses of dexamethasone and cessation of insulin in the 24 hours prior to the study [19]. They were then given insulin infusions at varying rates (0.01, 0.1 and 1 U/kg/h) in random order. Steady-state levels of insulin were measured and the rates of fall of glucose and ketones, as measured by β-hydroxybutyric acid and acetoacetate, observed with the different doses. The principal conclusions were as follows:

1 An infusion rate of 0.1 U/kg/h achieves a steady-state insulin concentration between 100 and 200 µU/mL (an increase between 90 and 112 µU/mL over baseline).

2 Logarithmic increases in infusion rates resulted in logarithmic increases in insulin concentration.

3 The effect of insulin on reducing ketones was maximal at 0.1 U/kg/h but the effect on reducing blood glucose had no such plateau effect; i.e. the rate of fall of blood glucose continues to increase with larger doses of insulin.

Unfortunately, an infusion rate of 0.05 U/kg/h was not tested but it can be deduced from the above that this lower rate of infusion would be likely to result in a steady-state concentration of insulin of ~55 µU/mL, which may well be sufficient to switch off ketogenesis (the principal aim of insulin therapy in the treatment of DKA) whilst reducing the rate of fall of blood glucose. This is supported by another study, also conducted in adults [20], and also quoted in the LWPES/BSPED guidelines, in which patients with newly diagnosed diabetes were admitted with DKA and treated with insulin at a rate of 1 mU/kg/min ($\equiv$0.06 U/kg/h). This resulted in a steady fall in blood glucose at an acceptable rate of 3.3 mmol/L/h and correction of the acidosis.

In some units it is considered important to control the rate of fall of blood glucose with the use of systems that involve the use of solutions of different strengths of dextrose, used at different rates depending upon circumstances, a situation that arguably increases the risk of error. Even so, in one such study [21], which was conducted in children, the recommended dose of 0.1 U/kg/h was used and the blood glucose fell initially, when no glucose was being infused, by approximately 33 mmol/L in the first 5 hours (6.6 mmol/h), a rate which is now regarded as being too rapid. Although there is little evidence to support it, a maximum of 5 mmol/L/h is recommended by the ISPAD guidelines (**E**) [17].

It is therefore clear that the evidence for the recommended dose of insulin is weak and has never been properly tested in children. It is possible that this dose *is* correct (although it may be different at different ages) but, as stated in the NICE guidelines, '*further research to investigate the effectiveness of different concentrations of . . . insulin infusion in the management of diabetic ketoacidosis*' is required (see above). Evidence-based medicine should ultimately be able to provide an answer.

Guidelines are widely quoted throughout this book and in many instances, the recommendations are clearly evidence based and have a high degree of validity. Nevertheless, in view of the fact that they are all consensus documents, they are always given an **E** grading. Whilst there is clearly a hierarchy of validity between **A** and **C**, an **E** grading does not necessarily mean that this is the lowest level since consensus documents do often contain systematic reviews or meta-analyses, which, under other circumstances, might be rated **A**. Having said that, some **C**-graded articles, particularly those that are case reports, may still carry quite a lot of weight if they contain, for instance, convincing genetic data.

Sources of data

Electronic databases, such as MEDLINE, have proved enormously helpful in searching for relevant studies. Not only do they make the searches much faster than previously, but they are inevitably more thorough. We have made use of all the available databases including:
• Allied & Complementary Medicine – 1985 to date
• British Nursing Index – 1994 to date
• CINAHL (R) – 1982 to date
• DH-DATA – 1983 to date
• EMBASE – 1974 to date
• King's Fund – 1979 to date
• MEDLINE – 1950 to date
• PsycINFO – 1806 to date.

These have all been available either via KA24, the National Health Service (NHS) portal available to NHS employees (accessible via http://www.hilo.nhs.uk/ to registered personnel) [22], or via PUBMED, a service of the National Library of Medicine and the National Institutes of Health (accessible via http://www.ncbi.nlm.nih.gov/entrez/query.fcgi?CMD=Pager&DB=pubmed).

In addition, the relevant Cochrane databases have been examined. These are a series of systematic reviews based on available publications and are also available via http://www.hilo.nhs.uk/ [22]. (This requires no special permissions.) Cochrane describes a systematic review as follows:

• To help identify which forms of health-care work, which do not and which are even harmful, Results from similar randomised trials need to be brought together. Trials need to be assessed and those that are good enough can be combined to produce both a more statistically reliable result and one that can be more easily applied in other settings. This combination of trials needs to be done in as reliable a way as possible. It needs to be systematic. A systematic review uses a predefined, explicit methodology. The methods used include steps to minimise bias in all parts of the process: identifying relevant studies, selecting them for inclusion and collecting and combining their data. Studies should be sought regardless of their results.

• A systematic review does not need to contain a statistical synthesis of the results from the included studies. This might be impossible if the designs of the studies are too different for an averaging of their results to be meaningful or if the outcomes measured are not sufficiently similar. If the results of the individual studies are combined to produce an overall statistic, this is usually called a meta-analysis. A meta-analysis can also be done without a systematic review, simply by combining the results from more than one trial. However, although such a meta-analysis will have greater mathematical precision than an analysis of any one of the component trials, it will be subject to any biases that arise from the study-selection process and may produce a mathematically precise, but clinically misleading, result.

The Cochrane databases deal mainly with adult practice and have little relevance to paediatrics. There is only one systematic review relating directly to children listed on their website [23]. Nevertheless, the principles of systematic reviews and meta-analyses are important and apply equally to children as to adults.

Summary and conclusions

Evidence-based medicine is becoming increasingly important in determining how best patients should be treated. There is an element of cost-effectiveness built into the system but this is not the principal aim of the process. Unfortunately, in paediatric practice, there is a certain paucity of studies in many areas and it has been necessary to rely on studies in adults which are then extrapolated into paediatrics. Whilst this is valid in some areas, it may not be so in others and one has to retain a certain degree of scepticism in doing so. The aim of this book is to present the data that are available in the hope that they will shed some light on why paediatricians treat their patients as they do and to highlight some of the areas where knowledge is lacking and which require further research.

References

1 Dickersin K, Straus SE, Bero LA. Increasing, not dictating, choice. *BMJ* 2007; **334**(Supplement Medical Milestones): s10.
2 The Cochrane Library. *Evidence for healthcare decision-making.* Available at: http://www3.interscience. wiley.com/cgi-bin/mrwhome/106568753/WhatAreSystematicReviews.html.
3 National Institute of Public Health. *First Annual Nordic Workshop on how to critically appraise and use evidence in decisions about healthcare.* Oslo, Norway, 1996.

4 Muir-Gray JA. *Evidence-Based Healthcare: How to Make Health Policy and Management Decisions.* Churchill Livingstone, London, 1997.

5 Sackett DL, Rosenberg WM, Gray JA *et al.* Evidence based medicine: what it is and what it isn't. *BMJ* 1996; **312**: 71–2.

6 Singh S. *Fermat's Last Theorem.* Clays Ltd., St Ives, UK, 1997.

7 Scottish Intercollegiate Guideline Network. *SIGN 50: A Guideline Developers' Handbook Section 6: Forming Guideline Recommendations.* Available at: http://www.sign.ac.uk/guidelines/fulltext/50/section6.html

8 NICE. *Type 1 Diabetes in Children and Young People: Full Guideline 2004.* Available at: http://www.nice.org.uk/page.aspx?o=CG015childfullguideline

9 American Diabetes Association. Summary of revisions for the 2007 clinical practice recommendations. *Diabetes Care* 2007; **30**(suppl 1): S3.

10 Grimshaw J, Russell I. Achieving health gain through clinical guidelines. I: developing scientifically valid guidelines. *Qual Health Care* 1993; **2**: 243–8.

11 Burgers JS, Grol R, Klazinga NS *et al.* Towards evidence-based clinical practice: an international survey of 18 clinical guideline programs. *Int J Qual Health Care* 2003; **15**: 31–45.

12 Craig ME, Hattersley A, Donaghue K. ISPAD Clinical Practice Consensus Guidelines 2006–2007: definition, epidemiology and classification. *Pediatr Diabetes* 2006; **7**: 343–51.

13 Hattersley A, Bruining J, Shield J *et al.* ISPAD Clinical Practice Consensus Guidelines 2006–2007: the diagnosis and management of monogenic diabetes in children. *Pediatr Diabetes* 2006; **7**: 352–60.

14 Russell B. *Marriage and Morals.* George Allen & Unwin, London, 1929.

15 Dunger DB, Sperling MA, Acerini CL *et al.* European Society for Paediatric Endocrinology/Lawson Wilkins Pediatric Endocrine Society consensus statement on diabetic ketoacidosis in children and adolescents. *Pediatrics* 2004; **113**: e133–40.

16 Edge JA. *BSPED Recommended DKA Guidelines.* Available at: http://www.bsped.org.uk/professional/guidelines/docs/BSPEDDKAApr04.pdf

17 Wolfsdorf J, Craig ME, Daneman D *et al.* ISPAD Clinical Practice Consensus Guidelines 2006–2007: Diabetic Ketoacidosis. *Pediatr Diabetes* 2007; **8**: 28–43.

18 NHMRC. *The Australian Clinical Practice Guidelines on the Management of Type 1 Diabetes in Children and Adolescents 2005.* Available at: http://www.chw.edu.au/prof/services/endocrinology/apeg/apeg_handbook_final.pdf

19 Schade DS, Eaton RP. Dose response to insulin in man: differential effects on glucose and ketone body regulation. *J Clin Endocrinol Metab* 1977; **44**: 1038–53.

20 Luzi L, Barrett EJ, Groop LC *et al.* Metabolic effects of low-dose insulin therapy on glucose metabolism in diabetic ketoacidosis. *Diabetes* 1988; **37**: 1470–7.

21 Grimberg A, Cerri RW, Satin-Smith M *et al.* The 'two bag system' for variable intravenous dextrose and fluid administration: benefits in diabetic ketoacidosis management. *J Pediatr* 1999; **134**: 376–8.

22 HILO (Health Information for London Online). KA24: Knowledge Access 24 hours. *KA24.* Available at: http://www.hilo.nhs.uk/

23 Clar C, Waugh N, Thomas S. Routine hospital admission versus out-patient or home care in children at diagnosis of type 1 diabetes mellitus. *Cochrane Database Syst Rev* 2003; Issue 3: Art no CD004099.

CHAPTER 2

Definition, epidemiology and classification of diabetes and structure of the diabetes team

Maria Craig, Sarah J Glastras & Kim Donaghue

Accurate knowledge is the basis of correct opinions; the want of it makes the opinions of most people of little value.

—Charles Simmons, American Writer (1924–)

Definition, epidemiology and classification

Diabetes mellitus is a group of metabolic diseases characterised by chronic hyperglycaemia resulting from defects in insulin secretion, insulin action, or both. The abnormalities in carbohydrate, fat and protein metabolism that are found in diabetes are due to deficient action of insulin on target tissues. If ketones are present in blood or urine, treatment is urgent, because ketoacidosis can evolve rapidly.

Diagnostic criteria for diabetes in childhood and adolescence

Diabetes in children usually presents with the characteristic symptoms of polyuria, polydipsia and weight loss, in association with glycosuria and ketonuria. In its most severe form ketoacidosis or, rarely, a non-ketotic hyperosmolar state may develop and lead to stupor, coma and, without treatment, death. The diagnosis is usually confirmed quickly by measurement of a markedly elevated blood glucose level. If ketones are also present in blood or urine, treatment is urgent. Waiting another day to confirm the hyperglycaemia is dangerous as ketoacidosis can evolve rapidly (**E**).

In the presence of mild symptoms, the diagnosis of diabetes should never be made on the basis of a single abnormal blood glucose value. Diagnosis may require continued observation with fasting and/or 2-hour postprandial blood glucose levels and/or an oral glucose tolerance test (OGTT) (**E**) [1, 2] (Table 2.1). In the absence of symptoms of diabetes, hyperglycaemia detected incidentally or under conditions of acute infection, trauma, circulation or other stress may be transitory and should not in itself be regarded as diagnostic of diabetes.

An OGTT should not be performed if diabetes can be diagnosed using fasting and random or postprandial criteria, as excessive hyperglycaemia can result. It is rarely indicated in making the diagnosis of type 1 diabetes mellitus (T1DM) in childhood and adolescence (**E**) [1]. If doubt remains, periodic retesting should be undertaken until the diagnosis is

Table 2.1 Criteria for the diagnosis of diabetes mellitus **(E)** [1, 2]

- Symptoms of diabetes plus casual plasma glucose concentration ≥11.1 mmol/L (200 mg/dL)*
  (Casual is defined as any time of day without regard to time since last meal.)
  or
- Fasting plasma glucose ≥7.0 mmol/L (≥126 mg/dL)
  (Fasting is defined as no caloric intake for at least 8 h.)
  or
- Two-hour post-load glucose ≥11.1 mmol/L (≥200 mg/dL) during an OGTT

The test should be performed as described by WHO [1], using a glucose load containing the equivalent of 75 g anhydrous glucose dissolved in water or 1.75 g/kg of body weight to a maximum of 75 g.

---

*Corresponding values (mmol/L) are ≥10.0 for venous whole blood and ≥11.1 for capillary whole blood and ≥6.1 for both venous and capillary whole blood.

established. In the absence of unequivocal hyperglycaemia with acute metabolic decompensation, these criteria should be confirmed by repeat testing on a different day.

Impaired glucose tolerance and impaired fasting glycaemia

Impaired glucose tolerance (IGT) and impaired fasting glycaemia (IFG) are intermediate stages in the natural history of disordered carbohydrate metabolism between normal glucose homeostasis and diabetes **(E)** [1, 2]. IFG and IGT are not interchangeable and represent different abnormalities of glucose regulation; IFG is a measure of disturbed carbohydrate metabolism in the basal state, whilst the IGT is a dynamic measure of carbohydrate intolerance after a standardised glucose load.

Patients with IFG and/or IGT are now referred to as having 'pre-diabetes', indicating their relatively high risk for development of diabetes **(A)** [3, 4]. Pre-diabetes can be observed as an intermediate stage in any of the disease processes given in Table 2.2. IFG and IGT may be associated with the metabolic syndrome, which includes obesity (especially abdominal or visceral obesity), dyslipidaemia of the high-triglyceride and/or low-high-density lipoprotein type and hypertension **(E)** [5].

Individuals who meet criteria for IGT or IFG may be euglycaemic in their daily lives as shown by normal or near-normal glycated haemoglobin levels, and those with IGT may manifest hyperglycaemia only when challenged with an OGTT. Recently, the European Diabetes Epidemiology Group has recommended revising the lower cut-off for IFG back to 6.1 mmol/L from the current value of 5.6 mmol/L due to the two- to fivefold increase in prevalence of IFG across the world **(E)** [6] but the American Diabetes Association (ADA) continues to recommend 5.6 mmol/L as the cut-off point for normal FPG [2].

Categories of fasting plasma glucose (FPG) are defined as follows [2]:
- FPG <5.6 mmol/L (100 mg/dL) = normal fasting glucose
- FPG 5.6–6.9 mmol/L (100–125 mg/dL) = IFG
- FPG ≥7.0 mmol/L (126 mg/dL) = provisional diagnosis of diabetes (The diagnosis must be confirmed, as described above in the section *Diagnostic criteria*.)

The corresponding categories for stimulated plasma glucose when the OGTT is used are as follows:
- 2-hour post-load glucose <7.8 mmol/L (140 mg/dL) = normal glucose tolerance
- 2-hour post-load glucose 7.8–11.1 mmol/L (140–199 mg/dL) = IGT
- 2-hour post-load glucose ≥11.1 mmol/L (200 mg/dL) = provisional diagnosis of diabetes (The diagnosis must be confirmed, as described above.)

Table 2.2 Aetiological classification of disorders of glycaemia

---

I Type 1
  Beta-cell destruction, usually leading to absolute insulin deficiency
  Autoimmune
  Idiopathic

II Type 2
  It may range from predominantly insulin resistance with relative insulin deficiency to a
    predominantly secretory defect with or without insulin resistance

III Other specific types
(a) Genetic defects of beta-cell development or function

Chromosome 12, HNF-1$_\alpha$	(MODY3)
Chromosome 7, glucokinase	(MODY2)
Chromosome 20, HNF-4$_\alpha$	(MODY1)
Chromosome 13, insulin promoter factor-1	(IPF-1; MODY4)
Chromosome 17, HNF-1ß	(MODY5)
Chromosome 2, *NeuroD1*	(MODY6)
carboxyl exter lipase (CEL) gene	(MODY7)
Mitochondrial DNA mutation	DIDMOAD (Wolfram)
Chromosome 11	PNDM
Chromosome 11	PNDM/TNDM
Chromosome 6	TNDM
Chromosome 2	Wolcott—Rallison
Chromosome X	IPEX
Chromosome 10	PNDM and cerebellar agenesis
Others	

(b) Genetic defects in insulin action
  Type A insulin resistance
  Leprechaunism
  Rabson–Mendenhall syndrome
  Lipoatrophic diabetes
  Others
(c) Diseases of the exocrine pancreas
  Pancreatitis
  Trauma/pancreatectomy
  Neoplasia
  Cystic fibrosis
  Haemochromatosis
  Fibrocalculous pancreatopathy
  Others
(d) Endocrinopathies
  Acromegaly
  Cushing syndrome
  Glucagonoma
  Phaeochromocytoma
  Hyperthyroidism
  Somatostatinoma
  Aldosteronoma
  Others
(e) Drug or chemical induced
  Vacor
  Pentamidine
  Nicotinic acid
  Glucocorticoids
  Thyroid hormone

Continued

Table 2.2 *Continued*

   Diazoxide
   β-adrenergic agonists
   Thiazides
   Dilantin
   Interferon alpha
   Others
(f) Infections
   Congenital rubella
   Enterovirus
   Cytomegalovirus
   Others
(g) Uncommon forms of immune-mediated diabetes
   'Stiff-man' syndrome
   Anti-insulin receptor antibodies
   Autoimmune polyendocrine syndromes (APS) I and II
   Others
(h) Other genetic syndromes sometimes associated with diabetes
   Down syndrome
   Klinefelter syndrome
   Turner syndrome
   DIDMOAD (Wolfram) syndrome
   Friedreich ataxia
   Huntington chorea
   Laurence–Moon–Biedl syndrome
   Myotonic dystrophy
   Porphyria
   Prader–Willi syndrome
   Others

IV Gestational diabetes

DIDMOAD, Diabetes insipidus, diabetes mellitus, optic atrophy and deafness; PNDM, permanent neonatal diabetes mellitus; TNDM, transient neonatal diabetes mellitus; IPEX, immune dysregulation, polyendocrinopathy, enteropathy X-linked syndrome.

Epidemiology of T1DM

Approximately 50–60% of individuals with T1DM are diagnosed before the age of 15 years (**B**) [7]. In most Western countries, T1DM accounts for over 90% of childhood and adolescent diabetes. However, T2DM is becoming more common and it accounts for a significant proportion of youth-onset diabetes in certain at-risk populations (**B**) [8, 9].

    T1DM incidence varies greatly between different countries, within countries, and between different ethnic populations (**B**) [10]. Epidemiological incidence studies define the 'onset of T1DM' by the date of the first insulin injection because of the variable time between the onset of symptoms and diagnosis (**B**) [10]. Annual incidence rates for childhood T1DM (0–14 yr age group) comparing different countries of the world are shown in Figure 2.1 (0.1–43.9/100,000) [10–13]. Gender differences in incidence are found in some, but not all, populations (**B**) [10, 14–17].

    Incidence rates show a close correlation with the frequency of human leucocyte antigen (HLA) susceptibility genes in the general population of white Caucasian ancestry; this locus confers approximately 50% of the genetic susceptibility to T1DM (**B**) [18–20] (see Chapter 3 for a more detailed discussion of this). In countries where the incidence of T1DM

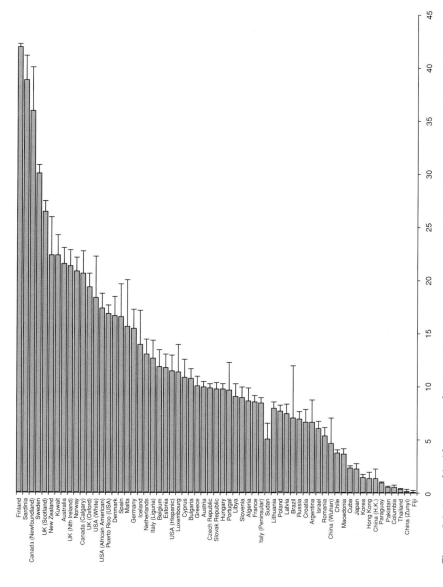

Figure 2.1 Annual incidence rates for T1DM (0–14 yr age group) comparing different countries in the world. (Modified from IDF Atlas 2003 [10, 11].)

is extremely low, HLA associations are different from those in white Caucasians [21]. In addition, a unique, slowly progressive form of T1DM is found in Japan (**B**) [22, 23].

Migrating populations may exhibit diabetes incidence rates closer to those of their new country compared with their country of origin [24, 25], although this is not universally the case [26], suggesting that the interplay between genetics and environmental factors is variable.

A well-documented rise in the incidence has been noted in many countries. From 1960 to 1996, there was a significant increase in 65% of countries and an upward trend in 32% (**B**) [27]. From 1995 to 1999, the average annual increase was 3.4% [10]. In Europe the average increase was 3.2% (95% CI 2.7–3.7) from 1989 to 1999, in keeping with the increases reported in other parts of the world (**B**) [10, 28, 29]. In some reports there has been a disproportionately greater increase in those under the age of 5 years (**B**) [10, 27, 30, 31]. The rising incidence is unlikely to have a strong genetic basis, as it has occurred over too short a time period [32]. Possible explanations include increased exposure to infections and wealth-related factors, such as lifestyle and nutrition [28, 33–35].

A seasonal variation in the presentation of new cases is well described, with the peak being in the autumn and winter months (**B**) [17, 30, 36]. Seasonality of birth has also been described in some countries, suggesting a perinatal environmental trigger [37, 38]. Higher incidence rates have been found in countries with colder climates (**B**) [10] and in colder areas of large nations, such as China [39].

Despite familial aggregation, there is no recognisable pattern of Mendelian inheritance. The risk of diabetes to an identical twin of a patient with T1DM is about 36% (**B**) [40] and for a sibling the risk is approximately 4% by age 20 years (**B**) [41, 42] and 9.6% by age 60 years (**B**) [43], compared with 0.5% for the general population. The risk is higher in siblings of probands diagnosed at younger age (**B**) [42, 44]. T1DM is two to three times more common in the offspring of diabetic men (3.6–8.5%) compared with diabetic women (1.3–3.6%) (**B**) [42, 44–49].

The age of onset of T1DM has decreased in many countries (**B**) [31, 50]. This has been accompanied by increased weight and linear growth prior to the onset of diabetes and the observation that children with T1DM are heavier and taller than their peers [34, 51]. These epidemiological findings suggest that insulin resistance is responsible for overloading the beta cell ('the accelerator hypothesis') (**B, C**) [33, 34, 51–53], although this hypothesis remains to be proven and is not universally accepted.

When the clinical presentation is typical of T1DM (often associated with diabetic ketoacidosis) but antibodies are absent, then the diabetes is classified as type 1B (idiopathic) [54]. This represents approximately 5% of T1DM in white populations but is more common in other parts of the world, such as Japan [22].

Classification
The aetiological classification recommended by the ADA (**E**) [2] and the WHO expert committee on the classification and diagnosis of diabetes (**E**) [1] is shown in Table 2.2 with minor modification.

Classifying types of diabetes
The differentiation between T1DM, T2DM and monogenic diabetes has important implications for both therapeutic decisions and educational approaches. Regardless of the type of diabetes, however, the child who presents with severe fasting hyperglycaemia, metabolic

derangements and ketonaemia will require insulin therapy initially to reverse the metabolic abnormalities [55].

Measurement of diabetes-associated autoantibody markers, for example ICA, GAD, IA2, IAA and/or HbA1c, may be helpful in some situations. However, there is currently insufficient evidence to support the routine use of HbA1c for the diagnosis of diabetes (**E**) [54].

Measurement of fasting insulin or C-peptide may be useful in the diagnosis of T2DM in children. Fasting insulin and C-peptide levels are usually normal or elevated, although not as elevated as might be expected for the degree of hyperglycaemia (**E**) [56]. If patients are insulin treated, measuring C-peptide when the glucose is sufficiently high (>8 mmol/L) to stimulate C-peptide will detect if endogenous insulin secretion is still occurring. This is rare outside the honeymoon period (2–3 yr) in children with T1DM (**E**).

The possibility of other types of diabetes should be considered in:
• the antibody-negative child who has a family history of diabetes consistent with autosomal dominant inheritance
• associated conditions such as deafness, optic atrophy or syndromic features
• marked insulin resistance
• those requiring little or no insulin outside the partial remission phase
• a history of exposure to drugs that are known to be toxic to beta cells or that cause insulin resistance.

The characteristic features of *T1DM* with *T2DM* and *monogenic diabetes* are compared in Table 2.3.

Type 2 diabetes mellitus
T2DM is rapidly increasing in children and adolescents (**B, E**) [8, 57]. There may be predominantly insulin resistance with relative insulin deficiency or a predominantly secretory defect (non-autoimmune mediated) with or without insulin resistance.

The possibility of T2DM should be considered in children and adolescents who are obese, have a strong family history of T2DM, come from an ethnic background at high risk for diabetes, produce little or no ketonuria and manifest signs of insulin resistance (acanthosis nigricans or polycystic ovarian syndrome) (Table 2.3).

The rising incidence of T2DM is associated with the epidemic of obesity. Lifestyle factors such as little exercise and overeating leading to obesity have profound effects. Whilst many indigenous ethnic groups are especially prone to T2DM (e.g. Pima Indians in Arizona, Cree–Ojibwe Indians in Canada, Pacific islanders, Australian Aborigines, Torres Strait islanders), the increased risk is now being seen in many populations (e.g. Indian, Pakistani and Bangladeshi communities originating from South Asia, Chinese, Africans, African-Americans, African-Caribbeans, Arabs and Hispanic-Americans) (**B**) [8].

T2DM is often asymptomatic but may present with ketosis and even mild-to-moderate ketoacidosis (**B**) [57]. It may be the underlying cause of hyperglycaemia associated with infections and severe illness in some patients (see section *Stress hyperglycaemia* below).

The long-term microvascular complications of diabetes occur at least as frequently as in T1DM (**B**) [58] and the onset may be earlier (**C**) [59, 60]. The risk of nephropathy appears to be greater in patients with early onset of T2DM (<20 yr of age) compared with adult-onset T2DM. However, based on limited data, the risk of retinopathy does not appear to be increased in youth-onset T2DM [58]. Abnormalities of liver function are found in up to half of youth with T2DM [61, 62]. Because T2DM may have a prolonged

Table 2.3 Clinical characteristics of T1DM, T2DM and monogenic diabetes in children and adolescents

Characteristic	Type 1	Type 2	Monogenic
Genetics	Polygenic	Polygenic	Monogenic
Age	Throughout childhood	Usually pubertal (or later)	Often postpubertal except MODY2 and neonatal diabetes
Onset	Most often acute, rapid	Variable; from slow, mild (often insidious) to severe	Variable
Associations Autoimmunity	Yes	No	No
Ketosis	Common	Rare	Rare in MODY, common in neonatal diabetes
Obesity	Reflects the background risk	Very common	Reflects the background risk
Acanthosis nigricans	No	Yes	No
Frequency (percentage of all diabetes in young people)	Usually 90%+	Most countries < 10% (Japan 60–80%)	?1–3%
Parent with diabetes	2–4%	80%	90%

asymptomatic phase, screening for complications should start at diagnosis or soon after (**E**) [63, 64]. The risks for macrovascular complications are also increased and reflect the underlying metabolic syndrome in T2DM.

Screening for T2DM

Population screening for T2DM in children and adolescents cannot be justified in some countries because of the low prevalence. In countries with higher incidence, such as Japan and Taiwan, annual school glycosuria screening programmes are in place [9, 65]. Targeted screening of youths is recommended at the point of medical contact if they are overweight *and* have any two risk factors listed below (**E**) [66, 67]. Testing may also be considered in other high-risk patients who have any of the risk factors (Table 2.4). Testing of high-risk subjects should be undertaken starting at age 10 years or at onset of puberty, whichever is earlier, and every 2 years thereafter (**E**) [56].

Table 2.4 Risk factors for T2DM – screening is recommended if any two risk factors are present

---

Overweight defined as either:
    BMI > 85th percentile for age and sex
    Weight for height > 85th percentile
    Weight > 120% of ideal (50th percentile) for height
A family history of T2DM in first- or second-degree relatives
An at-risk ethnic group:
    Native Americans
    African-Americans
    Hispanic-Americans
    Asians
    South Pacific islanders
Signs of insulin resistance or conditions associated with insulin resistance:
    Acanthosis nigricans
    Hypertension
    Dyslipidaemia
    Polycystic ovarian syndrome

BMI, body mass index.

Maturity-onset diabetes of the young

Maturity-onset diabetes of the young (MODY) was described as a disorder with the following characteristics: onset before 25 years of age, autosomal dominant inheritance and non-ketotic diabetes mellitus [68, 69]. These classical definitions given to MODY are no longer very helpful, as T2DM diabetes occurs in children and will often meet all these criteria (**B, C**) [63]. In addition, defining the molecular genetics has shown that there are marked differences between genetic subgroups within these old, broad categories making it much more appropriate to use the genetic subgroups, an approach that has been supported by the ADA and WHO in their guidelines on classification (**E**) (Table 2.2). There is great variation in the degree of hyperglycaemia, need for insulin and risk for future complications (**B**) [70] (see Chapter 13 for more details).

Stress hyperglycaemia

Stress hyperglycaemia has been reported in up to 5% of children presenting to an emergency department with acute illness or injury. Traumatic injuries, febrile seizures and elevated body temperature (>39 °C) were identified as the most common associated features [71]. The reported incidence of progression to overt diabetes varies from 0 to 32% (**B, C**) [72–77]. Children with incidental hyperglycaemia without a serious concomitant illness were more likely to develop diabetes than those with a serious illness [73]. Islet cell antibodies and insulin autoantibody testing had a high positive and negative predictive value for T1DM in children with stress hyperglycaemia [73].

Structure of the diabetes management team

Consensus guidelines on the management of diabetes in childhood and adolescence recommend that children and adolescents with diabetes should have frequent access to care by a multidisciplinary team (**E**) [55, 78–80]. The diabetes management team includes the child or adolescent, his or her family, paediatric endocrinologist or physician with specialist training in childhood diabetes, diabetes educator, dietitian and social worker or psychologist (Table 2.5). The aims of the diabetes management team are to provide education, initiate insulin replacement and blood glucose monitoring and provide nutritional planning and psychological support.

There have been no conclusive evidence-based studies validating the multidisciplinary team approach to diabetes management, as opposed to care provided by individual disciplines. However, many studies have demonstrated that a team approach improves diabetes outcomes. The largest study to date, the Diabetes Control and Complications Trial (DCCT), was a prospective, randomised multicentred clinical trial which convincingly showed that strict glycaemic control could be achieved by individualised treatment provided by a team of highly trained diabetes doctors, nurses, educators and dietitians (A) [87]. Their strategies included frequent contact via outpatient visits as well as regular telephone contact. The investigators aimed to educate patients and parents and empower them in diabetes management. The effectiveness of the diabetes management team in assisting patients to improve glycaemic control and preventing or delaying onset of diabetes complications in the DCCT has been the motivating factor in establishing the diabetes management team as a necessary component of diabetes care (B, E) [55, 79, 80, 87]. In the paediatric population, a multidisciplinary team approach to intensive management of T1DM has also been shown to improve glycaemic control (A, B) [88–91].

Involvement by the diabetes management team should begin at initial diagnosis of diabetes (E). This multidisciplinary approach has been shown to reduce hospital length of stay, as compared with management by an endocrinologist or general physician alone (B) [92]. Management by the multidisciplinary team at diagnosis may reduce the risk of microvascular disease at follow-up [84]. Many children and adolescents with newly diagnosed diabetes can be managed from diagnosis at home rather than in hospital (A) [93, 94] (Table 2.6). Initial ambulatory management does not lead to any disadvantages in terms of metabolic control, diabetes complications and subsequent hospitalisations or psychosocial adjustments. However, children who present with diabetic ketoacidosis at diagnosis must of necessity be managed in hospital until stabilisation (E) [55, 79, 80].

Ongoing review by the diabetes management team should be carried out regularly after diagnosis. More frequent visits to a multidisciplinary diabetes clinic were associated with lower HbA1c levels (three to four visits compared with one to two visits) (B) [89, 95]. Provision of a mobile diabetes education and care team to a rural area in Germany was associated with lower HbA1c levels, fewer hospitalisations and better quality of life in children with T1DM (B) [96]. Current guidelines suggest that there should be at least one major annual review where growth, blood pressure, puberty, associated conditions, nutrition and complications are assessed and managed (E) [78, 79]. Availability of a patient's HbA1c result at the time of the clinic visit improved glycaemic control (A) [97]. Diabetes management via telemedicine may provide a more time-effective way of delivering care to patient with diabetes. Telemedicine may offer the advantage of more frequent contact and result in improvement of glycaemic control, decreased insulin requirements and reduced number of hypoglycaemic events (A, B) [98–102] (see Chapter 14 for a more detailed discussion of this). However, regular phone contact with adolescents does not always improve glycaemic control (B) [103, 104].

Current guidelines recommend that the diabetes management team should be specially trained in the management of diabetes in children and adolescents [55, 78–80]. A child's

Table 2.5 Evidence for the role of the diabetes management team

Team member	Role	Evidence for effectiveness	Level of evidence
Diabetes specialist	To provide high-level medical care	(a) Specialist care was associated with higher levels of participation in diabetes self-care practices and better glycaemic control. (b) There was a higher incidence of neuropathy, overt nephropathy and coronary artery disease in those who did not receive ongoing care from an endocrinologist, diabetologist or diabetes clinic after diagnosis of T1DM in childhood.	**(B)** [81]
Diabetes educator	To teach and support children and families to manage the diabetes regimen and to become independent	(a) Clinic attendance, hospital admission and glycaemic control were improved in 154 children after institution of a diabetes educator. (b) There was a 50% reduction in length of hospitalisation at diagnosis 2 yr after employment of an educator and A1c levels were lower 1 and 3 yr after using a primary nurse managed in the team.	**(A)** [82, 83]
Dietitian	To provide specific diabetes-related dietary advice and education	(a) Dietitians have special training in applying and teaching about appropriate food choices and exercise. (b) Their expertise is utilised by 86% of consultant paediatric services caring for young people with diabetes in the UK.	**(C)**
Social worker	To support child and family and provide financial and community support as required	(a) Appropriate emotional support should be offered at diagnosis to all children with diabetes. (b) Intensive psychosocial education/support in the month following diagnosis led to better adherence to therapy, better family relations and better sociability. (c) Consultation with a social worker at diagnosis reduced retinopathy 6 yr later.	**(B, C)** [80, 84, 85]
Psychologist	To provide psychological assessment and management	(a) There was an improvement in glycaemic control from referral to psychologist and next clinic appointment	**(C)** [86]
Case ambassador	To encourage families to seek medical advice and remind or reschedule clinic appointments	(a) Their involvement increased visits made to the diabetes clinic. (b) When written material regarding specific issues pertaining to diabetes care was provided, there was also a significant reduction in hospital use and hypoglycaemic events.	**(A)** [82]

Table 2.6 Evidence for stabilisation in ambulatory versus in-hospital care

Study	Population	Intervention	Comparator	Outcome	Evidence level
Clar 2003	Six studies involving children with newly diagnosed T1DM. Total of 237 patients in the outpatient/home-care group (mean age 10–13 yr)	Home-based management at diagnosis	Inpatient stabilisation at diagnosis	No significant difference in glycaemic control, admission to hospital in first 2 yr, acute complications and cost	Cochrane systematic review (B) [93]
Srinivasan 2004	All children newly diagnosed with T1DM (n = 61) after introduction of programme compared with a pre-intervention cohort (n = 49)	Diabetes day-care programme	Inpatient stabilisation at diagnosis	Children receiving ambulatory stabilisation via a DCCP had a shorter initial stay in hospital and suffered no adverse events	(B) [94]
McEvilly 2005	400 children with diabetes	Diabetes home-care service	20-yr comparison between outpatient care now and inpatient care before (~1980)	Reduced readmission rates to hospital, HbA1c after stabilisation, diabetic ketoacidosis and cost	Historical comparison (C) [91]

age and stage of development affect management priorities such as age-specific glycaemic goals as well as issues in self-management. Glycaemic goals in very young children should take into account the unique risks of hypoglycaemia (see Chapter 5 for a more detailed discussion of this). The family unit is always an integral part of the management team. Whereas young children rely heavily on their families for diabetes care, middle- and high-school students should be expected to provide some of their own diabetes care while maintaining close supervision by their parents [55]. To date, there is a limited evidence base to support these recommendations regarding age-specific management and education.

Conclusion

Childhood diabetes is predominantly due to T1DM that needs prompt treatment to prevent the development of ketoacidosis. Other forms of diabetes are also found and may be more common than T1DM diabetes in certain populations. The incidence of T1DM varies significantly worldwide and is increasing by approximately 3% per year globally. The rising incidence is likely to have a multifactorial basis, with recent evidence suggesting that nutritional and lifestyle factors are important. Initial and ongoing care by a multidisciplinary diabetes team forms the standard for management of diabetes in children and adolescents.

References

1 Alberti K, Aschner P, Assal J-P *et al. Definition, Diagnosis and Classification of Diabetes Mellitus and its Complications. Report of a WHO Consultation Part 1: Diagnosis and Classification of Diabetes Mellitus.* Geneva, 1999. Available at: http://www.staff.ncl.ac.uk/philip.home/who_dmc.htm#Authors

2 American Diabetes Association. Diagnosis and classification of diabetes mellitus. *Diabetes Care* 2007; **30**(suppl 1): S42–7.

3 Harris R, Donahue K, Rathore SS *et al.* Screening adults for type 2 diabetes: a review of the evidence for the U.S. Preventive Services Task Force. *Ann Intern Med* 2003; **138**: 215–29.

4 Hoerger TJ, Harris R, Hicks KA *et al.* Screening for type 2 diabetes mellitus: a cost-effectiveness analysis. *Ann Intern Med* 2004; **140**: 689–99.

5 Alberti KG, Zimmet P, Shaw J. The metabolic syndrome – a new worldwide definition. *Lancet* 2005; **366**: 1059–62.

6 Forouhi NG, Balkau B, Borch-Johnsen K *et al.* The threshold for diagnosing impaired fasting glucose: a position statement by the European Diabetes Epidemiology Group. *Diabetologia* 2006; **49**: 822–7.

7 Vandewalle CL, Coeckelberghs MI, De Leeuw IH *et al.* Epidemiology, clinical aspects, and biology of IDDM patients under age 40 years. Comparison of data from Antwerp with complete ascertainment with data from Belgium with 40% ascertainment. The Belgian Diabetes Registry. *Diabetes Care* 1997; **20**: 1556–61.

8 Pinhas-Hamiel O, Zeitler P. The global spread of type 2 diabetes mellitus in children and adolescents. *J Pediatr* 2005; **146**: 693–700.

9 Wei JN, Sung FC, Lin CC *et al.* National surveillance for type 2 diabetes mellitus in Taiwanese children. *JAMA* 2003; **290**: 1345–50.

10 The DIAMOND Project Group. Incidence and trends of childhood Type 1 diabetes worldwide 1990–1999. *Diabet Med* 2006; **23**: 857–66.

11 International Diabetes Federation. *Diabetes Atlas*, 2nd edn. International Diabetes Federation, Brussels, 2003.

12 Green A, Patterson CC. Trends in the incidence of childhood-onset diabetes in Europe 1989–1998. *Diabetologia* 2001; **44**(suppl 3): B3–8.

13 Karvonen M, Viik-Kajander M, Moltchanova E *et al.* Incidence of childhood type 1 diabetes worldwide. Diabetes Mondiale (DiaMond) Project Group. *Diabetes Care* 2000; **23**: 1516–26.

14 Cucca F, Goy JV, Kawaguchi Y *et al*. A male-female bias in type 1 diabetes and linkage to chromosome Xp in MHC HLA-DR3-positive patients. *Nat Genet* 1998; **19**: 301–2.

15 Gale EA, Gillespie KM. Diabetes and gender. *Diabetologia* 2001; **44**: 3–15.

16 Karvonen M, Pitkaniemi M, Pitkaniemi J *et al*. Sex difference in the incidence of insulin-dependent diabetes mellitus: an analysis of the recent epidemiological data. World Health Organization DIAMOND Project Group. *Diabetes Metab Rev* 1997; **13**: 275–91.

17 Weets I, Kaufman L, Van der AB *et al*. Seasonality in clinical onset of type 1 diabetes in Belgian patients above the age of 10 is restricted to HLA-DQ2/DQ8-negative males, which explains the male to female excess in incidence. *Diabetologia* 2004; **47**: 614–21.

18 Barker JM. Clinical review: type 1 diabetes-associated autoimmunity: natural history, genetic associations, and screening. *J Clin Endocrinol Metab* 2006; **91**: 1210–17.

19 Gillespie KM, Bain SC, Barnett AH *et al*. The rising incidence of childhood type 1 diabetes and reduced contribution of high-risk HLA haplotypes. *Lancet* 2004; **364**: 1699–1700.

20 Kukko M, Virtanen SM, Toivonen A *et al*. Geographical variation in risk HLA-DQB1 genotypes for type 1 diabetes and signs of beta-cell autoimmunity in a high-incidence country. *Diabetes Care* 2004; **27**: 676–81.

21 Sugihara S, Sakamaki T, Konda S *et al*. Association of HLA-DR, DQ genotype with different beta-cell functions at IDDM diagnosis in Japanese children. *Diabetes* 1997; **46**: 1893–7.

22 Kawasaki E, Matsuura N, Eguchi K. Type 1 diabetes in Japan. *Diabetologia* 2006; **49**: 828–36.

23 Ohtsu S, Takubo N, Kazahari M *et al*. Slowly progressing form of type 1 diabetes mellitus in children: genetic analysis compared with other forms of diabetes mellitus in Japanese children. *Pediatr Diabetes* 2005; **6**: 221–9.

24 Raymond NT, Jones JR, Swift PG *et al*. Comparative incidence of Type I diabetes in children aged under 15 years from South Asian and White or Other ethnic backgrounds in Leicestershire, UK, 1989 to 1998. *Diabetologia* 2001; **44**(suppl 3): B32–6.

25 Shamis I, Gordon O, Albag Y *et al*. Ethnic differences in the incidence of childhood IDDM in Israel (1965–1993). Marked increase since 1985, especially in Yemenite Jews. *Diabetes Care* 1997; **20**: 504–8.

26 Neu A, Willasch A, Ehehalt S *et al*. Diabetes incidence in children of different nationalities: an epidemiological approach to the pathogenesis of diabetes. *Diabetologia* 2001; **44**(suppl 3): B21–6.

27 Onkamo P, Vaananen S, Karvonen M *et al*. Worldwide increase in incidence of Type I diabetes – the analysis of the data on published incidence trends. *Diabetologia* 1999; **42**: 1395–1403.

28 Haynes A, Bulsara MK, Bower C *et al*. Independent effects of socioeconomic status and place of residence on the incidence of childhood type 1 diabetes in Western Australia. *Pediatr Diabetes* 2006; **7**: 94–100.

29 Taplin CE, Craig ME, Lloyd M *et al*. The rising incidence of childhood type 1 diabetes in New South Wales, 1990–2002. *Med J Aust* 2005; **183**: 243–6.

30 EURODIABS ACE Study Group. Variation and trends in incidence of childhood diabetes in Europe. EURODIAB ACE Study Group. *Lancet* 2000; **355**: 873–6.

31 Karvonen M, Pitkaniemi J, Tuomilehto J. The onset age of type 1 diabetes in Finnish children has become younger. The Finnish Childhood Diabetes Registry Group. *Diabetes Care* 1999; **22**: 1066–70.

32 Viskari HR, Koskela P, Lonnrot M *et al*. Can enterovirus infections explain the increasing incidence of type 1 diabetes? *Diabetes Care* 2000; **23**: 414–16.

33 Betts P, Mulligan J, Ward P *et al*. Increasing body weight predicts the earlier onset of insulin-dependant diabetes in childhood: testing the 'accelerator hypothesis' (2). *Diabet Med* 2005; **22**: 144–51.

34 EURODIABS Study Group. Rapid early growth is associated with increased risk of childhood type 1 diabetes in various European populations. *Diabetes Care* 2002; **25**: 1755–60.

35 Patterson CC, Dahlquist G, Soltesz G *et al*. Is childhood-onset type I diabetes a wealth-related disease? An ecological analysis of European incidence rates. *Diabetologia* 2001; **44**(suppl 3): B9–16.

36 Levy-Marchal C, Patterson C, Green A. Variation by age group and seasonality at diagnosis of childhood IDDM in Europe. The EURODIAB ACE Study Group. *Diabetologia* 1995; **38**: 823–30.

37 Laron Z, Lewy H, Wilderman I *et al*. Seasonality of month of birth of children and adolescents with type 1 diabetes mellitus in homogenous and heterogeneous populations. *Isr Med Assoc J* 2005; **7**: 381–4.

38 Rothwell PM, Gutnikov SA, McKinney PA *et al*. Seasonality of birth in children with diabetes in Europe: multicentre cohort study. European Diabetes Study Group. *BMJ* 1999; **319**: 887–8.

39 Yang Z, Long X, Shen J *et al*. Epidemics of type 1 diabetes in China. *Pediatr Diabetes* 2005; **6**: 122–8.

40 Olmos P, A'Hern R, Heaton DA *et al.* The significance of the concordance rate for type 1 (insulin-dependent) diabetes in identical twins. *Diabetologia* 1988; **31**: 747–50.

41 Harjutsalo V, Podar T, Tuomilehto J. Cumulative incidence of type 1 diabetes in 10,168 siblings of Finnish young-onset type 1 diabetic patients. *Diabetes* 2005; **54**: 563–9.

42 Steck AK, Barriga KJ, Emery LM *et al.* Secondary attack rate of type 1 diabetes in Colorado families. *Diabetes Care* 2005; **28**: 296–300.

43 Lorenzen T, Pociot F, Hougaard P *et al.* Long-term risk of IDDM in first-degree relatives of patients with IDDM. *Diabetologia* 1994; **37**: 321–7.

44 Gillespie KM, Gale EA, Bingley PJ. High familial risk and genetic susceptibility in early onset childhood diabetes. *Diabetes* 2002; **51**: 210–14.

45 Dorman JS, Steenkiste AR, O'Leary LA *et al.* Type 1 diabetes in offspring of parents with type 1 diabetes: the tip of an autoimmune iceberg? *Pediatr Diabetes* 2000; **1**: 17–22.

46 el Hashimy M, Angelico MC, Martin BC *et al.* Factors modifying the risk of IDDM in offspring of an IDDM parent. *Diabetes* 1995; **44**: 295–9.

47 EURODIABS ACE Study Group. Familial risk of type I diabetes in European children. The Eurodiab Ace Study Group and The Eurodiab Ace Substudy 2 Study Group. *Diabetologia* 1998; **41**: 1151–6.

48 Lorenzen T, Pociot F, Stilgren L *et al.* Predictors of IDDM recurrence risk in offspring of Danish IDDM patients. Danish IDDM Epidemiology and Genetics Group. *Diabetologia* 1998; **41**: 666–73.

49 Warram JH, Krolewski AS, Gottlieb MS *et al.* Differences in risk of insulin-dependent diabetes in offspring of diabetic mothers and diabetic fathers. *N Engl J Med* 1984; **311**: 149–52.

50 Dahlquist G, Mustonen L. Analysis of 20 years of prospective registration of childhood onset diabetes time trends and birth cohort effects. Swedish Childhood Diabetes Study Group. *Acta Paediatr* 2000; **89**: 1231–7.

51 Hypponen E, Virtanen SM, Kenward MG *et al.* Obesity, increased linear growth, and risk of type 1 diabetes in children. *Diabetes Care* 2000; **23**: 1755–60.

52 Clarke SL, Craig ME, Garnett SP *et al.* Increased adiposity at diagnosis in younger children with type 1 diabetes does not persist. *Diabetes Care* 2006; **29**: 1651–3.

53 Kordonouri O, Hartmann R. Higher body weight is associated with earlier onset of Type 1 diabetes in children: confirming the 'Accelerator Hypothesis'. *Diabet Med* 2005; **22**: 1783–4.

54 World Health Organization. Diagnosis and classification of diabetes mellitus. *Diabetes Care* 2006; **29**(suppl 1): S43–8.

55 Silverstein J, Klingensmith G, Copeland K *et al.* Care of children and adolescents with type 1 diabetes: a statement of the American Diabetes Association. *Diabetes Care* 2005; **28**: 186–212.

56 American Diabetes Association. Type 2 diabetes in children and adolescents. American Diabetes Association. *Pediatrics* 2000; **105**: 671–80.

57 Pinhas-Hamiel O, Dolan LM, Zeitler PS. Diabetic ketoacidosis among obese African-American adolescents with NIDDM. *Diabetes Care* 1997; **20**: 484–6.

58 Krakoff J, Lindsay RS, Looker HC *et al.* Incidence of retinopathy and nephropathy in youth-onset compared with adult-onset type 2 diabetes. *Diabetes Care* 2003; **26**: 76–81.

59 Eppens MC, Craig ME, Cusumano J *et al.* Prevalence of diabetes complications in adolescents with type 2 compared with type 1 diabetes. *Diabetes Care* 2006; **29**: 1300–6.

60 Pavkov ME, Bennett PH, Knowler WC *et al.* Effect of youth-onset type 2 diabetes mellitus on incidence of end-stage renal disease and mortality in young and middle-aged Pima Indians. *JAMA* 2006; **296**: 421–6.

61 Nadeau KJ, Klingensmith G, Zeitler P. Type 2 diabetes in children is frequently associated with elevated alanine aminotransferase. *J Pediatr Gastroenterol Nutr* 2005; **41**: 94–98.

62 Roberts EA. Non-alcoholic fatty liver disease (NAFLD) in children. *Front Biosci* 2005; **10**: 2306–18.

63 American Diabetes Association. Type 2 diabetes in children and adolescents. *Diabetes Care* 2000; **23**: 381–9.

64 American Diabetes Association. Screening for type 2 diabetes. *Diabetes Care* 2004; **27**(suppl 1): S11–14.

65 Urakami T, Kubota S, Nitadori Y *et al.* Annual incidence and clinical characteristics of type 2 diabetes in children as detected by urine glucose screening in the Tokyo metropolitan area. *Diabetes Care* 2005; **28**: 1876–81.

66 Alberti G, Zimmet P, Shaw J *et al.* Type 2 diabetes in the young: the evolving epidemic: the international diabetes federation consensus workshop. *Diabetes Care* 2004; **27**: 1798–1811.

67 Pinhas-Hamiel O, Standiford D, Hamiel D *et al.* The type 2 family: a setting for development and treatment of adolescent type 2 diabetes mellitus. *Arch Pediatr Adolesc Med* 1999; **153**: 1063–7.

68 Fajans SS, Bell GI, Polonsky KS. Molecular mechanisms and clinical pathophysiology of maturity-onset diabetes of the young. *N Engl J Med* 2001; **345**: 971–80.

69 Owen K, Hattersley AT. Maturity-onset diabetes of the young: from clinical description to molecular genetic characterization. *Best Pract Res Clin Endocrinol Metab* 2001; **15**: 309–23.

70 Ehtisham S, Hattersley AT, Dunger DB *et al.* First UK survey of paediatric type 2 diabetes and MODY. *Arch Dis Child* 2004; **89**: 526–9.

71 Valerio G, Franzese A, Carlin E *et al.* High prevalence of stress hyperglycaemia in children with febrile seizures and traumatic injuries. *Acta Paediatr* 2001; **90**: 618–22.

72 Bhisitkul DM, Vinik AI, Morrow AL *et al.* Prediabetic markers in children with stress hyperglycemia. *Arch Pediatr Adolesc Med* 1996; **150**: 936–41.

73 Herskowitz-Dumont R, Wolfsdorf JI, Jackson RA *et al.* Distinction between transient hyperglycemia and early insulin-dependent diabetes mellitus in childhood: a prospective study of incidence and prognostic factors. *J Pediatr* 1993; **123**: 347–54.

74 Herskowitz RD, Wolfsdorf JI, Ricker AT *et al.* Transient hyperglycemia in childhood: identification of a subgroup with imminent diabetes mellitus. *Diabetes Res* 1988; **9**: 161–7.

75 Schatz DA, Kowa H, Winter WE *et al.* Natural history of incidental hyperglycemia and glycosuria of childhood. *J Pediatr* 1989; **115**: 676–80.

76 Shehadeh N, On A, Kessel I *et al.* Stress hyperglycemia and the risk for the development of type 1 diabetes. *J Pediatr Endocrinol Metab* 1997; **10**: 283–6.

77 Vardi P, Shehade N, Etzioni A *et al.* Stress hyperglycemia in childhood: a very high risk group for the development of type I diabetes. *J Pediatr* 1990; **117**: 75–7.

78 ISPAD. *Consensus Guidelines for the Management of Type 1 Diabetes Mellitus in Children and Adolescents.* Available at: http://www.diabetesguidelines.com/health/dkw/pro/guidelines/ispad/ispad.asp

79 NHMRC. *The Australian Clinical Practice Guidelines on the Management of Type 1 Diabetes in Children and Adolescents 2005.* Available at: http://www.chw.edu.au/prof/services/endocrinology/apeg/

80 NICE. *Type 1 Diabetes in Children and Young People: Full Guideline 2004.* Available at: http://www.nice.org.uk/page.aspx?o=CG015childfullguideline

81 Zgibor JC, Songer TJ, Kelsey SF *et al.* Influence of health care providers on the development of diabetes complications: long-term follow-up from the Pittsburgh Epidemiology of Diabetes Complications Study. *Diabetes Care* 2002; **25**: 1584–90.

82 Ahern JA, Ramchandani N, Cooper J *et al.* Using a primary nurse manager to implement DCCT recommendations in a large pediatric program. *Diabetes Educ* 2000; **26**: 990–4.

83 Cowan FJ, Warner JT, Lowes LM *et al.* Auditing paediatric diabetes care and the impact of a specialist nurse trained in paediatric diabetes. *Arch Dis Child* 1997; **77**: 109–14.

84 Donaghue KC, Craig ME, Chan AK *et al.* Prevalence of diabetes complications 6 years after diagnosis in an incident cohort of childhood diabetes. *Diabet Med* 2005; **22**: 711–18.

85 Galatzer A, Amir S, Gil R *et al.* Crisis intervention program in newly diagnosed diabetic children. *Diabetes Care* 1982; **5**: 414–19.

86 Gelfand K, Geffken G, Lewin A *et al.* An initial evaluation of the design of pediatric psychology consultation service with children with diabetes. *J Child Health Care* 2004; **8**: 113–23.

87 DCCT Research Group. The effect of intensive treatment of diabetes on the development and progression of long-term complications in insulin-dependent diabetes mellitus. The Diabetes Control and Complications Trial Research Group. *N Engl J Med* 1993; **329**: 977–86.

88 DCCT Research Group. Effect of intensive diabetes treatment on the development and progression of long-term complications in adolescents with insulin-dependent diabetes mellitus: Diabetes Control and Complications Trial. Diabetes Control and Complications Trial Research Group. *J Pediatr* 1994; **125**: 177–88.

89 Kaufman FR, Halvorson M, Carpenter S. Association between diabetes control and visits to a multi-disciplinary pediatric diabetes clinic. *Pediatrics* 1999; **103**: 948–51.

90 Lawson ML, Frank MR, Fry MK *et al.* Intensive diabetes management in adolescents with type 1 diabetes: the importance of intensive follow-up. *J Pediatr Endocrinol Metab* 2000; **13**: 79–84.

91 McEvilly A, Kirk J. Twenty years of a multidisciplinary paediatric diabetes home care unit. *Arch Dis Child* 2005; **90**: 342–5.

92 Levetan CS, Salas JR, Wilets IF *et al*. Impact of endocrine and diabetes team consultation on hospital length of stay for patients with diabetes. *Am J Med* 1995; **99**: 22–8.

93 Clar C, Waugh N, Thomas S. Routine hospital admission versus out-patient or home care in children at diagnosis of type 1 diabetes mellitus. *Cochrane Database Syst Rev* 2003; Issue no 3: Art No CD004099

94 Srinivasan S, Craig ME, Beeney L *et al*. An ambulatory stabilisation program for children with newly diagnosed type 1 diabetes. *Med J Aust* 2004; **180**: 277–80.

95 Nordly S, Mortensen HB, Andreasen AH *et al*. Factors associated with glycaemic outcome of childhood diabetes care in Denmark. *Diabet Med* 2005; **22**: 1566–73.

96 von Sengbusch S, Muller-Godeffroy E, Hager S *et al*. Mobile diabetes education and care: intervention for children and young people with Type 1 diabetes in rural areas of northern Germany. *Diabet Med* 2006; **23**: 122–7.

97 Cagliero E, Levina EV, Nathan DM. Immediate feedback of HbA1c levels improves glycemic control in type 1 and insulin-treated type 2 diabetic patients. *Diabetes Care* 1999; **22**: 1785–9.

98 d'Annunzio G, Bellazzi R, Larizza C *et al*. Telemedicine in the management of young patients with type 1 diabetes mellitus: a follow-up study. *Acta Biomed Ateneo Parmense* 2003; **74**(suppl 1): 49–55.

99 Farmer A, Gibson OJ, Tarassenko L *et al*. A systematic review of telemedicine interventions to support blood glucose self-monitoring in diabetes. *Diabet Med* 2005; **22**: 1372–8.

100 Gelfand K, Geffken G, Halsey-Lyda M *et al*. Intensive telehealth management of five at-risk adolescents with diabetes. *J Telemed Telecare* 2003; **9**: 117–21.

101 Izquierdo RE, Knudson PE, Meyer S *et al*. A comparison of diabetes education administered through telemedicine versus in person. *Diabetes Care* 2003; **26**: 1002–7.

102 Liesenfeld B, Renner R, Neese M *et al*. Telemedical care reduces hypoglycemias and improves glycemic control in children and adolescents with type 1 diabetes. *Diabetes Technol Ther* 2000; **2**: 561–7.

103 Howells L, Wilson AC, Skinner TC *et al*. A randomized control trial of the effect of negotiated telephone support on glycaemic control in young people with Type 1 diabetes. *Diabet Med* 2002; **19**: 643–8.

104 Lawson ML, Cohen N, Richardson C *et al*. A randomized trial of regular standardized telephone contact by a diabetes nurse educator in adolescents with poor diabetes control. *Pediatr Diabetes* 2005; **6**: 32–40.

CHAPTER 3

Aetiology of type 1 diabetes mellitus – genetics, autoimmunity and trigger factors

Loredana Marcovecchio, David B. Dunger,
Mark Peakman & Keith W. Taylor

A thing is not proved just because no one has ever questioned it. What has never been gone into impartially has never been properly gone into. Hence scepticism is the first step toward truth. It must be applied generally, because it is the touchstone.
— Denis Diderot, French author, encyclopaedist and philosopher (1713–1784)

It is now well established that type 1 diabetes mellitus (T1DM) results from a combination of a genetic predisposition and autoimmune processes that result in destruction of the beta cells of the pancreas and cause absolute insulin deficiency. However, not everyone who has this genetic predisposition develops T1DM and it is also thought that some additional factor is required to trigger the autoimmune responses that cause the beta-cell destruction. This chapter presents the evidence that is currently available to define that genetic predisposition, the immunological processes that occur to cause beta-cell destruction and the trigger factors that may provide the necessary spark.

Genetics of T1DM

Loredana Marcovecchio and David Dunger

T1DM is an autoimmune disease with genetic and environmental factors implicated in its aetiology. The role of genetic factors in the susceptibility to T1DM is strongly supported by family and twin studies (**B**) [1, 2]. The familial clustering of T1DM is well known, with 10–13% of newly diagnosed cases having a first-degree relative with T1DM and a 15-fold increased risk of developing the disease for a sibling (5–6%) of a patient with T1DM when compared to the general population (0.4%) (**B**) [2]. The family recurrence of T1DM varies depending on which relative is affected, with a higher risk for the siblings than for the offspring or parents of a patient with T1DM (**B**) [2, 3]. Furthermore, the risk for an offspring is higher when the father (6–9%) is affected than when the mother (1.3–4.0%) is the index case, and this difference might be related to imprinted genes or to a protective role of maternal environmental factors during pregnancy (**B**) [3].

In T1DM the concordance rate for monozygotic twins ranges between 21 and 70%, while for dizygotic twins it is 0–13% (**B**) [2]. The progression rate to T1DM for monozygotic

Table 3.1 Examples of HLA haplotypes and genotypes associated with susceptibility for or protection against T1DM

	DR alleles	DQ alleles	OR-r (CI)
High-risk haplotypes	DR4: DRB1*0401	A1*0301, B1*0302 (DQ8)	8.3 (7.2–9.6)
	DR4: DRB1*0405	A1*0301, B1*0302	6.6 (5.3–8.3)
	DR4: DRB1*0402	A1*0301, B1*0302	4.0 (3.0–5.5)
	DR4: DRB1*0404	A1*0301, B1*0302	3.5 (3.0–4.1)
	DR3: DRB1*0301	A1*0501, B1*0201 (DQ2)	4.1 (3.7–4.6)
Protective haplotypes	DR2: DRB1*15	A1*01, B1*06 (DQ6)	0.0 (0.0–0.1)
	DR5: DRB1*11	A1*0501, B1*0301	0.1 (0.1–0.2)
	DR6: DRB*14	A1*01, B1*05	0.1 (0.1–0.2)
	DR7: DRB*07	A1*0201, B1*0303	0.1 (0.1–0.2)
	DR4: DRB*0407	A1*0301, B1*0301	0.2 (0.1–0.4)
	DR/DQ haplotype 1	**DR/DQ haplotype 2**	**OR-r (CI)**
Genotypes	DR4/DQ8	DR3/DQ2	47.2 (26.7–83.3)
	DR4/DQ8	DR4/DQ8	11.9 (6.1–23.1)
	DR3/DQ2	DR3/DQ2	10.4 (6.0–18.0)
	DR2/DQ6	DR2/DQ6	0.1 (0.0–0.3)

OR-r (CI), odds ratios (confidence intervals), calculated relative to the *DQB1*5-DRB1*01* reference haplotype (OR = 1).
Data from Koeleman BP *et al.*, 2004 [7].

twins is greater than 50% if the index twin develops diabetes before the age of 5 years, while it is less than 10% if the diagnosis is made after the age of 25 years (**A, B**) [4, 5]. The absence of a 100% concordance between monozygotic twins, however, suggests that other factors, such as environmental triggers, are implicated (**B**) [2].

Multiple genetic loci contributing to T1DM risk have been identified but not all have been confirmed. They provide both susceptibility and protection (**B**) [6]. The human leucocyte antigen (HLA) complex (*IDDM1* locus) was the first susceptibility locus to be associated with T1DM and it confers about 40–50% of the inherited risk (**B**) [6]. The HLA genes, located within the major histocompatibility complex on the chromosome 6p21, are highly polymorphic and have an important role in the modulation of the immune system (Figure 3.1). The risk for T1DM is mostly associated with class II genes, particularly with *HLA-DRB1*, *DQA1* and *DQB1* (**B**) [1, 6–8] (Table 3.1). The high-risk haplotypes *DR3/DQ2* (*DRB1*0301-DQA1*0501-DQB1*0201*) and *DR4/DQ8* (*DRB1*0401, *0402, *0405-DQA1*0301-DQB1*0201*) are carried by more than 90% of white Caucasian individuals with T1DM and by fewer than 40% of normal controls. The highest risk is associated with *DR3/DR4* heterozygosity, which is found in almost 50% of children who develop diabetes before the age of 5 years, in 20–30% of adults presenting with diabetes and in only 2.4% of the general population (**B**) [2]. However, the HLA high-risk genotypes seem to be uncommon in children with permanent neonatal diabetes and in those diagnosed before the age of 6 months, who are therefore more likely to have a non-autoimmune form of diabetes, often related to activating mutations in the *Kir6.2* (*KCNJ11*) and *SUR1* genes (**A**) [9–11].

The different HLA haplotypes are also associated with the pattern of autoantibodies, with insulin autoantibodies (IAA) and IA-2 particularly frequent in patients with the *DR4-DQ8* haplotype and GAD-65 more common in patients with the *DR3-DQ2* haplotype and the

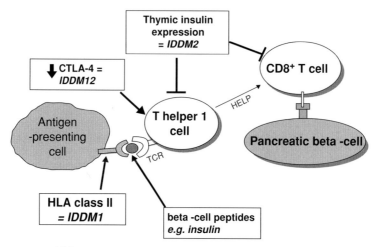

Figure 3.1 A model for immune pathogenesis in T1DM: role of the susceptibility *loci IDDM1*, *IDDM2* and *IDDM12*.

highest probability to be autoantibody negative for patients without *DR3* and *DR4* (**B**) [12]. Some HLA alleles can also confer protection from diabetes and among them the best known is *HLA-DQ6* (*HLA-DQB1*0602*), carried by fewer than 1% of subjects with T1DM compared to 20% of the general population (**B**) [2].

The second known susceptibility locus for T1DM is *IDDM2* on chromosome 11p15.5, which includes the variable number of tandem repeats (*VNTR*) region located in the promoter of the insulin gene and contributes about 10% to disease susceptibility (**B**) [2]. There are three main classes of *VNTR* alleles, categorised on the basis of the number of repeats: class I (26–63 repeats), class II (approximately, 80 repeats) and class III (140–200 repeats). Variation in the number of repeats affects the expression of the insulin gene in the thymus and pancreas and the placental expression of the insulin-like growth factor 2 gene [13]. The class III alleles determine the highest insulin levels within the thymus and confer a dominant protection against T1DM, while homozygosity for class I alleles is associated with the lowest insulin expression and the highest risk for the disease. The association between insulin expression within the thymus and diabetes susceptibility is thought to be related to a dose-dependent effect of insulin in modifying the selection of potentially damaging autoreactive T cells and/or inducing insulin-specific regulatory T cells (i.e. high insulin levels in the thymus lead to deletion of the damaging cells and induction of regulatory ones) [13] (Figure 3.1). The susceptibility related to *VNTR* polymorphisms shows race-dependent differences, with a greater effect in white Caucasians than in black Caucasians and no effect in the Japanese population (**A**) [14]. Furthermore, in some studies a parent-of-origin effect has been described, with protection deriving from the paternally transmitted allele (**A**) [15].

The third susceptibility locus in T1DM (*IDDM12*) is located on chromosome 2q33 and encodes a co-stimulatory molecule, called cytotoxic T lymphocyte antigen 4 (*CTLA-4*), which is expressed on the surface of activated T cells (**B**) [16, 17] and plays a critical role in the response to antigens through a negative regulation of T-cell activation. Different polymorphisms in the *CTLA-4* gene have been associated with T1DM and they are located in the 3' untranslated, promoter (−319C > T) and coding regions (+49A/G) (**B**) [17].

Some of these polymorphisms are associated with reduced stability of the RNA or alterations in the splicing mechanism with a reduced expression of *CTLA-4* on the cell surface (Figure 3.1). Recently, evidence for a role of *CTLA-4* in other autoimmune endocrinopathies, particularly Grave's disease and hypothyroidism, has also been found (**A**) [18]. As for *IDDM2*, also for the *IDDM12* locus there is an ethnic heterogeneity in susceptibility to T1DM (**B**) [19].

A fourth human susceptibility locus, protein tyrosine phosphatase non-receptor type 22 (*PTPN22*), on chromosome 1p13, has recently been reported (**B, A**) [20, 21]. This locus contains the gene encoding for a lymphocyte-specific phosphatase implicated in a negative regulation of T-cell development and activation.

Recently, convincing statistical support has also been found for two other regions: the IL2RA/CD25 on chromosome 10p15.1, encoding the alpha chain of the IL-2 receptor, and the interferon-induced helicase 1 gene region (*IFIH1*/MDA5) on chromosome 2q24.3 (**A**) [22, 23].

Other loci have been associated with T1DM, but for most of them the related gene has not been identified yet and different results have been often found in different populations (Table 3.2) [24–30]. Linkage and association analyses have been the two main approaches used to identify T1DM susceptibility genes but the main barrier in their mapping results from small sample sizes and the heterogeneity of the populations analysed in different genome-wide scans (**C**). In order to facilitate the identification of genes implicated in T1DM with a good statistical power, a collection of DNA samples from 8000 subjects with T1DM and the same number of controls has now been underway as part of the UK Genetic Resource Investigating Diabetes (GRID) study (**A**) [31]. Furthermore, a T1DM consortium has also been established with the aim of collecting and analysing thousands of DNA samples from affected sibling pairs (**A**) [24].

Immunology of T1DM

Mark Peakman

T1DM has all of the hallmarks of an autoimmune disorder; indeed, it is often referred to as the prototypic organ-specific autoimmune disease (Table 3.3). What exactly does this mean? In short, it implies that in a patient with the disease the immune system has become sufficiently dysregulated to attack and destroy healthy islet beta cells. This process takes between a few months and several years and is the end result of a complex interplay of host genetic and environmental factors, which are becoming increasingly better understood.

Pathology of the islet in T1DM

Healthy human islets of Langerhans are composed of a core of some 80% beta cells (making the glucose-regulating hormone insulin), with a mantle of other endocrine cell types, producing glucagon, somatostatin and pancreatic polypeptide (alpha, delta and PP cells, respectively) making up the remainder. Histologically, the islets of Langerhans at diagnosis of T1DM have a mixture of appearances:
• Some islets are small, without beta cells and have no inflammatory cells.
• Others have numerous beta cells surrounded by infiltrating activated T (CD4 and CD8) and B lymphocytes and various antigen-presenting cells (APCs) of the immune system (an appearance termed insulitis) [41].
• Some islets appear normal.

Table 3.2 T1DM susceptibility loci with LOD scores as observed in genome linkage scans

Locus	Location	Candidate gene	LOD [reference]
IDDM1	6p21	*HLA DR/DQ*	116.4 [24]
IDDM2	11p15	*Insulin VNTR*	1.87 [24]
IDDM3	15q26		2.5 [25]
IDDM4	11q13	*ZFM1, LRP5, FADD*	3.4 [26]
IDDM5	6q25	*SUMO4, MnSOD*	1.96 [27]
IDDM6	18q12-q21	*JK, ZNF236, BCL-2*	1.1 [26]
IDDM7	2q33	*NEUROD, IL1B, HOXD8, GAD1, GALNT3*	3.34 [24]
IDDM8	6q27		1.8 [27]
IDDM9	3q22-25		3.4 [28]
IDDM10	10p11-q11		3.21 [24]
IDDM11	14q24-q31	*ENSA, SEL1L*	4.0 [29]
IDDM12	2q31-q33	*CTLA-4*	3.34 [24]
IDDM13	2q34-q35	*IGFBP-2, IGFBP-5, IA-2, NRAMPI*	2.6 [27]
IDDM15	6q21		22.4 [24]
IDDM16	14q32	*IGH*	
IDDM17	10q25		2.38 [30]
IDDM18	5q33	*IL12B*	
	1p13	*PTPN22 (LYP)*	
	1q42		2.2 [27]
	2q24.3	*IFIH1 (MDA5)*	
	3p13-p14		1.52 [24]
	9q33-q34		2.20 [24]
	10p15	*IL2RA (CD45)*	
	12q14-q12		1.66 [24]
	16p12-q11.1		1.88 [24]
	16q22-q24		2.64 [24]
	17q25		1.81 [27]
	19q11		1.80 [27]
	19p13.3-p13.2		1.92 [24]

LOD scores are mostly from the recent four genome-wide linkage scans in 1435 multiplex families (USA, UK and Scandinavia) [24]. As this analysis did not show significant linkage for some loci previously identified, a LOD value from a different reference is reported, when available.
LOD, logarithm of odds.

Table 3.3 Evidence that T1DM is an autoimmune disease

Criteria	Reference
Major	
Presence of circulating autoantibodies against targets in the beta cell	[32]
Presence of circulating, activated T cells directed against targets in the beta cell	[33, 34]
Clinical response to immune suppression	[35–37]
Coexistence of other autoimmune diseases (thyroiditis and the Addison disease)	[38]
Inclusion of T1DM in autoimmune polyendocrine syndromes (APS I, II)	[38]
Minor	
Existence of relevant spontaneous animal model (NOD mouse)	[39]
Passive transfer of disease using T lymphocytes from diabetic NOD mouse to naïve mouse	[39]
Association between T1DM and possession of HLA genes	[40]

NOD, non-obese diabetic.

It is probable that these appearances reflect stages of a process during which the immune cells travel between islets in a 'seek, destroy, move on' operation ('flitting insulitis'). This immune system's 'target-and-destroy' operation is exquisitely specific – only the beta cells are damaged, whilst the other endocrine cells remain intact and functional.

Islet cell autoantibodies

Islet cell autoantibodies are the defining immunological feature of T1DM. There are three proteins that constitute the major target autoantigens for these autoantibodies:
• insulin (IAA)
• glutamic acid decarboxylse 65 (GAD-65 autoantibodies, GADA)
• tyrosine phosphatase-like molecule called IA-2 (IA-2A)

Insulin is the only islet autoantigen specifically localised to the beta cells. GAD-65 and IA-2 may also be found in other islet cell types and in the central and peripheral nervous system. Although each individual autoantibody may only be present in a half to three-quarters of children at the time of development of T1DM, typically 90–95% of these will have at least one of the autoantibodies. Insulin autoantibodies are more prevalent in children than in adults, whilst the reverse is true of GADA (A) [32].

The technology to detect these three types of islet cell autoantibodies is now widely available in clinical immunology laboratories, begging the question as to when their measurement might be useful clinically. In the vast majority of cases T1DM is diagnosed clinically in children because of the classical history and laboratory findings. Rarely in children, but more commonly in adults, the disease may evolve slowly or have an unusual presentation and autoantibodies are useful as a confirmation. However, the detection of islet cell autoantibodies is emerging as being especially important in disease prediction. From studies on individuals at risk of developing T1DM (e.g. first-degree relatives of patients), it has become clear that apparently healthy people can have islet cell autoantibodies – up to 10% of relatives are positive for IAA, GADA or IA-2A when tested. Through the prospective follow-up of such individuals for 5–10 years, a very clear pattern of disease risk has emerged, in which some of these relatives do indeed progress to diabetes, the risk increasing with the number of autoantibodies present (B) [42]. Thus it would appear that the breadth and intensity of the autoimmune response, as reflected in the number of different autoantibodies produced, determines whether anti-islet immunity develops into clinical disease. These pioneering studies have now been translated into the general population (A) [43]. (This is important for screening purposes, as 90% of new diabetic patients do not have relatives with the disease.) Although far fewer of the general public are autoantibody positive, those who are have a disease risk determined by the number of autoantibodies present. Combinations of autoantibodies and genetic markers (e.g. the high-risk HLA gene *DQB1*0302*) can be used to increase the specificity of prediction. Although disease prediction through islet cell autoantibody detection was initially an academic exercise, it has become the lynchpin of strategies for the development of new approaches to disease prevention (see below) and is being increasingly developed and refined.

The immune pathogenesis of T1DM

Advances in immunological understanding in the last 30 years, since the first descriptions of HLA and autoantibody associations with T1DM, have led to a much clearer view of how beta cells might undergo damage, although many questions remain. The fact that islet cell

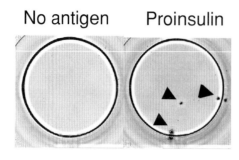

No antigen   Proinsulin

Figure 3.2 Visualising beta-cell-specific autoreactive T cells in T1DM. Here, the circulating lymphocytes from a patient have been stimulated with peptide from proinsulin, representing a known target in the beta cell. CD4$^+$ T cells reacting against the peptide produce interferon gamma, visualised here through an immunochemical technique termed the enzyme-linked cellular immunospot assay. Each spot (arrowed) represents a CD4$^+$ T cell responding to proinsulin. Such cells are present at low frequency (1/20,000–1/100,000) in patients and are generally absent in non-diabetic individuals.

autoantibodies cannot induce diabetes by passive transfer into animals, and do not transfer disease to the unborn fetus despite being occasionally present in cord blood, argues strongly against autoantibodies *per se* being responsible for beta-cell damage. Rather, T lymphocytes recognising islet autoantigens are widely considered to be the agents responsible for beta-cell destruction [44]. Indirect evidence for this derives from the fact that therapeutic agents directed against T cells can preserve beta-cell mass (see below), at least for as long as the therapy is given. There are also several case reports in which T1DM has arisen in non-diabetic individuals a few months or years after receiving bone marrow grafts (for haematological malignancy) from siblings with T1DM, despite the recipients having undergone ablation of their own immune system as part of the conditioning regimen (**C**) [45, 46]. This inadvertent 'passive transfer' of the agents that cause diabetes can be prevented by depletion of mature T cells from the graft, strongly implying that memory T cells reactive against islet targets remain for many years after diabetes diagnosis and can be reactivated in the new host, with diabetes as the outcome.

Confirmation that such T cells can be found has come from analysis of T-cell responses in peripheral blood, showing that during the late stages of disease (no studies have as yet looked at the pre-diabetic period) there are CD4 helper T cells present in the blood that recognise islet autoantigens, such as proinsulin, GAD-65 and IA-2 (**A**) [33, 34]. These T cells secrete pro-inflammatory cytokines, such as interferon gamma and tumour necrosis factor alpha, in response to this stimulation, thus categorising T1DM as a disease driven by type 1 helper T cell (T$_H$1) cells (Figure 3.2) [33, 47]. These cytokines in themselves can have damaging effects on islet beta cells. However, the presence of CD8$^+$ T cells in the insulitis also implies that T$_H$1 cells drive the generation of cytotoxic T cells that recognise islet components, and these cells would be capable of direct damage to beta cells through the release of cytokines and toxic granules (e.g. perforin and granzymes). CD8 T cells have proved a greater challenge to study, but recent advances have also demonstrated islet-reactive cytotoxic T cells in the peripheral blood (**B**) [48]. Thus the most favoured pathogenic scenario suggests that the combined efforts of T$_H$1 and CD8 T cells conspire to kill beta cells (Figure 3.3).

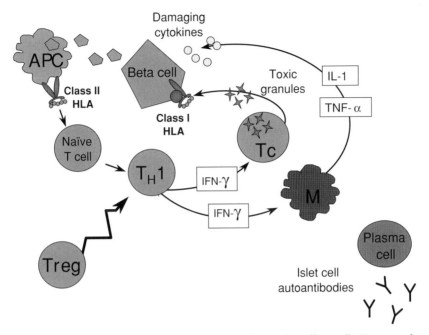

Figure 3.3 Probable steps involved in immune system destruction of beta cells. Damage to beta cells (possibly through effects of islet-tropic viruses) leads to uptake of beta-cell autoantigens by antigen-presenting cells (APCs) and transport to the local lymph node for presentation to naïve CD4 T cells. As a result of the associated inflammation, a Th1 response is dominant, leading to induction of beta-cell autoantigen-specific CD4 T cells that may also drive cytotoxic CD8 T-cell generation (Tc) or, after migration to islets, activation of tissue macrophages (M). In concert, these cells promote islet damage through release of cytokines (IL-1, interleukin-1; tumour necrosis factor-alpha, TNF-α) and toxic granules. Plasma cells producing islet cell autoantibodies are generated as a consequence but have little or no direct pathogenic role. Failure of regulatory mechanisms (Treg) allows the process to be initiated and perpetuated. (Reproduced from Hyöty and Taylor [65] with permission.)

It remains to be established what mechanisms in the host are operative to allow these cells to become activated from naïve precursors and expand in sufficient numbers to cause such tissue damage. In theory, potentially autoreactive T cells are deleted in the thymus during fetal and neonatal development. For those that might escape and have the potential to cause autoimmune disease, there should be peripheral mechanisms of control. Thymic deletion might fail if the key autoantigens, such as insulin, are not available in the thymus to allow the deletion of T cells that react against them. It is interesting to note, therefore, that the polymorphism in the *INS* gene that is associated with increased diabetes susceptibility appears to give reduced levels of thymic insulin mRNA, as discussed above **(B)** [49]. Thymic insulin mRNA levels are also reduced in the absence of the *AIRE* gene (for autoimmune regulator) which is the genetic abnormality underlying the autoimmune polyendocrine syndrome type 1 (APS-1), of which autoimmune diabetes is a feature **(A)** [38, 50]. Peripheral mechanisms of regulation might also fail, and there are reports in the literature that an important population of regulatory T cells (the CD4$^+$CD25$^+$ regulatory T cell (Treg) subset) is defective in T1DM patients **(A)** [51]. Moreover, as mentioned, T1DM is associated with a polymorphism in the gene encoding *CTLA-4*, a negative regulator of immune responses that is expressed by some Tregs (**B**) [17].

Under unfavourable circumstances, therefore, such as incomplete thymic deletion of insulin-reactive T cells or impaired peripheral regulation, activation of autoreactive T_H1 cells could ensue under at least two possible circumstances. The first of these would arise if there were mimicry between a pathogen and a beta-cell autoantigen, such that the immune response to the microbe induced T_H1 cells with cross-reactivity with the beta cell. Although an attractive theory, there is very little evidence to support this pathogenic scenario in man. A second possibility is termed bystander activation. Here, an islet-tropic pathogen induces an inflammatory response and limited islet damage that leads to presentation of some beta-cell autoantigens in the local lymph node. Poor islet-specific regulation, and/or availability of T cells that have not been deleted in the thymus, could favour the initiation of an autoimmune response, which leads to further beta-cell damage, and a slowly evolving, vicious cycle.

The piece of the jigsaw that is missing in these schemes is the role of HLA molecules in T1DM development. The genes encoding these confer by far the highest genetically determined disease risk, yet the mechanism through which HLA molecules confer protection or susceptibility is not known. Since HLA molecules present antigenic peptides to T cells, it is most likely that HLA exerts its effect during thymic selection or during the activation of autoreactive T cells in the periphery.

Diabetes prevention and cure

As discussed, advances in the use of genes and autoantibodies to predict diabetes make it feasible to identify individuals who are pre-diabetic. Current protocols for this can predict future diabetes in first-degree relatives of diabetic probands such that 40–50% will develop the disease within 5 years. This opens up the possibility of interfering in the disease process at a relatively early stage. Two pioneering multicentre studies have demonstrated the feasibility of this. In one (the US-based Diabetes Prevention Trials), either low-dose parenteral insulin (**A**) [52] or daily oral insulin (**A**) [53] was administered to high-risk individuals, with screening of over 100,000 first-degree relatives required to achieve the requisite number of participants. The rationale for these studies was a series of experiments in animal models demonstrating that insulin administration by a number of different routes could prevent diabetes progression, possibly by restoration of tolerance to this key autoantigen or by allowing beta-cell recovery [54]. The parenteral study showed no therapeutic effect. Likewise, at first analysis, the oral insulin study also showed no effect of therapy. However, a significant beneficial treatment effect was seen in a subgroup of subjects with high titre IAA that received oral insulin, suggesting that the approach works best in the presence of definite insulin-specific autoimmunity. In another study of similar scale, the European Nicotinamide Diabetes Intervention Trial (ENDIT), nicotinamide was administered as a beta-cell protectant, but without success (**A**) [55].

Although disappointing, these landmark studies have important sequelae. First, the outcome of the oral insulin study is of great potential interest, and a repeat study is already planned. Second, these studies have provided proof of concept that multicentre efforts, with sophisticated screening algorithms, can achieve appropriately powered recruitment targets and reach designated end points. As a direct result, an initiative called Diabetes TrialNet (http://www.diabetestrialnet.org/) has been established. The aim is to achieve rapid throughput of clinical intervention strategies in T1DM, at both the preventive (pre-diabetic) and the intervention (at diagnosis) stages. Interventions that are effective at diagnosis in preserving residual beta-cell mass are also of potential importance, since they may reduce insulin requirements, enhance glycaemic control and delay initiation and progression of complications. There is considerable interest in agents that might achieve this and monoclonal anti-CD3 antibody has emerged from two independent studies (**A, B**) [35, 36, 55] as a therapy that after a single administration preserves beta-cell function for 12–24 months (CD3 is a surface molecule present on all T cells). The anti-CD3 therapy does not deplete the immune system of T cells, rather T cell function is transiently modulated, possibly leading to enhanced Treg function. Other immunosuppressive agents with similarly acceptable toxicity profiles are also in clinical trials.

It seems probable that immune suppression alone will not be the only approach required to cure or prevent T1DM. Like any complex human disease, combinations of therapeutic approaches, each aimed at a different aspect of the disease process, will be needed to obtain any long-lasting impact on the disease. It is clear from the discussion above regarding the outcome of bone marrow transplantation from diabetic donors, as well as the outcome of twin–twin pancreas transplants (in which the recipient twin with T1DM destroyed the new islets in the donor pancreas from their non-diabetic co-twin a short period after engraftment (**C**)) [56], that autoreactive T cells capable of driving the T1DM process are long-lived and capable of reactivation. One approach to achieving long-lasting therapeutic effects is therefore to induce or promote the activity of beta-cell antigen-specific Tregs. This can be achieved in animal models through administration of beta-cell antigens in 'tolerogenic' regimes, and this approach, termed antigen-specific immunotherapy, is an active area of clinical research [57] (see also [37, 39, 40]).

In summary, through numerous avenues of clinical, animal and laboratory research over the last four decades, the immune pathogenesis of T1DM has been unravelled. Absolute knowledge and certainty are lacking, but there is sufficient progress for empirical intervention studies to be contemplated, designed and implemented.

Trigger factors for T1DM

Ken Taylor

It is now generally accepted that a combination of genetic and environmental factors is responsible for T1DM in children. The genetics of this form of diabetes is discussed elsewhere in this chapter. This short review will consider some of the more important extraneous agents that are thought to be involved in inducing the disease especially in genetically susceptible children. They are best classified under the headings:
- toxic
- nutritional
- infective

Such factors are discussed in relation to specific effects on the B cells of pancreatic islets, which may lead to insulin deficiency.

Toxic factors

Although toxic factors may seem rather unlikely to be important triggers for initiating diabetes among children, they should not be entirely discounted. A host of toxic chemicals is known that may damage the insulin-producing cells of the islets of Langerhans in animals and, clearly, this may be the case sometimes in man. The nitroso-compound streptozotocin used in treating tumours of the islets is in this category. Epidemiological studies have however suggested that the onset of T1DM in children may be related to an excess of nitrates in food or drinking water (**B**) [58, 59]. Nitrates could be a precursor of nitroso-compounds. The present status of these agents is unclear in the induction of most cases of childhood diabetes. Their effect may be additive to other factors.

Nutritional factors

Cow's milk proteins

The finding that breast-feeding as opposed to cow's milk feeding in infancy appeared to protect children from diabetes led to theories that breast milk proteins from a different species might have diabetogenic properties (**B**) [60]. It was postulated that antibodies to cow's milk proteins might cross-react with islet cell membrane proteins so as to induce damage. The role of milk proteins in triggering diabetes is at present very controversial [61]. There are many other dietary factors that may influence the rate of development of the disease, without initiating it. They are reviewed elsewhere [61].

Infections

Early work on the seasonal incidence of diabetes has been interpreted as indicating an infective aetiology for the disease [62]. Very recently, clustering analyses of the newly diagnosed have reinforced this view (**B**) [63, 64].

Infections can act in two ways to promote the full clinical expression of childhood diabetes. They can act non-specifically to reduce glucose tolerance, and thus to exacerbate a developing diabetes. Alternatively, they may act specifically on the B cells of islets at various stages of a destructive process. This is the case with some viruses. Bacterial infections by contrast may frequently diminish carbohydrate tolerance temporarily.

Virus infections and diabetes

A large number of viruses have been reported to be diabetogenic in man and animals. They include both RNA and DNA viruses. In most instances effects on the islets of Langerhans have been reported. They are discussed in detail in reviews elsewhere [65, 66].

However, only a few of these viruses seem relevant to childhood diabetes. These are mumps, rubella and certain members of the enterovirus group (coxsackie and echoviruses). Other viruses that have occasionally been associated with childhood diabetes include rotavirus, cytomegalovirus and retrovirus [65].

Mumps
An association between mumps infection and diabetes has been suggested for well over a hundred years, (**C**) [67] and there are many case reports in the literature that support this. More systematic analysis of mumps in large surveys has confirmed the association of the two diseases (**C**) [68]. Only a very small number of cases of newly diagnosed diabetes seemed directly attributable to mumps, in the period before MMR vaccines were in use [68].

Rubella
The link between the congenital rubella syndrome and the later development of diabetes was first pointed out by Menser and her colleagues in Australia many years ago (**B**) [69].

Follow-up on the children revealed that diabetes, sometimes of an insulin-requiring type, appeared in up to 25% of cases analysed and often after long intervals of time. This work has been confirmed elsewhere [70]. Islet cell antibodies may be present. This form of diabetes shows that intrauterine infection may be a major risk factor for diabetes in children.

Enteroviruses

Much attention has been focused on enterovirus infection, which has now been shown to be associated with the onset of diabetes in children frequently and under a wide variety of circumstances. The earliest suggestions for the involvement of enteroviruses in childhood diabetes were derived from studies carried out by Gamble and his colleagues 40 years ago [71]. Despite methodological criticisms of earlier work, using more discriminatory techniques, the work has been recently confirmed for a particular enterovirus strain (**B**) [72]. More modern methods using polymerase chain reaction technology have again underlined the association between enterovirus infections and the onset of diabetes in children in Sweden, Germany, Australia and Japan, in many though not all cases. The very low numbers of virus copies that may be present at diagnosis have contributed to the problem.

Several other lines of evidence underline the association of enterovirus infection with the onset of childhood diabetes. Thus, enterovirus isolated from the pancreas of child diabetics was diabetogenic in animals on two separate occasions, thus fulfilling Koch's postulates (**C**) [73, 74]. Typical insulin-deficiency diabetes may accompany acute enterovirus infections. There are a number of case reports (**C**) [75]. In such cases, islet cell antibodies have been identified in several instances. Familial diabetes involving several members of the same family and accompanying enterovirus infection has been encountered [76]. An enterovirus (echovirus 6) was identified in identical infant twins, who had acquired diabetes simultaneously (**C**) [77]. Importantly, the enterovirus genome has been identified in the pancreas of diabetic children, post-mortem in some cases, but not in controls (**B**) [78]. Much recent work has shown that human islets of Langerhans maintained in tissue culture are susceptible to attack by appropriate strains of enteroviruses, where they may replicate and interfere with islet function, through cytokines (**C**) [79].

Long-term effects of enterovirus infection in relation to childhood diabetes. It has been suggested that enterovirus infection during pregnancy may be an important contributory factor for triggering childhood diabetes (**B**) [80]. This work needs confirmation.

Perhaps the most significant development in examining the role of enteroviruses in the genesis of diabetes lies in recent prospective studies in groups of children with the genetic propensity for acquiring diabetes (**B**) [81]. Such children in Finland have been followed until they acquire islet cell antibodies or until they become diabetic – a process continuing over months or years. These children exhibit enterovirus infections more than controls, and these infections seem associated with the development of islet cell antibodies (**C**) [82, 83]. Following infections at intervals of time, the children become permanently diabetic. This is illustrated in Figure 3.4.

These important studies have very recently been confirmed in the United States [84].

Summary

Various factors, toxic, nutritional and infective, are considered as agents for the induction of childhood diabetes. Of these, viruses appear to be the most plausible candidates. It is

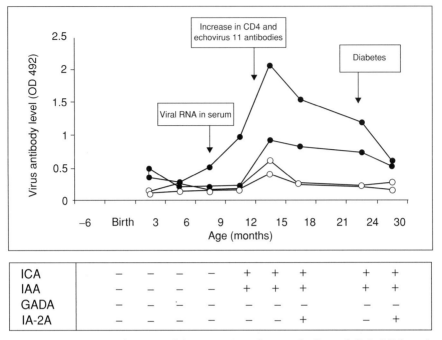

		−6	Birth	3	6	9	12	15	18	21	24	30
ICA		−	−	−	−	+	+	+		+	+	
IAA		−	−	−	−	+	+	+		+	+	
GADA		−	−	−	−	−	−	−		−	−	
IA-2A		−	−	−	−	−	−	+		−	+	

Figure 3.4 Enterovirus infections and the appearance of autoantibodies and clinical diabetes in a child participating in the Finnish Diabetes Prediction and Prevention (DIPP) trial. Enterovirus antibody levels against different enterovirus antigens as measured by EIA from serial serum samples are shown in the upper panel. Twofold or greater increases between the samples were considered to be significant. The presence or absence of autoantibodies during the follow-up is indicated by (+/−) in the lower panel. Levels of coxsackie virus B4 IgG are shown by ● and B4 IgA by ○. Levels of echovirus 11 IgG are shown by ◆ and IgA by ◇. (Reproduced from Hyöty and Taylor [65] with permission.)

now certain that enteroviruses are associated with the onset of diabetes in children in many instances. Growing evidence indicates that they may have a major role as trigger factors in child diabetes. Final proof of their suspected clinical importance might have to await clinical trials of vaccines or antiviral agents, nevertheless.

References

1 Hirschhorn JN. Genetic epidemiology of type 1 diabetes. *Pediatr Diabetes* 2003; **4**: 87–100.
2 Redondo MJ, Fain PR, Eisenbarth GS. Genetics of type 1A diabetes. *Recent Prog Horm Res* 2001; **56**: 69–89.
3 Warram JH, Krolewski AS, Kahn CR. Determinants of IDDM and perinatal mortality in children of diabetic mothers. *Diabetes* 1988; **37**: 1328–34.
4 Kumar D, Gemayel NS, Deapen D *et al.* North-American twins with IDDM. Genetic, etiological, and clinical significance of disease concordance according to age, zygosity, and the interval after diagnosis in first twin. *Diabetes* 1993; **42**: 1351–63.
5 Redondo MJ, Rewers M, Yu L *et al.* Genetic determination of islet cell autoimmunity in monozygotic twin, dizygotic twin, and non-twin siblings of patients with type 1 diabetes: prospective twin study. *BMJ* 1999; **318**: 698–702.
6 Pociot F, McDermott MF. Genetics of type 1 diabetes mellitus. *Genes Immun* 2002; **3**: 235–49.

7 Koeleman BP, Lie BA, Undlien DE *et al.* Genotype effects and epistasis in type 1 diabetes and HLA-DQ trans dimer associations with disease. *Genes Immun* 2004; **5**: 381–8.

8 Lambert AP, Gillespie KM, Thomson G *et al.* Absolute risk of childhood-onset type 1 diabetes defined by human leukocyte antigen class II genotype: a population-based study in the United Kingdom. *J Clin Endocrinol Metab* 2004; **89**: 4037–43.

9 Babenko AP, Polak M, Cave H *et al.* Activating mutations in the ABCC8 gene in neonatal diabetes mellitus. *N Engl J Med* 2006; **355**: 456–66.

10 Edghill EL, Dix RJ, Flanagan SE *et al.* HLA genotyping supports a nonautoimmune etiology in patients diagnosed with diabetes under the age of 6 months. *Diabetes* 2006; **55**: 1895–8.

11 Gloyn AL, Pearson ER, Antcliff JF *et al.* Activating mutations in the gene encoding the ATP-sensitive potassium-channel subunit Kir6.2 and permanent neonatal diabetes. *N Engl J Med* 2004; **350**: 1838–49.

12 Kulmala P, Savola K, Reijonen H *et al.* Genetic markers, humoral autoimmunity, and prediction of type 1 diabetes in siblings of affected children. Childhood Diabetes in Finland Study Group. *Diabetes* 2000; **49**: 48–58.

13 Kelly MA, Rayner ML, Mijovic CH *et al.* Molecular aspects of type 1 diabetes. *Mol Pathol* 2003; **56**: 1–10.

14 Undlien DE, Hamaguchi K, Kimura A *et al.* IDDM susceptibility associated with polymorphisms in the insulin gene region: a study of blacks, Caucasians and orientals. *Diabetologia* 1994; **37**: 745–9.

15 Pugliese A, Awdeh ZL, Alper CA *et al.* The paternally inherited insulin gene B allele (1,428 FokI site) confers protection from insulin-dependent diabetes in families. *J Autoimmun* 1994; **7**: 687–94.

16 Nistico L, Buzzetti R, Pritchard LE *et al.* The *CTLA-4* gene region of chromosome 2q33 is linked to, and associated with, type 1 diabetes. Belgian Diabetes Registry. *Hum Mol Genet* 1996; **5**: 1075–80.

17 Ueda H, Howson J, Esposito L *et al.* Association of the T-cell regulatory gene CTLA4 with susceptibility to autoimmune disease. *Nature* 2003; **423**: 506–11.

18 Ban Y, Tozaki T, Taniyama M *et al.* Association of a CTLA-4 3' untranslated region (CT60) single nucleotide polymorphism with autoimmune thyroid disease in the Japanese population. *Autoimmunity* 2005; **38**: 151–3.

19 Marron MP, Raffel LJ, Garchon HJ *et al.* Insulin-dependent diabetes mellitus (IDDM) is associated with CTLA4 polymorphisms in multiple ethnic groups. *Hum Mol Genet* 1997; **6**: 1275–82.

20 Bottini N, Musumeci L, Alonso A *et al.* A functional variant of lymphoid tyrosine phosphatase is associated with type I diabetes. *Nat Genet* 2004; **36**: 337–8.

21 Smyth D, Cooper JD, Collins JE *et al.* Replication of an association between the lymphoid tyrosine phosphatase locus (LYP/PTPN22) with type 1 diabetes, and evidence for its role as a general autoimmunity locus. *Diabetes* 2004; **53**: 3020–3.

22 Smyth DJ, Cooper JD, Bailey R *et al.* A genome-wide association study of nonsynonymous SNPs identifies a type 1 diabetes locus in the interferon-induced helicase (IFIH1) region. *Nat Genet* 2006; **38**: 617–19.

23 Vella A, Cooper JD, Lowe CE *et al.* Localization of a type 1 diabetes locus in the IL2RA/CD25 region by use of tag single-nucleotide polymorphisms. *Am J Hum Genet* 2005; **76**: 773–9.

24 Concannon P, Erlich HA, Julier C *et al.* Type 1 diabetes: evidence for susceptibility loci from four genome-wide linkage scans in 1,435 multiplex families. *Diabetes* 2005; **54**: 2995–3001.

25 Field LL, Tobias R, Magnus T. A locus on chromosome 15q26 (IDDM3) produces susceptibility to insulin-dependent diabetes mellitus. *Nat Genet* 1994; **8**: 189–94.

26 Davies JL, Kawaguchi Y, Bennett ST *et al.* A genome-wide search for human type 1 diabetes susceptibility genes. *Nature* 1994; **371**: 130–6.

27 Cox NJ, Wapelhorst B, Morrison VA *et al.* Seven regions of the genome show evidence of linkage to type 1 diabetes in a consensus analysis of 767 multiplex families. *Am J Hum Genet* 2001; **69**: 820–30.

28 Laine AP, Turpeinen H, Veijola R *et al.* Evidence for linkage to and association with type 1 diabetes at the 3q21 region in the Finnish population. *Genes Immun* 2006; **7**: 69–72.

29 Field LL, Tobias R, Thomson G *et al.* Susceptibility to insulin-dependent diabetes mellitus maps to a locus (IDDM11) on human chromosome 14q24.3-q31. *Genomics* 1996; **33**: 1–8.

30 Babu SR, Conant GC, Eller E *et al.* A second-generation genome screen for linkage to type 1 diabetes in a Bedouin Arab family. *Ann N Y Acad Sci* 2004; **1037**: 157–160.

31 UK GRID Project. *UK GRID: Genetic Resource Investigating Diabetes.* Available at: http://www-gene.cimr.cam.ac.uk/ucdr/grid.shtml

32 Bingley P, Bonifacio E, Mueller P. Diabetes Antibody Standardization Program: first assay proficiency evaluation. *Diabetes* 2003; **52**: 1128–36.

33 Arif S, Tree TI, Astill T *et al.* Autoreactive T cell responses show proinflammatory polarization in diabetes but a regulatory phenotype in health. *J Clin Invest* 2004; **113**: 451–63.

34 Peakman M, Stevens EJ, Lohmann T *et al.* Naturally processed and presented epitopes of the islet cell autoantigen IA-2 eluted from HLA-DR4. *J Clin Invest* 1999; **104**: 1449–57.

35 Herold K, Hagopian W, Auger J *et al.* Anti-CD3 monoclonal antibody in new-onset type 1 diabetes mellitus. *N Engl J Med* 2002; **346**: 1692–8.

36 Keymeulen B, Vandemeulebroucke E, Ziegler A *et al.* Insulin needs after CD3-antibody therapy in new-onset type 1 diabetes. *N Engl J Med* 2005; **352**: 2598–608.

37 Bougnères PF, Landais P, Boisson C *et al.* Limited duration of remission of insulin dependency in children with recent overt type I diabetes treated with low-dose cyclosporin. *Diabetes* 1990; **39**: 1264–72.

38 Anderson M. Autoimmune endocrine disease. *Curr Opin Immunol* 2002; **14**: 760–4.

39 Atkinson MA, Leiter EH. The NOD mouse model of type 1 diabetes: as good as it gets? *Nat Med* 1999; **5**: 601–4.

40 Todd JA, Wicker LS. Genetic protection from the inflammatory disease type 1 diabetes in humans and animal models. *Immunity* 2001; **15**: 387–95.

41 Gepts W, Lecompte PM. The pancreatic islets in diabetes. *Am J Med* 1981; **70**: 105–15.

42 Bingley PJ, Williams AJ, Gale EA. Optimized autoantibody-based risk assessment in family members Implications for future intervention trials. *Diabetes Care* 1999; **22**: 1796–1801.

43 Bingley PJ, Bonifacio E, Williams AJ *et al.* Prediction of IDDM in the general population: strategies based on combinations of autoantibody markers. *Diabetes* 1997; **46**: 1701–10.

44 Tree T, I, Peakman M. Autoreactive T cells in human type 1 diabetes. *Endocrinol Metab Clin North Am* 2004; **33**: 113–33.

45 Lampeter EF, Homberg M, Quabeck K *et al.* Transfer of insulin-dependent diabetes between HLA-identical siblings by bone marrow transplantation. *Lancet* 1993; **341**: 1243–4.

46 Lampeter EF, McCann SR, Kolb H. Transfer of diabetes type 1 by bone-marrow transplantation. *Lancet* 1998; **351**: 568–9.

47 Adorini L, Gregori S, Harrison LC. Understanding autoimmune diabetes: insights from mouse models. *Trends Mol Med* 2002; **8**: 31–8.

48 Pinkse G, Tysma O, Bergen C *et al.* Autoreactive CD8 T cells associated with beta cell destruction in type 1 diabetes. *Proc Natl Acad Sci U S A* 2005; **102**: 18425-30.

49 Pugliese A, Zeller M, Fernandez A, Jr, *et al.* The insulin gene is transcribed in the human thymus and transcription levels correlated with allelic variation at the INS VNTR-IDDM2 susceptibility locus for type 1 diabetes. *Nat Genet* 1997; **15**: 293–7.

50 Anderson M, Venanzi E, Klein L *et al.* Projection of an immunological self shadow within the thymus by the aire protein. *Science* 2002; **298**: 1395–1401.

51 Lindley S, Dayan C, Bishop A *et al.* Defective suppressor function in CD4+CD25+ T-cells from patients with type 1 diabetes. *Diabetes* 2005; **54**: 92–9.

52 Diabetes Prevention Trial – Type 1 Diabetes Study Group. Effects of insulin in relatives of patients with type 1 diabetes mellitus. *N Engl J Med* 2002; **346**: 1685–91.

53 Skyler J, Krischer J, Wolfsdorf J *et al.* Effects of oral insulin in relatives of patients with type 1 diabetes: the Diabetes Prevention Trial – type 1. *Diabetes Care* 2005; **28**: 1068–76.

54 Shoda L, Young D, Ramanujan S *et al.* A comprehensive review of interventions in the NOD mouse and implications for translation. *Immunity* 2005; **23**: 115–26.

55 Gale EAM, Bingley PJ, Emmett CL *et al.* European Nicotinamide Diabetes Intervention Trial (ENDIT): a randomised controlled trial of intervention before the onset of type 1 diabetes. *Lancet* 2004; **363**: 925–31.

56 Sibley RK, Sutherland DE, Goetz F *et al.* Recurrent diabetes mellitus in the pancreas iso- and allograft A light and electron microscopic and immunohistochemical analysis of four cases. *Lab Invest* 1985; **53**: 132–44.

57 Peakman M, Dayan CM. Antigen-specific immunotherapy for autoimmune disease: fighting fire with fire? *Immunology* 2001; **104**: 361–6.

58 Dahlquist GG, Blom LG, Persson LA *et al.* Dietary factors and the risk of developing insulin dependent diabetes in childhood. *BMJ* 1990; **300**: 1302–6.

59 Parslow RC, McKinney PA, Law GR *et al.* Incidence of childhood diabetes mellitus in Yorkshire, northern England, is associated with nitrate in drinking water: an ecological analysis. *Diabetologia* 1997; **40**: 550–6.

60 Borch-Johnsen K, Joner G, Mandrup P *et al.* Relation between breast-feeding and incidence rates of insulin dependent diabetes mellitus: a hypothesis. *Lancet* 1984; **2**: 1083–6.

61 Akerblom HK, Knip M. Putative environmental factors in Type 1 diabetes. *Diabetes Metab Rev* 1998; **14**: 31–67.

62 Gamble DR, Taylor KW. Seasonal incidence of diabetes mellitus. *BMJ* 1969; **3**: 631–3.

63 McNally RJQ, Feltbower RG, Parker L *et al.* Space-time clustering analyses of type 1 diabetes among 0- to 29-year-olds in Yorkshire, UK. *Diabetologia* 2006; **49**: 900–4.

64 Zhao HX, Moyeed RA, Stenhouse EA *et al.* Space-time clustering of childhood Type 1 diabetes in Devon and Cornwall, England. *Diabet Med* 2002; **19**: 667–72.

65 Hyöty H, Taylor KW. The role of viruses in human diabetes. *Diabetologia* 2002; **45**: 1353–61.

66 Jun HS, Yoon JW. The role of viruses in type I diabetes: two distinct cellular and molecular pathogenic mechanisms of virus-induced diabetes in animals. *Diabetologia* 2001; **44**: 271–85.

67 Harris H. A case of diabetes mellitus quickly following mumps. *Boston Med Surg J* 1898; **40**: 465–9.

68 Gamble DR. Relation of antecedent illness to development of diabetes in children. *BMJ* 1980; **281**: 99–101.

69 Menser MA, Dods L, Harley JD. A twenty-five-year follow-up of congenital rubella. *Lancet* 1967; **2**: 1347–50.

70 Ginsberg-Fellner F. The inter-relationships of congenital rubella (CR) and insulin dependent diabetes mellitus (IDDM). *Pediatr Res* 1980; **14**: 572.

71 Gamble DR, Kinsley ML, FitzGerald MG *et al.* Viral antibodies in diabetes mellitus. *BMJ* 1969; **3**: 627–30.

72 Frisk G, Tuvemo T. Enterovirus infections with beta-cell tropic strains are frequent in siblings of children diagnosed with type 1 diabetes children and in association with elevated levels of GAD65 antibodies. *J Med Virol* 2004; **73**: 450–9.

73 Champsaur H, Dussaix E, Samolyk D *et al.* Diabetes and Coxsackie virus B5 infection. *Lancet* 1980; **1**: 251.

74 Yoon JW, Austin M, Onodera T *et al.* Isolation of a virus from the pancreas of a child with diabetic ketoacidosis. *N Engl J Med* 1979; **300**: 1173–9.

75 Szopa TM, Titchener PA, Portwood ND *et al.* Diabetes mellitus due to viruses – some recent developments. *Diabetologia* 1993; **36**: 687–95.

76 Nelson PG, Arthur LJ, Gurling KJ *et al.* Familial juvenile-onset diabetes. *BMJ* 1977; **2**: 1126.

77 Smith CP, Clements GB, Riding MH *et al.* Simultaneous onset of type 1 diabetes mellitus in identical infant twins with enterovirus infection. *Diabet Med* 1998; **15**: 515–17.

78 Ylipaasto P, Klingel K, Lindberg AM *et al.* Enterovirus infection in human pancreatic islet cells, islet tropism in vivo and receptor involvement in cultured islet beta cells. *Diabetologia* 2004; **47**: 225–39.

79 Olsson A, Johansson U, Korsgren O *et al.* Inflammatory gene expression in Coxsackievirus B-4-infected human islets of Langerhans. *Biochem Biophys Res Commun* 2005; **330**: 571–6.

80 Dahlquist GG, Ivarsson S, Lindberg B *et al.* Maternal enteroviral infection during pregnancy as a risk factor for childhood IDDM A population-based case-control study. *Diabetes* 1995; **44**: 408–13.

81 Hyöty H, Hiltunen M, Knip M *et al.* A prospective study of the role of coxsackie B and other enterovirus infections in the pathogenesis of IDDM Childhood Diabetes in Finland DiMe Study Group. *Diabetes* 1995; **44**: 652–7.

82 Hiltunen M, Hyöty H, Knip M *et al.* Islet cell antibody seroconversion in children is temporally associated with enterovirus infections Childhood Diabetes in Finland DiMe Study Group. *J Infect Dis* 1997; **175**: 554–60.

83 Sadeharju K, Lönnrot M, Kimpimäki T *et al.* Enterovirus antibody levels during the first two years of life in prediabetic autoantibody-positive children. *Diabetologia* 2001; **44**: 818–23.

84 Stene LC, Hyöty H, Olkarinen S. Enteroviral RNA detected in children positive for islet autoantibodies predicts progression to Type 1 diabetes, DAISY study. *Diabetes* 2006; **55**: A20.

CHAPTER 4

Type 1 diabetes mellitus – management

Joanne J. Spinks, Julie A. Edge, Krystyna Matyka & Shital Malik

A lie told often enough becomes the truth.
—Vladimir I. Lenin, Russian Communist politician and revolutionary (1870–1924)

Repetition does not transform a lie into a truth.
　　　　　　　　　　　　　　—Franklin D. Roosevelt, *radio address, October 26, 1939*
　　　　　　　　　　　　　　　　　　32nd president of US (1882–1945)

Diabetic ketoacidosis

Joanne Spinks and Julie Edge

Introduction

Diabetic ketoacidosis (DKA) is the leading cause of morbidity and mortality in children with type 1 diabetes mellitus (T1DM) (**B**) [1]. Most cases of DKA occur in children with established T1DM at a frequency of 1–10% per patient per year (**A**) [2–4] and are usually associated with inadvertent or deliberate insulin omission (**B**) [5, 6]. DKA at onset of T1DM is more common in younger children (**A**) [7, 8] and the frequency varies widely between 15 and 67% in Europe and North America (**A**) [9, 10]. It occurs in approximately 25% at onset of T2DM [11].

Pathophysiology

Absolute or relative insulin deficiency combined with counter-regulatory hormone excess causes glycogenolysis, gluconeogenesis and impaired peripheral glucose utilisation, with resultant hyperglycaemia [12]. Osmotic diuresis, electrolyte loss and dehydration follow, leading to poor tissue perfusion and lactic acidosis. Lipolysis with ketone body (β-hydroxybutyrate and acetoacetate) production causes ketonaemia and metabolic acidosis. Progressive dehydration and acidosis exaggerate stress hormone production and establish a self-perpetuating cycle of progressive metabolic decompensation.

The clinical manifestations are polyuria, polydipsia, dehydration, weight loss, vomiting, abdominal pain, Kussmaul respiration to buffer acidosis and progressive obtundation leading to coma. In younger children DKA may often be misdiagnosed as respiratory or abdominal disease.

The biochemical criteria for diagnosis include hyperglycaemia with ketonuria and ketonaemia. Severity is defined by the degree of the acidosis, varying from mild (venous pH <7.30 and bicarbonate concentration 10–15 mmol/L) to moderate (pH <7.2 and bicarbonate 5–10 mmol/L) to severe (pH <7.1 and bicarbonate <5 mmol/L) (**E**) [13]. Partially

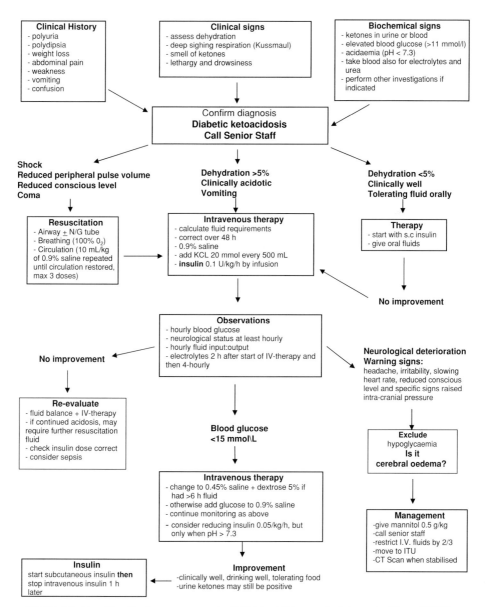

Figure 4.1 Algorithm for the management of DKA in children and adolescents. (From BSPED Consensus statement for the management of DKA [14].)

treated children may have only modestly elevated blood glucose levels, sometimes less than 11 mmol/L.

Management

Management is described according to the guidelines produced by the British Society of Paediatric Endocrinology and Diabetes (Figure 4.1) **(E)** [14]. Further evidence-based guidelines produced by the International Society of Pediatric and Adolescent Diabetes have been published in 2007 [14a]. These are general guidelines for management and each child requires frequent reassessment with modification of treatment as appropriate to suit the individual. The algorithm should be used together with the following essential notes (Figure 4.1).

General issues
The child with DKA should be cared for in a unit that has:
• a specialist/consultant paediatrician with training and expertise in the management of DKA
• experienced nursing staff trained in monitoring and management
• a clear protocol
• access to laboratories for frequent evaluation of biochemical variables (**E**) [13].
   Children with signs of severe DKA or those with signs of, or at risk of, cerebral oedema (including <5 yr of age, new onset) should be considered for treatment in a high dependency or intensive care unit (**C**) [15].

Resuscitation
DKA is a medical emergency and, in common with other emergencies, resuscitation should follow the 'ABC' pattern. The airway should be secured and a nasogastric tube should be inserted and left on free drainage if the child is semiconscious or vomiting. One hundred per cent oxygen should be given and intravenous access established. If the child is in shock, 10 mL/kg 0.9% saline should be given as a bolus and repeated to a maximum of 30 mL/kg.

Clinical assessment
A clinical evaluation to confirm the diagnosis should be made. The child should be weighed and the severity of dehydration assessed. The extent of dehydration is often overestimated and there is rarely a fluid deficit of over 10%. Conscious level should be assessed along with any signs or symptoms of cerebral oedema.

Fluid management
DKA is characterised by severe depletion of water and electrolytes from both the intracellular and the extracellular fluid compartments. The objectives of fluid and electrolyte therapy are to restore the circulating volume in order to enhance clearance of glucose and ketones by the kidneys and to replace sodium and water deficit cautiously to reduce the risk of cerebral oedema.

Fluid rate
Once the circulating volume has been restored, ongoing fluid requirement can be calculated as follows:

Fluid requirement = Maintenance + fluid deficit − resuscitation fluid given

   Deficit should be replaced evenly over 48 hours [16] and should never exceed 10% body weight (**E**). Urinary losses should not be added to the calculation of replacement fluids unless these are excessive and preventing rehydration.

Fluid type
There are theoretical advantages to the use of colloids over crystalloids in resuscitation, but no data comparing the two in DKA. Solutions used should never be more dilute than

0.45% saline, since such fluids may lead to a rapid osmolar change and movement of fluid into the intracellular space. After resuscitation, fluid replacement should be with 0.9% saline for at least 4–6 hours (**C, E**) [16–19]. Thereafter, a solution that has a tonicity equal to or greater than 0.45% saline with added potassium chloride should be used (**C**) [16–18, 20]. It has been suggested that a low serum sodium level or failure of serum sodium to rise after glucose levels fall may be a sign of impending cerebral oedema [18, 21, 22], and in such cases it may be prudent to increase the sodium content of the fluid and reduce the infusion rate, although this has not been shown to affect outcome [18]. The use of large amounts of 0.9% saline has been associated with the development of a hyperchloraemic acidosis.

Insulin therapy

The primary aim of insulin therapy is to reverse metabolic acidosis by inhibiting ketogenesis [23]. Intravenous insulin should be commenced 1–2 hours after starting fluid-replacement therapy, as there is some evidence that insulin therapy within the first hour of treatment increases the risk of cerebral oedema (**B**) [24]. An intravenous bolus should not be used (**C**) [24]. The dose of insulin recommended in all international guidelines is 0.1 U/kg/h, which achieves steady-state plasma insulin levels of around 100–200 µU/mL within 60 minutes, and is effective (**B**) [25]. However, there is a body of opinion that a dose of 0.05 U/kg/h is sufficient to reverse the metabolic abnormalities and overcome any insulin resistance whilst reducing the blood glucose at a steadier rate (see Chapter 1 for a more detailed discussion of this). Some DKA management guidelines do modify their insulin recommendations to the effect that lower doses may be appropriate in younger children, although there is no research evidence to support this, and the ISPAD guidelines recommend 0.1 U/kg/h. This dose of insulin should continue until resolution of acidosis. Once the blood glucose falls to 14 mmol/L, glucose should be added to rehydration fluid to prevent hypoglycaemia.

Potassium replacement

Total body potassium deficits of 3–6 mmol/kg have been demonstrated in adults with DKA [26, 27], but at presentation plasma potassium levels may be normal, increased or decreased [28]. The plasma potassium concentration may decrease abruptly on administration of insulin and correction of the acidosis, which may predispose the patient to cardiac arrhythmias [29]. Potassium should be added to the intravenous fluids at a concentration of 40 mmol/L after initial volume expansion, with subsequent replacement based on 2–4 hourly plasma potassium measurements (**E**). If the patient is hyperkalaemic, potassium replacement can be deferred until urine output is documented, although this may not be necessary in children.

Phosphate replacement

Although total body phosphate depletion occurs in DKA [26, 27], prospective studies have shown no clinical benefit from phosphate replacement (**A**) [30–32].

Bicarbonate therapy

Insulin and fluid therapy reverse acidosis by prevention of ketoacid production and improvement in tissue perfusion and renal function (**A**). Controlled trials have shown no clinical benefit from bicarbonate administration (**B**) [33–35]. Bicarbonate therapy may cause paradoxical central nervous system acidosis [36, 37] and hypokalaemia [36, 38, 39] and has been implicated in the development of cerebral oedema [21]. Only patients

Table 4.1 Factors associated with an increased risk of cerebral oedema

Epidemiological factors	Features at presentation	Treatment variables
Younger age (C) [42]	More severe acidosis (C) [24, 43]	Bicarbonate therapy (C) [21, 44]
New onset diabetes (B) [1, 42]	Higher plasma urea (C) [21]	Greater volumes of fluid in the first 4 h (B) [24]
Longer duration of symptoms (C) [45]	Greater hypocapnia adjusting for degree of acidosis (C) [21, 46]	Insulin therapy within the first hour of fluid treatment (B) [24]

with severe acidaemia (pH <6.9) in whom decreased cardiac contractility and peripheral vasodilatation will further impair tissue perfusion may benefit from cautious alkali therapy.

Monitoring

Successful management of DKA requires meticulous monitoring of clinical and biochemical parameters so that necessary adjustments to treatment can be made (E). Vital signs, neurological observations, fluid balance and capillary blood glucose measurements should be recorded hourly along with 2–4 hourly blood gas, electrolyte and ketone measurements. Continuous electrocardiographic monitoring to assess T waves for evidence of hyper- or hypokalaemia should occur. Monitoring for signs and symptoms of cerebral oedema should also be carried out (see below).

Transition to subcutaneous insulin therapy and oral fluids

Oral intake should be introduced only when substantial clinical improvement has occurred. The transition to subcutaneous insulin therapy should occur only when the ketoacidosis has resolved, as measured by blood rather than urine ketone measurements, and oral intake is tolerated.

Mortality and morbidity

The mortality rate from DKA in children is 0.15–0.30% (B) [1, 40], with cerebral oedema accounting for 60–90% of DKA deaths [21, 41]. Other causes of morbidity and mortality include hypo/hyperkalaemia, hypophosphataemia, hypoglycaemia, aspiration pneumonia, pulmonary oedema, adult respiratory distress syndrome, pneumothorax, thrombosis-related problems, disseminated intravascular coagulation, sepsis, rhabdomyolysis, acute renal failure and acute pancreatitis (C).

Cerebral Oedema

This potentially devastating complication of DKA has a mortality of approximately 25% with 35% of survivors left with permanent neurological damage (B, C) [21, 41]. The pathophysiology is not well understood, but recent case-control studies have started to identify risk factors already present on admission and certain aspects of DKA treatment that may cause or accelerate the development of cerebral oedema (Table 4.1).

Table 4.2 Proposed criteria for the diagnosis of cerebral oedema*

Diagnostic criteria	Abnormal motor or verbal response to pain Decorticate or decerebrate posture Cranial nerve palsy Abnormal neurogenic respiratory pattern
Major criteria	Altered mentation/fluctuating level of consciousness Sustained heart rate deceleration (decrease more than 20 beats/min) not attributable to improved intravascular volume or sleep state Age-inappropriate incontinence
Minor criteria	Vomiting Headache Lethargy or not easily arousable Diastolic blood pressure > 90 mmHg Age < 5yr

*From [51].

It has also been suggested that an attenuated rise in plasma sodium may be a risk factor for the development of cerebral oedema (C) [18, 21, 22] but it is unclear if this is actually a consequence of cerebral oedema rather than a causative factor and may merely reflect the effect of cerebral oedema on renal salt handling.

Pathophysiology

A number of mechanisms have been proposed and recent studies with newer imaging techniques are beginning to unravel the pathways of events leading to brain swelling [47, 48]. Previous hypotheses postulating osmotically mediated fluid shifts driven by the retention of intracellular osmolytes in the brain during rehydration form the basis for the current fluid management standards in DKA. However, recent findings suggest that the predominant mechanism of cerebral oedema may be cerebral ischaemia with resultant activation of ion transporters in the endothelial cells of the blood–brain barrier leading to reperfusion injury [48].

Management

Cerebral oedema usually develops 4–12 hours after treatment has started but can occur before any treatment (**B, C**) [21, 49, 50]. It is possible that quick intervention after early symptoms may reduce mortality and morbidity, so early recognition may be critical. A method of clinical diagnosis for the early detection of cerebral oedema has been proposed (Table 4.2). One diagnostic criterion, two major criteria or one major and two minor criteria had a sensitivity of 92% and a false-positive rate of only 4% in predicting cerebral oedema when used retrospectively (**C**) [51]. Furthermore, a large UK prospective study identified headache and bradycardia as features which should prompt early review [52].

As soon as cerebral oedema is suspected, mannitol 0.5 g/kg or 3% saline 5–10 mL/kg over 30 minutes should be given (**C**) [45, 53]. Intubation and ventilation may be necessary for the patient with impending respiratory failure but aggressive hyperventilation has been associated with a poorer outcome and is not recommended (**C**) [54, 55]. A cranial computed tomography scan is useful to exclude other possible intracerebral causes of neurological deterioration especially thrombosis or haemorrhage that may benefit from specific therapy.

There are no intervention studies with a large enough power to detect a real reduction in the incidence of cerebral oedema and so currently the only definitive method to prevent cerebral oedema is to prevent DKA itself.

Prevention of DKA

Increased public awareness of signs and symptoms of diabetes can lead to earlier diagnosis before progression to DKA in those of new-onset diabetes (**B**) [56]. A cause for the episode of DKA should be identified in those with established diabetes particularly those with recurrent DKA. Insulin omission can be prevented by schemes that provide education, psychosocial evaluation and treatment combined with adult supervision of insulin administration (**B**) [5, 6].

Ongoing insulin management

Krystyna Matyka and Shital Malik

Overall Introduction

The optimum management of a child with diabetes is a complicated issue. Children can develop diabetes from 0 to 18 years and come from many different backgrounds in cultural, sociodemographic and developmental terms. Management therefore needs to be individually tailored and will likely change, as the child grows in both physiological and emotional terms. This will require a good deal of clinical experience from the clinician as well as a good multidisciplinary team that will nurture the family and get to know its strengths and weaknesses.

As a result of this immense 'natural' variability, the study of management interventions is fraught with problems as it becomes difficult to standardise interventions which can then be workable in a clinical situation. Children need to be studied within circumscribed age groups that will define both physiological and emotional parameters and social and cultural issues will need to be considered. Adequate numbers of children need to be investigated to allow the study to have enough power to be interpreted and this is difficult unless multicentre studies are performed which will then introduce inter-centre confounders. As a result, a review of the data available for the day-to-day management of diabetes in childhood highlights significant deficiencies and there are few good quality, randomised controlled trials to guide clinical practice.

Insulin regimens

The optimal insulin regimen for paediatric patients with T1DM remains controversial. In 1995, the Hvidøre study group, an international multicentre group comprising 21 centres from 17 countries in Europe, Japan and North America, performed a survey on the quality of care in its respective institutions and a follow-up survey was performed in 1998 [57, 58]. Of 2873 children (age 0–18 yr) surveyed in 1995, 872 adolescents (11–18 yr) were restudied in 1998. Although the use of multiple injection regimens increased from 42 to 71%, this did not lead to an improvement in glycaemic control as judged by glycated haemoglobin concentrations (**B**). Although there was a tendency towards an increase in the rate of severe hypoglycaemia in the group of children/adolescents on intensive insulin regimens, this did not reach statistical significance, perhaps due to the low number of events recorded [57].

Very few randomised clinical trials of insulin regimens are available for children and adolescents. Even observational studies in this age group are few in number and are usually from single centres or countries. We found 19 studies on insulin regimens (excluding continuous subcutaneous insulin infusion, CSII) over a 10-year period from 1996 to 2006. Of these only 8 were true comparative studies, while the rest were observational studies and the majority involved the use of insulin analogues (Table 4.3). These studies will be examined with respect to age group studied.

Preschool children

There are very few studies based on preschool children, reflecting the ethical problems of research in this age group of children. One observational study has examined the effectiveness of postprandial insulin lispro in five toddlers with diabetes (C) [67]. This study showed that postprandial rapid-acting insulin administration results in blood glucose values as good as, or better than, those obtained with the same dose of soluble insulin given before the meal and no different from those seen with preprandial rapid-acting insulin. The possibility of reducing or omitting the short-acting insulin when the child does not eat offered an important potential advantage. Another observational study of flexible insulin therapy, adjusting doses of rapid-acting insulin based on carbohydrate content of food, found that although glycaemic control improved, there was a significant reduction in frequency of severe hypoglycaemia, although interestingly this benefit occurred only in the 57% of patients who were normal weight as opposed to overweight (C) [68] (for a more detailed discussion of the particular problems associated with the very young, see Chapter 8).

Prepubertal children

The majority of studies in school-aged children have been open randomised crossover studies and again although there have been some benefits of using analogue insulins compared to human insulins, there has been little demonstrable improvement in glycated haemoglobin [59–62, 65]. One study found that there were some improvements in post-meal glucose excursions when comparing rapid-acting analogues and soluble insulin (B) [60]. Other studies examined the potential consequences of giving rapid-acting analogue after food compared with either regular human insulin or rapid-acting insulin before meals (B) [59, 65]. Neither study showed a worsening in glycaemic control with postmeal dosing, and treatment satisfaction was equally high for both patients and carers. However, neither of these studies was of long duration and one lasted only 6 weeks [65].

Schober [62] compared insulin glargine and neutral protamine Hagedorn (NPH) insulin in 349 children and adolescents, aged 5–16 years, with T1DM. Although fasting blood glucose levels decreased significantly more in the insulin glargine group than in the NPH insulin group ($p = 0.02$), there were no significant differences in HbA1c (B).

Studies in adolescents

There has been a small number of studies of insulin regimens in adolescents and most have examined the benefits of analogue therapy. Studies of rapid-acting insulin suggest that there may be improvements in both postprandial glucose excursions and a reduction of nocturnal hypoglycaemia. A large ($n = 463$) crossover, open-label study comparing mealtime insulin lispro for 4 months with soluble insulin for 4 months concluded that insulin lispro significantly improved postprandial glycaemic control and reduced episodes

Table 4.3 Randomised studies of insulin regimen (excluding CSII) in children since 1996

Author and country	Study type	Age (yr)	Number	Comparators	Outcomes
Tupola/Finland, 2001 **(C)** [59]	Open randomised crossover study	Median age 6.2	24	• Postprandial insulin lispro vs premeal soluble • 3-mo duration in each arm	No significant differences in: • postmeal glucose excursions • HbA1c • rate of hypoglycaemia
Deeb/USA, 2001 **(B)** [60]	Randomised open crossover study	2.9–11.4	61	• Insulin lispro pre- or postmeal vs soluble insulin premeal • 3-mo duration of each treatment	• Improved postmeal glucose on premeal lispro • No significant differences in rate of hypoglycaemia or HbA1c between three treatment arms
Ford-Adams/UK, 2003 **(C)** [61]	Open crossover study	7–11	23	• Insulin lispro vs soluble insulin on a three-times-daily insulin regimen • 4-mo treatment in each arm	• Postmeal blood glucose levels were lower on insulin lispro • Between 22.00 and 04.00 hr, the prevalence of hypoglycaemia was lower on lispro than on soluble insulin ($p = 0.01$) • No differences in HbA1c
Schober/Austria, 2002 **(B)** [62]	Open-label, randomised study	5–16	349	• Insulin glargine vs NPH as part of MDI regimen • 6-mo duration	• Fasting glucose lower with glargine than with NPH ($p = 0.02$)

Study	Study type	Age	N	Intervention	Results
Holcombe/USA, 2002 **(B)** [63]	Crossover open-label study	9–18	463	• Insulin lispro vs regular insulin as part of MDI regimen • 4 mo in each treatment arm	• Lispro before breakfast and evening meal led to significantly lower mean 2-h postprandial blood glucose levels compared with soluble • No differences in HbA1c • Lower incidence of hypoglycaemia episodes per patient per 30 d with insulin lispro ($p = 0.023$)
Murphy/UK, 2003 **(A)** [64]	Randomised crossover trial	12–18	28	• Insulin glargine + lispro vs NPH insulin + soluble as part of MDI regimen • 16 wk in each arm	• Nocturnal hypoglycaemia was 43% lower on glargine + lispro • No difference in HbA1c or self-reported hypoglycaemia
Danne/Germany, 2003 **(B)** [65]	Open randomised crossover trial	6–12 13–17	42 34	• Preprandial vs postprandial injections of insulin aspart as part of MDI regimen • 6 wk in each arm	• No difference in HbA1c or rate of hypoglycaemia • Treatment satisfaction was equally high
Mortensen/Denmark, 2006 **(B)** [66]	Randomised, open-label, parallel-group study	Adolescents	167	• Insulin aspart with meals plus NPH insulin at bedtime vs premixed human insulin at breakfast, soluble insulin at lunch and dinner and NPH at bedtime • 4-mo duration	• No difference in HbA1c or rate of hypoglycaemia

Table 4.4 Randomised studies of CSII in children since 1996

Author and country	Study type	Age (yr)	Number	Comparators	Outcomes
Kaufman/USA, 2000 **(C)** [71]	Randomised crossover – 4-wk study	7–10	10	• Nocturnal CSII vs morning NPH and mealtime lispro • 4-wk duration	• CSII led to decrease in average ($p <$ 0.001), breakfast ($p < 0.0001$) and 3 a.m. ($p < 0.003$) glucose • Decreased fear of hypoglycaemia
Weintrob/Israel, 2003–2004 **(C)** [72, 73]	Randomised open crossover study	9.4–13.9	23	• CSII using lispro vs MDI (using NPH and soluble insulin) • 3.5 mo	• HbA1c and frequency of severe hypoglycaemia equivalent between the two groups • Higher treatment satisfaction with CSII • Using CGMS there was a longer duration of within target glucose on CSII, smaller area under curve for nocturnal hypoglycaemia and higher rate of hyperglycaemic episodes
DiMeglio/USA, 2004 **(C)** [74]	Randomised, open-label, prospective study	1.8–4.7	42	• 21 children randomised to CSII • 21 children remained on prior regimen (very varied) • 6-mo study	• Reduction in HbA1c in both groups during study • No significant between group difference in HbA1c at 6 mo • No difference in rate of severe hypoglycaemia but significant increase in meter-detected hypoglycaemia on CSII ($p < 0.05$)

Doyle/USA, 2004 **(B)** [75]	Randomised prospective study	8–21	32	• CSII using aspart vs MDI (using glargine and aspart) • 16-wk study	• HbA1c at 16 wk vs baseline: HbA1c reduced at 16 wk on CSII: 7.2 ± 1.0% vs 8.1 ± 1.2% on MDI ($p < 0.05$) Premeal glucose decreased on CSII ($p < 0.01$)
Tubiana-Rufi/France, 2004 **(C)** [76]	Open-label, randomised crossover, multicentre study	4.6 ± 2.2	27	• Comparing lispro vs soluble insulin on CSII • 16-wk study	• No difference in HbA1c • Prandial glucose excursion lower with lispro ($p < 0.01$ at dinner) • Higher midnight and 3 a.m. glucose values with lispro ($p < 0.05$) • Parental preference for lispro
Wilson/USA, 2005 **(C)** [77]	Randomised, controlled, feasibility study	1.7–6.1	19	• 9 on CSII • 10 on MDI • 12 mo	• No differences in: HbA1c diabetes quality of life CSII felt to be safe in very young children

of nocturnal hypoglycaemia (**B**) [63]. However, no differences in HbA1c were observed. Another study examined insulin aspart injected at mealtimes with NPH insulin at bedtime versus a human insulin regimen: premixed human insulin at breakfast, soluble insulin at lunch and evening meal and NPH insulin at bedtime. One hundred and sixty-seven adolescents took part in the study that used a parallel group design (**B**) [66]. After 4 months there were no significant differences in HbA1c between the two groups.

Only one RCT of the use of glargine in adolescents was found (**A**) [64]. Murphy compared insulin glargine plus insulin lispro versus NPH insulin plus soluble insulin as part of a multiple injection regimen. The results showed that nocturnal hypoglycaemia was significantly reduced (43%) with insulin glargine. Postprandial glucose excursions were also lower after breakfast and lunch, but again there were no significant differences in HbA1c [64].

Free mixing

With the advent of intensive insulin regimens the need to mix insulin in syringes rather than using insulin pens has decreased remarkably. However there remains a number of children and adolescents for whom an increase in the frequency of insulin injections is not suitable. Recent studies have looked at the possibility of mixing rapid-acting insulin analogues with insulin glargine in the same syringe (**C**) [69, 70]. These studies suggest that these insulins can be mixed with no detrimental effect on insulin action, provided they are used immediately.

Continuous subcutaneous insulin infusion

We found 18 studies on CSII over a 10-year period. Of these only 6 were randomised interventional studies (Table 4.4) and all of them studied only small numbers of children [71, 72, 74–77]. One study reported data from the same cohort in two individual papers: one of overall control and one discussing data from continuous glucose monitoring system (CGMS) recordings (**B**) [73]. Only Doyle (**B**) [75] found an improvement in HbA1c on CSII compared to an analogue multiple daily injection (MDI) regimen. The other studies showed little difference in either glycaemic control or rate of hypoglycaemia. Interestingly, in contrast to the studies of insulin regimen, the majority of these studies were performed in very young children. Preschool children appear to be especially concerning in terms of overall management and some of these studies looked to see if CSII could be safely used in this age group (**B**) [74].

A number of observational 'before-and-after' studies have examined HbA1c and rate of hypoglycaemia, often looking retrospectively through case records, and have found that improved glycaemic control can be achieved without a concomitant rise in rate of hypoglycaemia (**C**) [78, 79]. However, observational studies are difficult to interpret as other variables that may impact on diabetic control will not have been standardised.

Hypoglycaemia and insulin regimen

The impact on rates of hypoglycaemia using analogue insulins has been examined in only a few studies. A large study of 463 children aged 9–18 years showed a lower prevalence of hypoglycaemic episodes per patient per 30 days seen with insulin lispro (4.02 ± 4.5 vs 4.37 ± 4.5, respectively; $p = 0.023$) and significantly fewer hypoglycaemic episodes between midnight and 6 a.m. (1.0 ± 1.9 vs 1.7 ± 2.6; $p < 0.001$) (**B**) [63]. Two studies using rapid-acting analogues as part of a basal bolus regimen have found no differences in the rate of hypoglycaemia between analogues and regular human insulin (**B, C**) [59, 60]. Another study compared insulin lispro and soluble insulin as part of a three-times-daily insulin regimen, with isophane insulin as background. The prevalence of low blood glucose concentrations in the early part of the night was lower with analogue insulins (**C**) [61].

Glucose monitoring

Regular home blood glucose monitoring (HBGM) is felt to be an essential part of day-to-day diabetes management. The American Diabetes Association has recommended that patients with T1DM test their blood glucose a minimum of two times each day and need to be taught how to make adjustments to their diabetes management regimen in light of the results (**E**).

Glucose monitoring and glycaemic control

There are few robust data on how useful HBGM may be. A few recent studies have examined factors, including frequency of HBGM, which may predict glycaemic control in children attending paediatric diabetes services [3, 80, 81]. One of these studies, of 300 children, has found that frequency of HBGM was the only modifiable predictor of HbA1c. Children performing one or fewer blood tests per day had an average HbA1c of 9.1 ± 0.34% compared to a value of 8.0 ± 0.31% in those performing five or more blood tests (**C**) [81]. From these data it is not possible to decide whether HBGM improves glycaemic control or whether those children who were more compliant with their diabetes management, and hence are more likely to have better glycaemic control, may have been doing more HBGM. Another study of 415 subjects aged 0–34 years found that frequency of HBGM also predicted severe hypoglycaemia: a finding that was independent of intensive insulin therapy and glycaemic control (**C**) [80].

There appear to be fewer studies of how well patients respond to blood glucose results performed at home. One study has examined responses to hypoglycaemia (glucose <3.3 mmol/L) and hyperglycaemia (>13.2 mmol/L) using a telephone 24-hour recall interview questionnaire, with both a group of 125 adolescents and their parents (**C**) [82]. The authors found that adolescents failed to respond appropriately in 38% episodes of hypoglycaemia and 29% episodes of hyperglycaemia. Episodes of hypoglycaemia were more appropriately managed when the adolescents were supervised by their parents but, interestingly, episodes of hyperglycaemia were more likely to be inappropriately managed when adolescents were supervised by parents. The authors suggested that health-care professionals may underestimate adolescents' ability to respond to HBGM results. Parents may have more of a problem as more diabetes education is aimed at adolescents rather than parents at a time of life when adolescents are taking more responsibility for their diabetes care.

A number of patients feel that HBGM is unnecessary, as they can 'feel' what their blood glucose may be. This was examined in a small ($n = 6$) group of well-controlled children with diabetes aged from 6 to 15 years. Subjects were asked to estimate their blood glucose prior to performing HBGM over a period of a month. Blood glucose varied from 1.7 to 16.6 mmol/L. Children were accurate in 42% of readings and only slightly inaccurate in 37% (**C**) [83]. However, there was a dangerous misestimation in 19% of readings that would have had implications for management and safety.

Continuous glucose monitoring

In recent years continuous glucose monitoring has become available as an important clinical tool.

Continuous glucose monitoring system

The CGMS system includes a glucose-oxidase-based platinum electrode that is inserted into the subcutaneous tissue. Glucose oxidase catalyses the oxidation of glucose in the interstitial fluid generating an electrical current. This is carried by a cable to a pager-sized monitor that provides a glucose reading every 5 minutes for a maximum of 72 hours. Glucose data are stored in the memory and are subsequently downloaded – no real-time display is provided.

Studies of CGMS have highlighted the limitations of conventional HBGM [84, 85]. A study of 56 children aged 2–18 years compared 3 days of CGMS monitoring with 10–15 values from HBGM over the same time period. Interestingly, examining average daily blood glucose concentrations using CGMS and HBGM values, it was demonstrated that standard premeal HBGM provides a reasonably accurate reflection of control. Yet standard measures missed significant postmeal hyperglycaemia with 50% of values going above 16.5 mmol/L, even in young people on rapid-acting analogues. In addition, 68% of subjects had at least one episode of asymptomatic nocturnal hypoglycaemia and 12 children (21%) had asymptomatic hypoglycaemia on all three nights (C) [84]. Unfortunately, there are few data examining the benefit of regular CGMS monitoring on long-term glycaemic control. One small study of 11 subjects randomised five children to CGMS and had six controls (C) [86]. Children in the CGMS group used six 3-day sensors over a 30-day period and both groups used HBGM four times a day. HbA1c was measured at baseline, 1 month and 3 months. Glycaemic control improved in both groups but was significant only between the groups at 1 month and lost significance again at 3 months. This is too small a study to be clinically informative and larger studies are needed.

More recently, real-time monitors, some of which transmit directly to the pumps, have been developed but there are no studies in children to show what advantages, if any, these have over the CGMS. Studies are also being conducted in children to investigate the possibility of linking glucose sensors directly to pumps in such a way as to enable them to act as an 'artificial pancreas' but the results of these studies will not be available for some while yet.

Glucowatch biographer

Although the CGMS may be useful as a clinic tool, patients would welcome a non-invasive glucose monitor that provides a real-time display as well as having alarms to alert the individual to both hyper- and hypoglycaemia. The Glucowatch biographer (GWB2) is shaped like a watch and uses iontophoresis to sample interstitial fluid from which the glucose is measured and displayed every 10 minutes for up to 13 hours. Although not as accurate as HBGM, it has been found to be useful and acceptable to patients and their families in early small studies (C) [87, 88]. However a recent multicentre parallel group study of 200 subjects aged 7–18 years found less satisfactory results (B) [89]. Those randomised to the GWB2 group were asked to use the watch at least twice a week, but as often as desired, over the 6-month period of the study. Those in the control group were given a GWB2 to use after the intervention period of the study. Over the course of the intervention period 16% of subjects averaged two uses of more than 8 hours per week and by 6 months 27% of subjects had stopped using the monitor completely. There was no change in HbA1c over time or between the two groups. Some of the reasons for not using the GWB2 included local skin reactions in 76%, the monitor alarmed too often in 47% and did not provide accurate glucose readings in 33%.

Hypoglycaemia

Hypoglycaemia is a common and much feared complication of the management of T1DM in childhood.

Prevalence

A large number of studies have examined the prevalence of episodes of severe hypoglycaemia [2, 3, 90–92]. These have taken place across the world in North America, Europe and Australia. A variety of definitions of severe hypoglycaemia has been used and prevalence rates have varied from 3.1 to 85.7 episodes per 100 patient-years. It is likely that there are numerous factors that have influenced the wide variation in results presented. Some of these variables have been highlighted by the epidemiological studies themselves. However it is important to note that these studies have not been scientifically designed to examine risk factors for hypoglycaemia – they have merely looked at statistical correlations and do not study important clinical variables known to influence risk of hypoglycaemia, such as physical activity and diet.

Risk factors

Young age has been consistently found to be a risk factor for hypoglycaemia. Insulin regimen may be a confounder, as a number of these studies, even the most recent, will present relatively old data. Many younger children will not have been on more intensive insulin regimens, as these are relatively new approaches to management of diabetes in preschool children. More recent data on intensive insulin regimens such as CSII do suggest that glycaemic control can be tightened without a concomitant rise in the risk of severe hypoglycaemia (see section 'continuous subcutaneous insulin infusion'). A recent large study of paediatric diabetes centres in Germany suggests that centre experience, based on the number of children attending a clinic service, also influences risk of hypoglycaemia (**B**) [92]. This suggests that good education and support of patients is important in minimising the risk of hypoglycaemia.

Nocturnal hypoglycaemia may be a separate entity. Studies suggest that up to 50% of episodes of severe hypoglycaemia occur during sleep. Other studies have shown that many children sleep through episodes of hypoglycaemia, which can be profound and prolonged (**B**) [93–95]. Studies of overnight counter-regulation have found that this is blunted during sleep in both healthy children and those with diabetes, a fact that may influence symptom recognition overnight (**B**) [96]. Recent studies have shown that daytime exercise may be a risk factor for overnight hypoglycaemia, but episodes of nocturnal hypoglycaemia may also occur after sedentary days (**B**) [97, 98].

Treatment of hypoglycaemia

Treatment of hypoglycaemia will depend on the severity. ISPAD consensus guidelines [99] suggest that mild hypoglycaemia, during which the individual is cooperative, can be treated with 5–15 g of oral fast-acting carbohydrate (**E**). More severe hypoglycaemia where the subject is unable to cooperate but is still conscious with an intact gag reflex should be treated with oral glucose gel. If the subject is unconscious, intramuscular glucagon should be given in the first instance (0.5 mg if less than 5 yr and 1.0 mg if older than 5 yr). If this is unsuccessful then intravenous 10% dextrose should be given at a dose of 1–2 mL/kg until a response is achieved. It is not apparent that there have been any studies that have informed these decisions.

Many episodes of hypoglycaemia are dealt with at home by parents and/or other adult carers. Recent studies have shown that low-dose glucagon given using an insulin syringe rather than the more frightening glucagon syringe can be effective in managing hypoglycaemia when a child is unwilling to take oral carbohydrate (**C**) [100, 101].

Avoidance of hypoglycaemia

There are very few studies that have examined interventions designed to prevent hypoglycaemia. A review of studies examining insulin regimens has already been presented (see section 'insulin regimen').

Other approaches which have been used to prevent hypoglycaemia have included family education. In a study of Scandinavian subjects, 332 children with T1DM were randomised, in a 1:1:1 controlled study, to receive either an educational package (videotapes and brochures) aimed at informing subjects about hypoglycaemia or a more generic package about diabetes, or traditional treatment only. In families that were given the hypoglycaemia package, there was a significant reduction in the yearly prevalence of severe hypoglycaemia from 42 to 27%, with no change in either control group [102].

References

1 Edge JA, Ford-Adams ME, Dunger DB. Causes of death in children with insulin dependent diabetes 1990–96. *Arch Dis Child* 1999; **81**: 318–23.
2 Rewers A, Chase HP, Mackenzie T *et al.* Predictors of acute complications in children with type 1 diabetes. *JAMA* 2002; **287**: 2511–18.
3 Rosilio M, Cotton JB, Wieliczko MC *et al.* Factors associated with glycemic control. A cross-sectional nationwide study in 2,579 French children with type 1 diabetes. The French Pediatric Diabetes Group. *Diabetes Care* 1998; **21**: 1146–53.
4 Smith CP, Firth D, Bennett S *et al.* Ketoacidosis occurring in newly diagnosed and established diabetic children. *Acta Paediatr* 1998; **87**: 537–41.
5 Golden MP, Herrold AJ, Orr DP. An approach to prevention of recurrent diabetic ketoacidosis in the pediatric population. *J Pediatr* 1985; **107**: 195–200.
6 Flood RG, Chiang VW. Rate and prediction of infection in children with diabetic ketoacidosis. *Am J Emerg Med* 2001; **19**: 270–3.
7 Komulainen J, Kulmala P, Savola K *et al.* Clinical, autoimmune, and genetic characteristics of very young children with type 1 diabetes. Childhood Diabetes in Finland (DiMe) Study Group. *Diabetes Care* 1999; **22**: 1950–5.
8 Pinkey JH, Bingley PJ, Sawtell PA *et al.* Presentation and progress of childhood diabetes mellitus: a prospective population-based study. The Bart's-Oxford Study Group. *Diabetologia* 1994; **37**: 70–4.
9 Komulainen J, Lounamaa R, Knip M *et al.* Ketoacidosis at the diagnosis of type 1 (insulin dependent) diabetes mellitus is related to poor residual beta cell function. Childhood Diabetes in Finland Study Group. *Arch Dis Child* 1996; **75**: 410–15.
10 Levy-Marchal C, Papoz L, de Beaufort C *et al.* Clinical and laboratory features of type 1 diabetic children at the time of diagnosis. *Diabet Med* 1992; **9**: 279–84.
11 American Diabetes Association. Type 2 diabetes in children and adolescents. American Diabetes Association. *Diabetes Care* 2000; **23**: 381–9.
12 Foster DW, McGarry JD. The metabolic derangements and treatment of diabetic ketoacidosis. *N Engl J Med* 1983; **309**: 159–69.

13 Dunger DB, Sperling MA, Acerini CL *et al.* ESPE/LWPES consensus statement on diabetic ketoacidosis in children and adolescents. *Arch Dis Child* 2004; **89**: 188–94.

14 BSPED. *BSPED Consensus statement for the management of DKA.* Available at: www.bsped.org.uk/ professional/guidelines/docs/BSPDDKAApr04.pdf

14a Wolfsdorf J, Craig ME, Daneman D *et al. Pediatr Diabetes* 2007; **8**: 28–43.

15 Monroe KW, King W, Atchison JA. Use of PRISM scores in triage of pediatric patients with diabetic ketoacidosis. *Am J Manag Care* 1997; **3**: 253–8.

16 Harris GD, Fiordalisi I. Physiologic management of diabetic ketoacidemia: a 5-year prospective pediatric experience in 231 episodes. *Arch Pediatr Adolesc Med* 1994; **148**: 1046–52.

17 Adrogue HJ, Barrero J, Eknoyan G. Salutary effects of modest fluid replacement in the treatment of adults with diabetic ketoacidosis: use in patients without extreme volume deficit. *JAMA* 1989; **262**: 2108–113.

18 Harris GD, Fiordalisi I, Harris WL *et al.* Minimizing the risk of brain herniation during treatment of diabetic ketoacidemia: a retrospective and prospective study. *J Pediatr* 1990; **117**: 22–31.

19 Mel JM, Werther GA. Incidence and outcome of diabetic cerebral oedema in childhood: are there predictors? *J Paediatr Child Health* 1995; **31**: 17–20.

20 Rother KI, Schwenk WF. Effect of rehydration fluid with 75 mmol/L of sodium on serum sodium concentration and serum osmolality in young patients with diabetic ketoacidosis. *Mayo Clin Proc* 1994; **69**: 1149–53.

21 Glaser N, Barnett P, McCaslin I *et al.* Risk factors for cerebral edema in children with diabetic ketoacidosis. The Pediatric Emergency Medicine Collaborative Research Committee of the American Academy of Pediatrics. *N Engl J Med* 2001; **344**: 264–9.

22 Hale PM, Rezvani I, Braunstein AW *et al.* Factors predicting cerebral edema in young children with diabetic ketoacidosis and new onset type I diabetes. *Acta Paediatr* 1997; **86**: 626–31.

23 Luzi L, Barrett EJ, Groop LC *et al.* Metabolic effects of low-dose insulin therapy on glucose metabolism in diabetic ketoacidosis. *Diabetes* 1988; **37**: 1470–7.

24 Edge JA, Jakes RW, Roy Y *et al.* The UK case-control study of cerebral oedema complicating diabetic ketoacidosis in children. *Diabetologia* 2006; **49**: 2002–9.

25 Kitabchi AE. Low-dose insulin therapy in diabetic ketoacidosis: fact or fiction? *Diabetes Metab Rev* 1989; **5**: 337–63.

26 Atchley DW, Loeb RF, Richards DW *et al.* On diabetic ketoacidosis: a detailed study of electrolyte balances following the withdrawal and reestablishment of insulin therapy. *J Clin Invest* 1933; **12**: 297–326.

27 Nabarro JD, Spencer AG, Stowers JM. Metabolic studies in severe diabetic ketosis. *Q J Med* 1952; **21**: 225–48.

28 Adrogue HJ, Lederer ED, Suki WN *et al.* Determinants of plasma potassium levels in diabetic ketoacidosis. *Medicine (Baltimore)* 1986; **65**: 163–72.

29 DeFronzo RA, Felig P, Ferrannini E *et al.* Effect of graded doses of insulin on splanchnic and peripheral potassium metabolism in man. *Am J Physiol* 1980; **238**: E421–7.

30 Becker DJ, Brown DR, Steranka BH *et al.* Phosphate replacement during treatment of diabetic ketosis. Effects on calcium and phosphorus homeostasis. *Am J Dis Child* 1983; **137**: 241–6.

31 Fisher JN, Kitabchi AE. A randomized study of phosphate therapy in the treatment of diabetic ketoacidosis. *J Clin Endocrinol Metab* 1983; **57**: 177–80.

32 Keller U, Berger W. Prevention of hypophosphatemia by phosphate infusion during treatment of diabetic ketoacidosis and hyperosmolar coma. *Diabetes* 1980; **29**: 87–95.

33 Green SM, Rothrock SG, Ho JD *et al.* Failure of adjunctive bicarbonate to improve outcome in severe pediatric diabetic ketoacidosis. *Ann Emerg Med* 1998; **31**: 41–8.

34 Hale PJ, Crase J, Nattrass M. Metabolic effects of bicarbonate in the treatment of diabetic ketoacidosis. *BMJ (Clin Res Ed)* 1984; **289**: 1035–8.

35 Okuda Y, Adrogue HJ, Field JB *et al.* Counterproductive effects of sodium bicarbonate in diabetic ketoacidosis. *J Clin Endocrinol Metab* 1996; **81**: 314–20.

36 Assal JP, Aoki TT, Manzano FM *et al.* Metabolic effects of sodium bicarbonate in management of diabetic ketoacidosis. *Diabetes* 1974; **23**: 405–11.

37 Ohman JL, Jr, Marliss EB, Aoki TT *et al.* The cerebrospinal fluid in diabetic ketoacidosis. *N Engl J Med* 1971; **284**: 283–90.

38 Lever E, Jaspan JB. Sodium bicarbonate therapy in severe diabetic ketoacidosis. *Am J Med* 1983; **75**: 263–8.

39 Soler NG, Bennett MA, Dixon K *et al.* Potassium balance during treatment of diabetic ketoacidosis with special reference to the use of bicarbonate. *Lancet* 1972; **2**: 665–7.

40 Curtis JR, To T, Muirhead S *et al.* Recent trends in hospitalization for diabetic ketoacidosis in Ontario children. *Diabetes Care* 2002; **25**: 1591–6.

41 Edge JA, Hawkins MM, Winter DL *et al.* The risk and outcome of cerebral oedema developing during diabetic ketoacidosis. *Arch Dis Child* 2001; **85**: 16–22.

42 Rosenbloom AL. Intracerebral crises during treatment of diabetic ketoacidosis. *Diabetes Care* 1990; **13**: 22–33.

43 Durr JA, Hoffman WH, Sklar AH *et al.* Correlates of brain edema in uncontrolled IDDM. *Diabetes* 1992; **41**: 627–32.

44 Bureau MA, Begin R, Berthiaume Y *et al.* Cerebral hypoxia from bicarbonate infusion in diabetic acidosis. *J Pediatr* 1980; **96**: 968–73.

45 Bello FA, Sotos JF. Cerebral oedema in diabetic ketoacidosis in children. *Lancet* 1990; **336**: 64.

46 Mahoney CP, Vlcek BW, DelAguila M. Risk factors for developing brain herniation during diabetic ketoacidosis. *Pediatr Neurol* 1999; **21**: 721–7.

47 Cameron FJ, Kean MJ, Wellard RM *et al.* Insights into the acute cerebral metabolic changes associated with childhood diabetes. *Diabet Med* 2005; **22**: 648–53.

48 Glaser NS, Wootton-Gorges SL, Marcin JP *et al.* Mechanism of cerebral edema in children with diabetic ketoacidosis. *J Pediatr* 2004; **145**: 164–171.

49 Fiordalisi I, Harris GD, Gilliland MG. Prehospital cardiac arrest in diabetic ketoacidemia: why brain swelling may lead to death before treatment. *J Diabetes Complications* 2002; **16**: 214–19.

50 Lawrence SE, Cummings EA, Gaboury I *et al.* Population-based study of incidence and risk factors for cerebral edema in pediatric diabetic ketoacidosis. *J Pediatr* 2005; **146**: 688–92.

51 Muir AB, Quisling RG, Yang MC *et al.* Cerebral edema in childhood diabetic ketoacidosis: natural history, radiographic findings, and early identification. *Diabetes Care* 2004; **27**: 1541–6.

52 Edge JA, Flint J, Roy Y *et al.* Can cerebral oedema be identified before the reduction in conscious level? *Pediatr Diabetes* 2004; **5**(suppl 1): 48.

53 Curtis JR, Bohn D, Daneman D. Use of hypertonic saline in the treatment of cerebral edema in diabetic ketoacidosis (DKA). *Pediatr Diabetes* 2001; **2**: 191–4.

54 Marcin JP, Glaser N, Barnett P *et al.* Factors associated with adverse outcomes in children with diabetic ketoacidosis-related cerebral edema. *J Pediatr* 2002; **141**: 793–7.

55 Tasker RC, Lutman D, Peters MJ. Hyperventilation in severe diabetic ketoacidosis. *Pediatr Crit Care Med* 2005; **6**: 405–11.

56 Vanelli M, Chiari G, Ghizzoni L *et al.* Effectiveness of a prevention program for diabetic ketoacidosis in children: an 8-year study in schools and private practices. *Diabetes Care* 1999; **22**: 7–9.

57 Holl RW, Swift PG, Mortensen HB *et al.* Insulin injection regimens and metabolic control in an international survey of adolescents with type 1 diabetes over 3 years: results from the Hvidore study group. *Eur J Pediatr* 2003; **162**: 22–9.

58 Mortensen HB, Hougaard P. Comparison of metabolic control in a cross-sectional study of 2,873 children and adolescents with IDDM from 18 countries. The Hvidore Study Group on Childhood Diabetes. *Diabetes Care* 1997; **20**: 714–20.

59 Tupola S, Komulainen J, Jaaskelainen J *et al.* Post-prandial insulin lispro vs. human regular insulin in prepubertal children with Type 1 diabetes mellitus. *Diabet Med* 2001; **18**: 654–8.

60 Deeb LC, Holcombe JH, Brunelle R *et al.* Insulin lispro lowers postprandial glucose in prepubertal children with diabetes. *Pediatrics* 2001; **108**: 1175–9.

61 Ford-Adams ME, Murphy NP, Moore EJ *et al.* Insulin lispro: a potential role in preventing nocturnal hypoglycaemia in young children with diabetes mellitus. *Diabet Med* 2003; **20**: 656–60.

62 Schober E, Schoenle E, Van Dyk J *et al.* Comparative trial between insulin glargine and NPH insulin in children and adolescents with type 1 diabetes mellitus. *J Pediatr Endocrinol Metab* 2002; **15**: 369–76.

63 Holcombe JH, Zalani S, Arora VK *et al.* Comparison of insulin lispro with regular human insulin for the treatment of type 1 diabetes in adolescents. *Clin Ther* 2002; **24**: 629–38.

64 Murphy NP, Keane SM, Ong KK *et al.* Randomized cross-over trial of insulin glargine plus lispro or NPH insulin plus regular human insulin in adolescents with type 1 diabetes on intensive insulin regimens. *Diabetes Care* 2003; **26**: 799–804.

65 Danne T, Aman J, Schober E *et al.* A comparison of postprandial and preprandial administration of insulin aspart in children and adolescents with type 1 diabetes. *Diabetes Care* 2003; **26**: 2359–64.

66 Mortensen H, Kocova M, Teng LY *et al.* Biphasic insulin aspart vs. human insulin in adolescents with type 1 diabetes on multiple daily insulin injections. *Pediatr Diabetes* 2006; **7**: 4–10.

67 Rutledge KS, Chase HP, Klingensmith GJ *et al.* Effectiveness of postprandial Humalog in toddlers with diabetes. *Pediatrics* 1997; **100**: 968–72.

68 Alemzadeh R, Berhe T, Wyatt DT. Flexible insulin therapy with glargine insulin improved glycemic control and reduced severe hypoglycemia among preschool-aged children with type 1 diabetes mellitus. *Pediatrics* 2005; **115**: 1320–4.

69 Fiallo-Scharer R, Horner B, McFann K *et al.* Mixing rapid-acting insulin analogues with insulin glargine in children with type 1 diabetes mellitus. *J Pediatr* 2006; **148**: 481–4.

70 Kaplan W, Rodriguez LM, Smith OE *et al.* Effects of mixing glargine and short-acting insulin analogs on glucose control. *Diabetes Care* 2004; **27**: 2739–40.

71 Kaufman FR, Halvorson M, Kim C *et al.* Use of insulin pump therapy at nighttime only for children 7–10 years of age with type 1 diabetes. *Diabetes Care* 2000; **23**: 579–82.

72 Weintrob N, Benzaquen H, Galatzer A *et al.* Comparison of continuous subcutaneous insulin infusion and multiple daily injection regimens in children with type 1 diabetes: a randomized open crossover trial. *Pediatrics* 2003; **112**: 559–64.

73 Weintrob N, Schechter A, Benzaquen H *et al.* Glycemic patterns detected by continuous subcutaneous glucose sensing in children and adolescents with type 1 diabetes mellitus treated by multiple daily injections vs continuous subcutaneous insulin infusion. *Arch Pediatr Adolesc Med* 2004; **158**: 677–84.

74 DiMeglio LA, Pottorff TM, Boyd SR *et al.* A randomized, controlled study of insulin pump therapy in diabetic preschoolers. *J Pediatr* 2004; **145**: 380–4.

75 Doyle EA, Weinzimer SA, Steffen AT *et al.* A randomized, prospective trial comparing the efficacy of continuous subcutaneous insulin infusion with multiple daily injections using insulin glargine. *Diabetes Care* 2004; **27**: 1554–8.

76 Tubiana-Rufi N, Coutant R, Bloch J *et al.* Special management of insulin lispro in continuous subcutaneous insulin infusion in young diabetic children: a randomized cross-over study. *Horm Res* 2004; **62**: 265–71.

77 Wilson DM, Buckingham BA, Kunselman EL *et al.* A two-center randomized controlled feasibility trial of insulin pump therapy in young children with diabetes. *Diabetes Care* 2005; **28**: 15–19.

78 McMahon SK, Airey FL, Marangou DA *et al.* Insulin pump therapy in children and adolescents: improvements in key parameters of diabetes management including quality of life. *Diabet Med* 2005; **22**: 92–6.

79 Plotnick LP, Clark LM, Brancati FL *et al.* Safety and effectiveness of insulin pump therapy in children and adolescents with type 1 diabetes. *Diabetes Care* 2003; **26**: 1142–6.

80 Allen C, LeCaire T, Palta M *et al.* Risk factors for frequent and severe hypoglycemia in type 1 diabetes. *Diabetes Care* 2001; **24**: 1878–81.

81 Levine BS, Anderson BJ, Butler DA *et al.* Predictors of glycemic control and short-term adverse outcomes in youth with type 1 diabetes. *J Pediatr* 2001; **139**: 197–203.

82 Johnson SB, Perwien AR, Silverstein JH. Response to hypo- and hyperglycemia in adolescents with type I diabetes. *J Pediatr Psychol* 2000; **25**: 171–8.

83 Uchigata Y, Kawatahara M, Ohsawa M *et al.* Characteristics and learning effects of the predictability of the self-monitored blood glucose level in children with type 1 diabetes. *Diabetes Res Clin Pract* 2004; **65**: 79–83.

84 Boland E, Monsod T, Delucia M *et al.* Limitations of conventional methods of self-monitoring of blood glucose: lessons learned from 3 days of continuous glucose sensing in pediatric patients with type 1 diabetes. *Diabetes Care* 2001; **24**: 1858–62.

85 Kaufman FR, Gibson LC, Halvorson M *et al.* A pilot study of the continuous glucose monitoring system: clinical decisions and glycemic control after its use in pediatric type 1 diabetic subjects. *Diabetes Care* 2001; **24**: 2030–4.

86 Chase HP, Kim LM, Owen SL *et al.* Continuous subcutaneous glucose monitoring in children with type 1 diabetes. *Pediatrics* 2001; **107**: 222–6.

87 Chase HP, Roberts MD, Wightman C *et al.* Use of the GlucoWatch biographer in children with type 1 diabetes. *Pediatrics* 2003; **111**: 790–4.

88 Hathout E, Patel N, Southern C *et al.* Home use of the GlucoWatch G2 biographer in children with diabetes. *Pediatrics* 2005; **115**: 662–6.

89 Chase HP, Beck R, Tamborlane W *et al.* A randomized multicenter trial comparing the GlucoWatch Biographer with standard glucose monitoring in children with type 1 diabetes. *Diabetes Care* 2005; **28**: 1101–6.

90 Craig ME, Handelsman P, Donaghue KC *et al.* Predictors of glycaemic control and hypoglycaemia in children and adolescents with type 1 diabetes from NSW and the ACT. *Med J Aust* 2002; **177**: 235–8.

91 Vanelli M, Cerutti F, Chiarelli F *et al.* Nationwide cross-sectional survey of 3560 children and adolescents with diabetes in Italy. *J Endocrinol Invest* 2005; **28**: 692–9.

92 Wagner VM, Grabert M, Holl RW. Severe hypoglycaemia, metabolic control and diabetes management in children with type 1 diabetes in the decade after the Diabetes Control and Complications Trial – a large-scale multicentre study. *Eur J Pediatr* 2005; **164**: 73–9.

93 Beregszaszi M, Tubiana-Rufi N, Benali K *et al.* Nocturnal hypoglycemia in children and adolescents with insulin-dependent diabetes mellitus: prevalence and risk factors. *J Pediatr* 1997; **131**: 27–33.

94 Matyka KA, Wigg L, Pramming S *et al.* Cognitive function and mood after profound nocturnal hypoglycaemia in prepubertal children with conventional insulin treatment for diabetes. *Arch Dis Child* 1999; **81**: 138–42.

95 Porter PA, Keating B, Byrne G *et al.* Incidence and predictive criteria of nocturnal hypoglycemia in young children with insulin-dependent diabetes mellitus. *J Pediatr* 1997; **130**: 366–72.

96 Jones TW, Porter P, Sherwin RS *et al.* Decreased epinephrine responses to hypoglycemia during sleep. *N Engl J Med* 1998; **338**: 1657–62.

97 Admon G, Weinstein Y, Falk B *et al.* Exercise with and without an insulin pump among children and adolescents with type 1 diabetes mellitus. *Pediatrics* 2005; **116**: e348–55.

98 Tsalikian E, Mauras N, Beck RW *et al.* Impact of exercise on overnight glycemic control in children with type 1 diabetes mellitus. *J Pediatr* 2005; **147**: 528–34.

99 ISPAD. *ISPAD Clinical Practice Consensus Guidelines 2006–2007: Diabetic ketoacidosis.* Available at: http://www.ispad.org/FileCenter/10-Wolfsdorf_Ped_Diab_2007,8.28-43.pdf

100 Hartley M, Thomsett MJ, Cotterill AM. Mini-dose glucagon rescue for mild hypoglycaemia in children with type 1 diabetes: the Brisbane experience. *J Paediatr Child Health* 2006; **42**: 108–11.

101 Haymond MW, Schreiner B. Mini-dose glucagon rescue for hypoglycemia in children with type 1 diabetes. *Diabetes Care* 2001; **24**: 643–5.

102 Nordfeldt S, Johansson C, Carlsson E *et al.* Prevention of severe hypoglycaemia in type I diabetes: a randomised controlled population study. *Arch Dis Child* 2003; **88**: 240–5.

CHAPTER 5

Type 1 diabetes mellitus in the very young child

Stuart Brink

> *I think we ought always to entertain our opinions with some measure of doubt. I shouldn't wish people dogmatically to believe any philosophy, not even mine.*
> —Bertrand Russell, British author, mathematician and philosopher (1872–1970)

Diagnosis

The diagnosis of type 1 diabetes mellitus (T1DM) in very young children under the age of 6 is relatively rare (**E**) [1] and often not considered by health-care providers or parents (**B**) [2]. Such youngsters frequently present after days or weeks of symptoms that were missed, in varying stages of diabetic ketoacidosis (DKA) with an increased risk of morbidity and mortality (**B**) [2]. Symptoms are similar to other age groups with insulin deficiency but more difficult to recognise: polyuria (often manifest as saturated nappies), excessive thirst and unexplained weight loss. Vomiting, when present, is often misinterpreted as gastroenteritis or other viral illness. Suspecting the diagnosis of T1DM in young children is critical in avoiding severe dehydration and ketoacidosis. In *any* ill child, polydipsia or weight loss should trigger a question about volume of urination no matter what the suspected cause and especially in the midst of apparent viral epidemics. If urinary volume appears to be increased, urinalysis for glycosuria (and ketonuria) should be performed and consideration given to blood glucose testing (**E**) [3–5]. However, there is no evidence that teaching efforts aimed specifically at health-care providers who care for such youngsters have been able to encourage such routine considerations of diabetes in very young children (**B**) [6] but there are some studies which suggest that this possibility should be reconsidered and could be successful (**B**) [7]. New-onset T1DM occurs as a random event in the vast majority of families (see Chapter 2). Therefore, a negative family history of diabetes does not exclude the diagnosis. Neonatal diabetes (**E**) [8] (strictly defined as diabetes occurring during the first month of life and lasting more than 2 wk) is even more rare but infants developing diabetes before the age of 6 months should have appropriate genetic testing for possible sulphonylurea and potassium-channel genetic mutations, as this may allow treatment with sulphonylurea oral agents instead of multiple insulin injections (see Chapter 13).

New diagnosis of symptomatic diabetes mellitus is one of the true paediatric endocrine emergencies especially if dehydration and DKA occur. The principles of the treatment of DKA are similar to those of older children and are reviewed in Chapter 4. Once ketoacidosis is brought under control, balancing of insulin and food with frequent blood glucose monitoring should take place for the next several days in preparation for ongoing out-patient/ambulatory treatment. In the very young where the diagnosis of T1DM is made sufficiently early and there is no significant clinical dehydration, subcutaneous insulin must be started on the day of diagnosis to avoid a rapid deterioration towards DKA. As long as the young child is able to eat and drink and caretakers are able to be taught about monitoring and feeding, in many parts of the world, expensive inpatient hospitalisation may be avoided (**B**) [9]. Telephone access and daily education and support are necessary for such outpatient management. There are several studies documenting that this is possible to accomplish safely. This provides benefits not only in saving health-care costs but also in avoiding the inevitable psychological trauma of hospitalisation for the child as well as the family (**B**) [9].

Treatment goals

There are no prospective, controlled or randomised clinical trials treating very young children. Major problems with making the diagnosis in very young children are compounded by the imprecision of insulin therapy, impossibility of exact control of nutrient intake and irregularities of daily life. Good glucose control often remains elusive (**C, E**) [10–12] especially when compared to older children, adolescents and adults. Despite these obvious clinical problems, the principles of T1DM management in young children remain similar to other age groups (**E**) [1, 13] – to obtain the best possible blood glucose control whilst minimising hypoglycaemia (**E**) [14, 15].

These general goals of therapy must take into account:
• age and size of the child
• insulin requirements:
  – C-peptide reserve
  – absorption and insulin kinetics – peak effect and duration of effect of the insulin being used
  – brittleness – determined by frequent blood glucose testing
• nutritional requirements for growth and well-being
• ethnic and family cultural traditions about feeding
• likes and dislikes
• developmental inconsistencies of a pre-school-age child's eating patterns
• unpredictable activity and sleep patterns
• likely need for more frequent blood glucose monitoring needs
• the types of insulin available
• psychosocial concerns including appropriate limit setting, how other members of the family can be helpful, babysitting and day-care issues and who assumes responsibility for diabetes care of the very young child.

Insulin therapy

There are no evidence-based clinical prospective studies comparing twice-a-day, short-acting and isophane (Neutral pH Hagedorn, NPH) insulins (so-called conventional therapy) with multi-dose, rapid-acting (lispro or aspart) and basal isophane or basal long-acting (glargine or detemir) insulins (so-called basal-bolus therapy) that show superior outcomes. However, there are several studies that document fewer hypoglycaemic episodes when utilising insulin analogues versus either animal-based or recombinant human short-acting insulin (**B**) [16], as well as glargine or detemir instead of isophane (NPH) as the basal insulin. Dogmatic use of one or another type of insulin regimen should be avoided.

Twice-daily insulin regimens are still used in many centres but, despite the lack of evidence, increasingly popular regimens use rapid-acting insulin analogues (lispro or aspart) for preprandial and presnack bolus coverage coupled with bedtime long-acting insulin analogues (glargine or detemir) as a multi-dose regimen designed to mimic insulin physiology and minimise hypoglycaemia. There is almost no paediatric experience with glulisine, the newest rapid-acting insulin analogue. Experience with the long-acting insulin analogues suggests that they may not last a full 24 hours in pre-school-age children and either a morning or lunchtime dose of isophane can be added or a second dose of (morning) long-acting analogue added to the bedtime dose. There is evidence to show that in older people HbA1c does not differ if glargine is given at bedtime, breakfast or lunchtime and therefore the timing should be based on detailed blood glucose patterns. Different intermediate- or long-acting insulin, such as lente or ultralente, may be of value, although these are becoming increasingly unavailable in many countries.

For toddlers, the benefits of aspart or lispro are:
• the feasibility of giving the insulin immediately before the child eats because of rapid insulin absorption (**B**) [17]
• a documented decrease in hypoglycaemia compared to short-acting human insulin (**A**) [18]
• ability to administer these analogues immediately *after*, instead of before, meals thus allowing parents to know how much food is ingested, thereby avoiding food conflicts in children with unpredictable eating habits (**B**) [17].

Insulin-pump therapy has been used successfully in many parts of the world (France (**C**) [19], the United States (**B, E**) [20–22] and the Netherlands (**B**) [23]) in very young children but is expensive and requires team expertise as well as commitment on the part of the family to be successful (**E**) [24]. Such insulin-pump therapy, even for the pre-school-age child with diabetes, is increasing, with a goal of providing more flexibility than basal-bolus insulin programmes and more importantly, less hypoglycaemia (**B**) [25–27].

Food advice

As with all other aspects of this topic, there are no prospective, controlled clinical trials addressing the issue of meal planning or specific dietary recommendations for young children with diabetes. The principles of dietary advice are similar to those of older children and are dealt with in detail in Chapter 8. There is increasing consensus, although no scientific evidence to support it in paediatrics, to recommend carbohydrate counting to enable increased flexibility and more accurate balancing of insulin-to-carbohydrate ratios. The few studies that have been published in adults usually refute earlier (more restrictive) dietary regimens as having no specific proof of benefit.

General recommendations (**E**) [3, 5, 14, 28, 29] are much more based upon common-sense approaches since scientific studies in the preschool child are virtually non-existent. Complex high-fibre carbohydrates, such as pasta, bran, whole-wheat breads and cereals, vegetables and fruit (rather than juice), are encouraged with a general carbohydrate intake of approximately 50–55% of total calories coming from such complex carbohydrates.

Protein generally makes up 10–15% of total calories with fat comprising the remaining 30–35%.

Little children often eat in spurts; for weeks their appetite may be good and then they revert to being fussy. There is some behavioural paediatric literature about feeding choices and limit setting that applies to children with diabetes just as much as to those without diabetes but few controlled studies of what works or does not work except for the emphasis on individualised advice rather than dogma (**B**) [30]. While a variety of foods are important for proper provision of vitamins and minerals, battling over food should be avoidable with reasonable parental limit setting. With the newer rapid-acting analogues, some battles can be avoided since insulin may be given immediately after meals. As with most other childhood behavioural issues, positive reinforcement is superior to negative (**E**) [31]. Grandparents frequently need special encouragement to understand these principles of dietary management because of the tendency for them to overindulge.

Special events such as holiday or religious feast meals and birthdays as well as day-care or nursery-school parties require special organisation with adjustments to activity and/or insulin worked into the plans. Parents can be taught how to make such adjustments themselves by using blood glucose monitoring to help learn and get feedback on their choices. Mealtime interactions relate directly to dietary adherence as well as to glycaemic control, and specific behavioural interventions are useful in improving glycaemic outcome (**B**) [32].

Ice cream, long considered a forbidden food for people with diabetes, is a part of many cultures, especially in the warm summer months, and is popular with young children. Studies (**C**) [33] report that the glycaemic effect of potatoes is higher than that of ice cream and so there is no reason to eliminate ice cream from the meal plan of youngsters with diabetes. Because of the high-fat content of most ice creams, the glycaemic effects may be more prolonged than other types of foods and therefore may be an ideal food to counterbalance prolonged activity, such as a day at the beach or following several hours of sustained activities. Similarly, when offered as a bedtime snack, ice cream's glycaemic effect, delayed because of the fat content and slower gastrointestinal absorption, may also be an ideal food to help decrease nocturnal hypoglycaemia (**E**) [28].

Activity

Activity holds the same importance for toddlers as it does for older children but is even more difficult to quantify. Planning a certain amount, duration or intensity of activity on a day-to-day basis is an exercise in futility since little children are too unpredictable. It is therefore almost impossible prospectively to increase food and/or decrease insulin for such activity bursts but experience with blood glucose monitoring may help carers to learn how best to approach such changes (**E**) [34].

Health-care providers for the very young

An interdisciplinary team approach (**E**) [35, 36] is often recommended not only to assist teaching at diagnosis but also to follow up education and treatment adjustments with little evidence-based data to support such recommendations. The coordinated efforts of paediatric diabetes specialists, nurses and educators, dietitians, social workers and psychologists working together with family physicians and paediatricians remains an impossible ideal in many parts of the world. Such teams obviously increase health-care costs but must be balanced against the hoped-for improvement in outcome. However, there is abundant anecdotal evidence indicating that highly motivated, experienced, single-handed professionals can provide successful care even without the benefit of interdisciplinary teams.

Parent and carer education

As with other aspects of the care of the very young, the principles of treatment are similar to those of older children but are heavily influenced by the greater dependence of this group on their caregivers.

The principles of 'survival' followed by 'continuing' education are discussed in detail in Chapter 9. Special attention should be drawn to involving not just mothers but also fathers and other family members. Sometimes mothers assume all the care of the child with diabetes and fathers are inadvertently excluded from such care. Not only does this cause additional caretaker burdens for mothers but it may set up a pattern so that fathers never fully participate in the children's diabetes care because of their lack of full training and experience. This may also contribute to an attitude that the diabetes treatment itself is not so important, otherwise fathers would also participate (**E**) [37].

Helping to understand these new and often frightening tasks is a critical part of what the diabetes team must provide in the initial weeks after diagnosis. The child is no longer perceived as healthy and the psychological loss of this healthy child may be an important emotional factor to consider in how parents deal with the diagnosis (**C, B, E**) [38–40]. Initial-stage education for parents of young children, as with anyone else newly diagnosed with diabetes, is based on the concept that parents are in a state of shock or bereavement and must come to grips with the diagnosis before substantial learning retention is possible (**B**) [41].

Parents must be the central focus of educational and supervisory efforts when children under 5 years of age are diagnosed since they provide nearly all the needed care (**C, E**) [29, 42–45]. Awareness of specific ethnic and cultural patterns, which have an influence on parental roles and care provision, must also be acknowledged, as must the needs of child care and nursery staff. While most of the education is directed at parents, the young child with diabetes must not be forgotten. Pre-school-age children think concretely (**E**) [46]. They do not have future concepts on which to rely and a great deal of their information and behaviours are centred on the moment at hand. Explanations should be positive, short, unambiguous and specific to the immediate situation. Little children also believe their parents are omnipresent and omniscient. They may not understand why grown-ups, supposed to care and protect them, are now holding them down, inflicting pain with needles and lancets and saying 'no' to so many previously acceptable things. Unless carefully managed, they are likely to believe that they are being punished for being a 'bad child'. Body integrity is important developmentally in 3–5-year old children so that blood testing and insulin injections may easily become major battlegrounds. The very size of the lancet holders and syringes may be intimidating and out of proportion to the pain and discomfort of modern lancets and syringe needles.

Play therapy, utilising dolls or soft toys, can be helpful so that children can learn to 'care' for their dolls, 'inject' them with insulin, 'check' their glucose levels and help with other diabetes-related tasks. Colouring books, children's books incorporating diabetes into the story line and videos as well as CDs may help with this educational process. There is no rational way to explain this so that all young children will understand. The best approach is usually to be honest, provide information appropriate to the level of questioning and avoid unnecessary procrastination, with common sense as one's best guide coupled with open observation of the child's actual behaviour and comments.

Limit setting is important and should be carried out in a loving, caring, concerned fashion and consistent manner. Helping parents of young children to understand this helps them to understand why they must give injections and say 'no' to certain foods. Hugs, kisses and praise (E) [47] work positively when used liberally. Giving even very young children some choices, such as which fruit would they like, is a helpful strategy, particularly as a distraction from unpleasant experiences (B) [48]. Even little children can be educated to understand certain parts of their own diabetes care, such as explaining that sugar-free drinks are acceptable whereas sugar-containing ones are not. Praise is a powerful tool in encouraging children to wear medic alert bracelets and to say 'no' to offers of candy and sugar-containing foods (from well-meaning but uninformed adults). These requirements need to be explained to siblings at home, in neighbourhood playgroups and at nursery school.

Continuing education (E) [46, 49] follows the initial survival education. It should focus not only on technical aspects of diabetes care, updating meal plans and continued utilisation of blood glucose data but more on self-sufficiency with sick-day guidelines and with day-to-day insulin and food adjustments. In addition, paying particular attention to psychosocial needs and providing assistance with (parental) stress reduction may be valuable (C) [50]. Regularly scheduled outpatient follow-up is an accepted essential venue for such ongoing education and common sense (but no evidence base) suggests that these families benefit from an interdisciplinary team approach, if available. If not, then the diabetes specialist must assume the role of educator as well as doctor (E) [12]. The goal of continuing education includes reviewing basic concepts of diabetes treatment to be sure that when new information is available it is transmitted (e.g. new insulins) and to review previously taught concepts that may have been forgotten, mixed up or somehow lost in translation. Family weekend retreats or camping experiences are now being used in many parts of the world to bring such parents and families together with their children (with and without diabetes) so that experiences can be shared, ideas exchanged and sense of loneliness diminished (see Chapter 10). Group learning makes the learning process more varied and more interesting, and it potentially fosters positive behavioural changes designed to help in the overall management of diabetes (E) [51].

Over subsequent weeks and months, specific teaching can occur that focuses on individual needs, often supplemented by home learning using printed and media tools, such as Ragnar Hanas' *Type 1 Diabetes Mellitus* (E) [40] teaching guide, Peter Chase's '*Pink Panther' Type 1 Diabetes* manual (E) [52] and Jean Betschart's *Diabetes Care for Babies, Toddlers and Preschoolers* (E) [47]. Several of these manuals have been translated into different languages and are available in many countries or via Internet booksellers. Locally written manuals are also frequently available and provided by health-care providers. Local support groups, diabetes organisations and other Internet sources such as the Juvenile Diabetes Research Foundation (www.jdrf.org) and Children with Diabetes (accessible via www.childrenwithdiabetes.com) can also provide support and may help to minimise the isolation and fears reported by many parents and caregivers.

Monitoring of diabetes in the very young

A key rationale for frequent blood glucose monitoring is the provision of sufficient data upon which to make food and/or insulin adjustments. When pre- and postprandial blood glucose information is available, it can be analysed in logbooks or with computer down-loading of memory meters to identify patterns. Coupled with carbohydrate counting to allow estimation of insulin needs, such monitoring can help to determine if the chosen basal insulin regimen is working, if there is nocturnal hypoglycaemia – even if such hy-poglycaemia is asymptomatic – and whether or not sufficient insulin is being provided to cover prandial glycaemic excursions. The exact number of insulin injections is not a critical treatment factor but rather the decisions about age-specific glucose target goals preprandially, postprandially and overnight so that there can be optimal glucose control, growth and development, as well as minimising and avoiding hypoglycaemia (**E**) [53]. The concept of clear target setting and goals would seem to be very important for both parents (and caretakers) and health-care providers.

Blood glucose and ketone monitoring

The ISPAD Declaration of Kos (**E**) [54] and the 1995 ISPAD, IDF, ALAD and WHO Europe Consensus Guidelines (**E**) [55] reiterate the importance of monitoring equipment that should routinely be available around the world. Minimum monitoring of either urine or blood glucose might be a twice-a-day schedule before breakfast and the evening meal – the two times when most parents are more likely to make insulin and/or carbohydrate adjustments in relation to their next few hours of activity, food, etc. More sophisticated monitoring would involve testing at each meal and snack and learning how to use such data for more frequent food and insulin adjustments (**B, E**) [56, 57].

Urine ketone testing with appropriate testing strips is commonly taught for sick-day monitoring, whenever blood glucose levels are elevated above 13–14 mmol/L (approxi-mately 250 mg/dL). More recent availability of blood ketone test strips using small drops of capillary blood with a meter allow for accurate determination of ß-hydroxybutyric acid analysis. An added benefit of blood ß-hydroxybutyric acid testing is the potential for iden-tifying impending ketosis sooner than when urine specimens are utilised (**A**) [58] coupled with no longer having the need to obtain urine on demand.

Hypoglycaemia

Hypoglycaemia is extremely common and problematic in all children with T1DM (**B**) [59, 60]. Because young children do not always communicate in a manner that facilitates understanding how they are feeling, observation coupled with blood glucose confirma-tion helps to identify episodes of hypoglycaemia with a goal of minimising or preventing severe hypoglycaemia. It is unlikely that any injectable insulin regimen, even with insulin pumps, will totally avoid hypoglycaemia. Recent studies of continuous glucose monitoring document how frequently this occurs and how often such hypoglycaemia is unrecognised or extremely subtle (**C**) [61]. Particularly in pre-school-age children, it is a priority to avoid moderate hypoglycaemia (where assistance of others is required) and severe hypo-glycaemia (where there are convulsions and/or unconsciousness) (**E, B**) [62, 63]. Fear of hypoglycaemia, for either psychological reasons or legitimate safety reasons, is often the limiting step in achieving more optimal control (**E, C**) [62, 64] and sometimes leads to overfeeding or underinsulinisation (**B**) [62].

Safety and clinical risks of hypoglycaemia have been evaluated in several retrospective studies from Pittsburgh (**E, C**) [65] and Toronto (**C**) [66] and have suggested that the developing brain may be particularly susceptible not only to recurring and severe episodes but also to more subtle or asymptomatic hypoglycaemia because of how commonly it really occurs. Studies from Zurich, however, have documented worse long-term cognition problems related to hyperglycaemia rather than hypoglycaemia (**A**) [67] even in those with a history of convulsive hypoglycaemia. Studies from Yale (**B**) [25] suggest one of the most important benefits of insulin-pump use in very young children is the ability to titrate insulin needs more effectively with fewer episodes of hypoglycaemia and a decrease in severity of hypoglycaemia, even without a deterioration in HbA1c.

Treatment for hypoglycaemia follows the same general principles as for anyone else with diabetes-associated hypoglycaemia. For the most severe episodes, glucagon is given intramuscularly or subcutaneously and can be given anywhere in the body, in a dose appropriate for age and size (see Chapter 4). If given intramuscularly, this may speed up absorption time. Parents and anybody else responsible for supervising young children with diabetes should be taught how to use glucagon for such emergency situations. Because glucagon is not often used, it is wise to have an annual re-education to help relearn when and how it is used.

Monitoring goals

Normal premeal, postprandial and night-time values are impossible to obtain even in hospital or research facilities except during the honeymoon period (**B**) [68] particularly in very young children. Health-care providers must adapt targets to individual contexts and expectations within family circumstances. There is no evidence-based research to support any specific glucose target and, as with most aspects of diabetes management, individual team philosophy and individual parental philosophy are often the key factors. Research suggests that the average glucose value (or HbA1c as its surrogate) is more important than the daily variability of blood glucose levels in predicting, and preventing, complications (**A**) [69].

If moderate or severe hypoglycaemia occurs as a result of attempting to intensify insulin therapy, either the goals should be redefined or therapy modified (**C**) [66]. This is especially true if such hypoglycaemia is a recurring problem and seizures continue.

Glycated haemoglobin

There is no evidence-based research in children about optimum frequency of measurement of long-term glycaemia. There are consensus recommendations for HbA1c determinations offered by such organisations as the ADA (**E**) [5] and ISPAD (**E**) [3], suggesting that HbA1c measurements should be obtained a minimum of every 3–4 months. The Diabetes Control and Complications Trial (DCCT) [70] confirmed the importance of HbA1c and several paediatric studies (**B**) [71–73] confirm its relevance. In the DCCT not only were HbA1c tests done monthly but results were provided to patients and providers and utilised to adjust treatment goals and strategies. Capillary HbA1c measurements should be available

Table 5.1 Pre-school-age children and uncontrolled diabetes[†]

1.	Intercurrent infections – most frequent cause of DKA
2.	Leaking at insulin injections/technique problems
3.	Lipohypertrophy interfering with insulin absorption
4.	Failure to increase insulin for growth spurts/lack of medical follow-up with inadequate professional supervision/monitoring (poverty or parental guilt)
5.	*Abnormal counter-regulation
6.	Surgery or severe trauma
7.	*Cortisone-like medications (e.g. for asthma or urticaria)
8.	*Major emotional turmoil (e.g. parental divorce, child abuse or neglect, parental alcohol or drug abuse)
9.	Hypoglycaemia fears (and thus inadequate insulin provision)
10.	Insulin being bound and released sporadically by the body

[†] Adapted from Brink (E) [34].
*Most commonly associated with ketoacidosis if not properly treated.

for very young children so that venepuncture can be avoided. More recently, some diabetes specialists (**E**) [16] have recommended seeing very young patients every 4 weeks with HbA1c measurements every 4–8 weeks in an effort to be more proactive, identify problems, make more adjustments and focus on the psychosocial aspects of living with T1DM using the DCCT care model.

Poor glycaemic control

Uncontrolled diabetes can be caused by unavailability of insulin or test equipment, any kind of ongoing non-compliance (omitted insulin, dietary misinformation or errors), by being uneducated about goals of diabetes care or by illness, major emotional stress, surgery or trauma (**C**) [74]. Table 5.1 lists some specific clinical causes of uncontrolled diabetes in children less than 6 years with asterisks next to the ones that are commonly associated with ketoacidosis if not properly treated. While many cases of poorly controlled diabetes in older age groups can be corrected with intensive re-education and/or insulin adjustment, the difficulties of managing very young children often cannot be approached from as logical and rational a perspective. However, psychological or supervisory problems of parents or other adults may be identified and remediable steps be taken to help the situation. Psychosocial intervention often focuses on parenting issues, appropriate and consistent limit setting and ways to improve discipline, reinforce positive behaviour and reduce negative behaviour. Such problems are not diabetes specific but are often exaggerated because of the interplay between the behaviour and the diabetes management at issue.

Sick days caused by intercurrent illnesses in young children are handled in much the same way as in adolescents and school-age youngsters. Protocols for sick-day management usually suggest extra fluids and extra insulin, but vomiting and diarrhoea in young children may result in significant hypoglycaemia (see Chapter 7). Under such circumstances very small doses of glucagon can be used temporarily to boost glucose levels when nutrient intake is inadequate (**C**) [75]. Recurrent ketoacidosis is rare in this age group unless parental incompetence is the issue. Since parents are responsible for insulin administration, any episodes of recurring ketoacidosis reflect parental misunderstanding or neglect and demand immediate remediation.

Summary

In young children with diabetes, the availability of more frequent blood glucose monitoring, better analysis of such blood glucose results, more physiologic insulin delivery with either multi-dose insulin treatment algorithms or insulin pumps are increasingly utilised to achieve improved glucose control. More satisfactory HbA1c levels will help to prevent future glucose-associated long-term micro- and macrovascular complications. Interdisciplinary team efforts are utilised to assist not only with the complex educational needs for modern treatment of young children, but also with psychosocial issues that often influence outcomes significantly in this age group. Efforts to recognise and treat hypoglycaemia and especially to prevent or minimise such hypoglycaemia are equally important. Parents must be the focus for these medical, nursing, dietary, psychosocial and education efforts since they are the primary-care providers for young children. Emphasis on positive behaviour reinforcement, appropriate limit setting, stress reduction, conflict avoidance and common-sense flexibility should allow more youngsters to live better and happier lives without interference from severe hypoglycaemia, growth failure or the complications associated with long-term hyperglycaemia until better treatment options become available. If financial circumstances do not allow optimum management, efforts by health-care providers and government policy makers should ensure that minimum care recommendations are met initially but continue to improve standards of care since the long-term financial costs to the individual and to society far exceed the short-term costs of providing improved monitoring and treatment.

References

1 Brink S. Natural history and associated problems of type 1 diabetes in children less than 5 years old. *Pediatric and Adolescent Endocrinology.* S Karger AG, Basel, Switzerland, 1985.

2 Neu A, Willasch A, Ehehalt S *et al.* Ketoacidosis at onset of type 1 diabetes mellitus in children – frequency and clinical presentation. *Pediatr Diabetes* 2003; **4**: 77–81.

3 ISPAD. *ISPAD Clinical Practice Consensus Guidelines 2006–2007: Phases of Diabetes.* Available at: http://www.ispad.org/FileCenter/2-Couper_Ped_Diab_2007,8.44-47.pdf

4 NHMRC. *The Australian Clinical Practice Guidelines on the Management of Type 1Diabetes in Children and Adolescents,* 2005. Available at: www.chw.edu.au/prof/services/endocrinology/apeg/apeg_handbook_final.pdf

5 Silverstein J, Klingensmith G, Copeland K *et al.* Care of children and adolescents with type 1 diabetes: a statement of the American Diabetes Association. *Diabetes Care* 2005; **28**: 186–212.

6 Japan and Pittsburg Childhood Diabetes Research Groups. Coma at the onset of young insulin-dependent diabetes in Japan. *Diabetes* 1985; **34**: 1241–6.

7 Alexander V, on behalf of DiabNet Scotland. Reducing DKA: a practical approach. *J Pedtr Endocrinol Metab* 2002; **15**(suppl 2).

8 von Muhlendahl KE, Herkenhoff H. Long-term course of neonatal diabetes. *N Engl J Med* 1995; **333**: 704–8.

9 Siminerio LM, Charron-Prochownik D, Banion C *et al.* Comparing outpatient and inpatient diabetes education for newly diagnosed pediatric patients. *Diabetes Educ* 1999; **25**: 895–906.

10 Golden MP, Russell BP, Ingersoll GM *et al.* Management of diabetes mellitus in children younger than 5 years of age. *Am J Dis Child* 1985; **139**: 448–52.

11 Greene S. Diabetes in the pre-school child. *Diabetes Nutr Metab* 1999; **12**: 96–101.

12 Kushion W, Salisbury PJ, Seitz KW *et al.* Issues in the care of infants and toddlers with insulin-dependent diabetes mellitus. *Diabetes Educ* 1991; **17**: 107–110.

13 Kelnar CJDH. *Childhood and Adolescent Diabetes.* Chapman & Hall Medical, London, 1995.

14 Kaufman FR. Diabetes mellitus. *Pediatr Rev* 1997; **18**: 383–92.

15 Sperling M. Diabetes mellitus. In: Sperling MA, ed. *Pediatric Endocrinology*. WB Saunders, Philadelphia, 1997: 241–6.

16 Schober E, Schoenle E, Van Dyk J *et al.* Comparative trial between insulin glargine and NPH insulin in children and adolescents with type 1 diabetes mellitus. *J Pediatr Endocrinol Metab* 2002; **15**: 369–76.

17 Deeb LC, Holcombe JH, Brunelle R *et al.* Insulin lispro lowers postprandial glucose in prepubertal children with diabetes. *Pediatrics* 2001; **108**: 1175–9.

18 Brunelle BL, Llewelyn J, Anderson JH, Jr, *et al.* Meta-analysis of the effect of insulin lispro on severe hypoglycemia in patients with type 1 diabetes. *Diabetes Care* 1998; **21**: 1726–31.

19 Boselli E, Bougneres PF, Couprie C *et al.* Treatment of diabetes in children under 3 years of age: indications, methods and results. *Arch Fr Pediatr* 1987; **44**: 759–64.

20 DiMeglio LA, Pottorff TM, Boyd SR *et al.* A randomized, controlled study of insulin pump therapy in diabetic preschoolers. *J Pediatr* 2004; **145**: 380–4.

21 Kaufman FR, Halvorsan M, Miller D *et al.* Insulin pump therapy in the type 1 pediatric patient: indications and outcomes. *New perspectives in childhood diabetes and childhood obesity. 7th International ISPAD Course, Cosenza, Italy*. Editoriale Bios s.a.s., Pisa, Italy, 1999: 111–25.

22 Litton J, Rice A, Friedman N *et al.* Insulin pump therapy in toddlers and preschool children with type 1 diabetes mellitus. *J Pediatr* 2002; **141**: 490–5.

23 de Beaufort CE, Bruining GJ. Continuous subcutaneous insulin infusion in children. *Diabet Med* 1987; **4**: 103–8.

24 Fisher LK, Halvorson M. Future developments in insulin pump therapy: progression from continuous subcutaneous insulin infusion to a sensor-pump system. *Diabetes Educ* 2006; **32**: 47S–52S.

25 Dixon B, Peter CH, Burdick J *et al.* Use of insulin glargine in children under age 6 with type 1 diabetes. *Pediatr Diabetes* 2005; **6**: 150–4.

26 Hathout EH, Fujishige L, Geach J *et al.* Effect of therapy with insulin glargine (lantus) on glycemic control in toddlers, children, and adolescents with diabetes. *Diabetes Technol Ther* 2003; **5**: 801–6.

27 Weinzimer SA, Ahern JH, Doyle EA *et al.* Persistence of benefits of continuous subcutaneous insulin infusion in very young children with type 1 diabetes: a follow-up report. *Pediatrics* 2004; **114**: 1601–5.

28 Brink S. Pediatric and Adolescent Type 1 Diabetes Mellitus Meal Planning 1992: our best advice to prevent, postpone and/or minimize angiopathy. In: Weber B, Burger W, Danne T, eds. *Structural and Functional Abnormalities in Subclinical Diabetic Angiopathy*. S Karger AG, Basel, Switzerland, 1992: 156–69.

29 Etzwiler DD. Education and participation of patients and their families. *Pediatr Ann* 1983; **12**: 638–40, -42.

30 Powers SW, Byars KC, Mitchell MJ *et al.* Parent report of mealtime behavior and parenting stress in young children with type 1 diabetes and in healthy control subjects. *Diabetes Care* 2002; **25**: 313–18.

31 Connell JE. Pizazz in the pediatric population. *Diabetes Educ* 1991; **17**: 251–2, -4, -6.

32 Patton SR, Dolan LM, Powers SW. Mealtime interactions relate to dietary adherence and glycemic control in young children with type 1 diabetes. *Diabetes Care* 2006; **29**: 1002–6.

33 Nathan DM, Godine JE, Gauthier-Kelley C *et al.* Ice cream in the diet of insulin-dependent diabetic patients. *JAMA* 1984; **251**: 2825–7.

34 Brink SJ. The very young child with diabetes. In: Brink SJ, Serban V, eds. *Pediatric and Adolescent Diabetes*. Brumar, Timisoara, Romania, 2003: 189–232.

35 Brink SJ, Miller M, Moltz KC. Education and multidisciplinary team care concepts for pediatric and adolescent diabetes mellitus. *J Pediatr Endocrinol Metab* 2002; **15**: 1113–30.

36 Laffel LM, Brackett J, Ho J *et al.* Changing the process of diabetes care improves metabolic outcomes and reduces hospitalizations. *Qual Manag Health Care* 1998; **6**: 53–62.

37 Brink S. Preschool-age diabetes. In: Brink S, cd. *Pediatric and Adolescent Diabetes Mellitus*. Year Book Medical Publisher, Chicago, 1984: 3–31.

38 Galatzer A, Amir S, Gil R *et al.* Crisis intervention program in newly diagnosed diabetic children. *Diabetes Care* 1982; **5**: 414–19.

39 Hamman RF, Cook M, Keefer S *et al.* Medical care patterns at the onset of insulin-dependent diabetes mellitus: association with severity and subsequent complications. *Diabetes Care* 1985; **8**(suppl 1): 94–100.

40 Hanas R. *Type 1 Diabetes: A Guide for Children, Adolescents, Young Adults and Their Caregivers*. Marlow & Co., New York, 2005.

41 Delamater AM, Bubb J, Davis SG *et al.* Randomized prospective study of self-management training with newly diagnosed diabetic children. *Diabetes Care* 1990; **13**: 492–8.

42 Banion CR, Miles MS, Carter MC. Problems of mothers in management of children with diabetes. *Diabetes Care* 1983; **6**: 548–51.

43 Hatton DL, Canam C, Thorne S *et al.* Parents' perceptions of caring for an infant or toddler with diabetes. *J Adv Nurs* 1995; **22**: 569–77.

44 Laron Z. The role of education in the treatment of diabetic children. In: Laron Z, Pinelli L, eds. *Theoretical and Practical Aspects of the Treatment of Diabetic Children: 5th International ISPAD Course.* Editoriale Bios s.a.s., Cosenza, Italy, 1985: 115–18.

45 Lee PD. An outpatient-focused program for childhood diabetes: design, implementation, and effectiveness. *Tex Med* 1992; **88**: 64–8.

46 Piaget J. *The Child's Conception of the World.* Littlefield, New Jersey, 1965.

47 Betschart J. *Diabetes Care for Babies, Toddlers and Preschoolers: A Reassuring Guide.* John Wiley & Sons, New York, 1999.

48 Wysocki T, Huxtable K, Linscheid TR *et al.* Adjustment to diabetes mellitus in preschoolers and their mothers. *Diabetes Care* 1989; **12**: 524–9.

49 Karp MM. Education of diabetic children and adolescents. *Diabetes Rev* 1989; **2**: 10–14.

50 Streisand R, Swift E, Wickmark T *et al.* Pediatric parenting stress among parents of children with type 1 diabetes: the role of self-efficacy, responsibility, and fear. *J Pediatr Psychol* 2005; **30**: 513–21.

51 Brink SJ. Camping and psychosocial group programs for children and adolescents with IDDM. In: Lifshitz F, ed. *Pediatric Endocrinology: A Clinical Guide,* 3rd edn. Marcal Dekker, Inc., New York, 1996: 671–6.

52 Chase HP. *A First Book for Understanding Diabetes.* Chidren's Diabetes Foundation, Denver, Colorado, 2004.

53 Dorchy H. Insulin regimens and insulin adjustments in diabetic children, adolescents and young adults: personal experience. *Diabetes Metab* 2000; **26**: 500–7.

54 Weber B, Brink S, Bartsocas C *et al.* ISPAD declaration of Kos. International Study Group of Diabetes in Children and Adolescents. *J Paediatr Child Health* 1995; **31**: 156.

55 ISPAD, IDF, and WHO. *Consensus Guidelines for the Treatment of Insulin Dependent Diabetes Mellitus in Children and Adolescents,* Europe, 1995.

56 Bloomgarden ZT, Karmally W, Metzger MJ *et al.* Randomized, controlled trial of diabetic patient education: improved knowledge without improved metabolic status. *Diabetes Care* 1987; **10**: 263–72.

57 Brink SJ, Moltz KC. The message of the DCCT for children and adolescents. *Diabetes Spectrum* 1997; **10**: 259–67.

58 Laffel LM, Wentzell K, Loughlin C *et al.* Sick day management using blood 3-hydroxybutyrate (3-OHB) compared with urine ketone monitoring reduces hospital visits in young people with T1DM: a randomized clinical trial. *Diabet Med* 2006; **23**: 278–84.

59 Cox DJ, Kovatchev BP, Julian DM *et al.* Frequency of severe hypoglycemia in insulin-dependent diabetes mellitus can be predicted from self-monitoring blood glucose data. *J Clin Endocrinol Metab* 1994; **79**: 1659–62.

60 Daneman D, Frank M, Perlman K *et al.* Severe hypoglycemia in children with insulin-dependent diabetes mellitus: frequency and predisposing factors. *J Pediatr* 1989; **115**: 681–5.

61 Kaufman FR, Gibson LC, Halvorson M *et al.* A pilot study of the continuous glucose monitoring system: clinical decisions and glycemic control after its use in pediatric type 1 diabetic subjects. *Diabetes Care* 2001; **24**: 2030–4.

62 Cryer PE. Banting Lecture. Hypoglycemia: the limiting factor in the management of IDDM. *Diabetes* 1994; **43**: 1378–89.

63 White NH, Cleary PA, Dahms W *et al.* Beneficial effects of intensive therapy of diabetes during adolescence: outcomes after the conclusion of the Diabetes Control and Complications Trial (DCCT). *J Pediatr* 2001; **139**: 804–12.

64 Sullivan-Bolyai S, Deatrick J, Gruppuso P *et al.* Mothers' experiences raising young children with type 1 diabetes. *J Spec Pediatr Nurs* 2002; **7**: 93–103.

65 Becker DJ, Ryan CM. Hypoglycemia: a complication of diabetes therapy in children. *Trends Endocrinol Metab* 2000; **11**: 198–202.

66 Rovet JF, Ehrlich RM, Hoppe M. Intellectual deficits associated with early onset of insulin-dependent diabetes mellitus in children. *Diabetes Care* 1987; **10**: 510–15.

67 Schoenle EJ, Schoenle D, Molinari L *et al*. Impaired intellectual development in children with type I diabetes: association with HbA(1c), age at diagnosis and sex. *Diabetologia* 2002; **45**: 108–114.

68 Kiess W, Kapellen T, Siebler T *et al*. Practical aspects of managing preschool children with type 1 diabetes. *Acta Paediatr Suppl* 1998; **425**: 67–71.

69 Kilpatrick ES, Rigby AS, Atkin SL. The effect of glucose variability on the risk of microvascular complications in type 1 diabetes. *Diabetes Care* 2006; **29**: 1486–90.

70 Writing Team for the Diabetes Control and Complications Trial/Epidemiology of Diabetes Interventions and Complications Research Group. Effect of intensive therapy on the microvascular complications of type 1 diabetes mellitus. *JAMA* 2002; **287**: 2563–69.

71 Donaghue KC, Fung AT, Hing S *et al*. The effect of prepubertal diabetes duration on diabetes: microvascular complications in early and late adolescence. *Diabetes Care* 1997; **20**: 77–80.

72 Donaghue KC, Fairchild JM, Craig ME *et al*. Do all prepubertal years of diabetes duration contribute equally to diabetes complications? *Diabetes Care* 2003; **26**: 1224–9.

73 Rudberg S, Dahlquist G. Determinants of progression of microalbuminuria in adolescents with IDDM. *Diabetes Care* 1996; **19**: 369–71.

74 Golden MP, Herrold AJ, Orr DP. An approach to prevention of recurrent diabetic ketoacidosis in the pediatric population. *J Pediatr* 1985; **107**: 195–200.

75 Haymond MW, Schreiner B. Mini-dose glucagon rescue for hypoglycemia in children with type 1 diabetes. *Diabetes Care* 2001; **24**: 643–5.

CHAPTER 6

Adolescence and diabetes: clinical and social science perspectives

Alexandra Greene & Stephen Greene

Boys will be boys. And even that wouldn't matter if only we could prevent girls from being girls.
—Anthony Hope Hawkins, British author (1863–1933)

What a cunning mixture of sentiment, pity, tenderness, irony surrounds adolescence, what knowing watchfulness! Young birds on their first flight are hardly so hovered around.
—Georges Bernanos
French novelist and political writer (1888–1948)

Introduction

Adolescence is a critical period for the young person with diabetes. While the age of presentation of type 1 diabetes mellitus (T1DM) is decreasing in many countries, worldwide the adolescent period is still the commonest age for the newly diagnosed patient (**B**) [1]. It is also a time that frequently leads to deterioration in glycaemic control and, with it, the potential for disease complications. Many epidemiological studies have consistently documented this period of poor glycaemic control (**A, B**) [2–5]. The DIABAUD survey in 1998 across Scotland (**B**) [1] shows worsening glycaemic control with increasing age. A recent review of the outcome of young people with T1DM shows persisting poor control (**B**) [6] and personal information presented to the Scottish Study Group for the Care of the Young with Diabetes (SSGCYD) (Waugh *et al.*, November 2006) shows that glycaemic control deteriorates through older adolescence into early adult years, improving only in the third decade of age.

Clinical perspectives: why does glycaemic control deteriorate during adolescence?

Several factors appear to combine in preventing young people achieving tight glycaemic control (**A**) [2].

Physiological changes of puberty and diabetes
Physiological changes of glucose metabolism are seen in non-diabetic adolescents. There does appear to be increasing insulin 'resistance' and this can be reflected in changes in

fasting insulin levels when moving from childhood into puberty (**B**) [7]. There are also major changes in the insulin-like growth factor 1 (IGF-1)-binding protein and growth hormone concentration in association with the pubertal growth spurt (**B**) [8]. We have shown marked insulin resistance in non-diabetic young people in their response to a standard meal [9], raising the concern over emerging T2DM phenotype in a large percentage of the young population. This, taken together with the emerging 'epidemic' of obesity in the young (**B**) [10] and true clinical T2DM in adolescence (**E**) [11], is of concern to the T1DM population where in theory the two insulin problems may coexist. Body composition changes, with an increase in the percentage of body fat reflecting both the insulin resistance and the hormonal changes of puberty, may also relate to a change in glucose metabolism. These physiological changes in glucose metabolism appear to be heightened in adolescents with T1DM. There appears to be an apparent need for an increase in insulin dosage to maintain a similar level of glycaemia moving from childhood to adolescence. IGF-1 decreases significantly in the puberty years and there are major increases in IGF-binding protein and growth hormone concentration (**B**) [8]. Body composition changes can be quite marked in the young with diabetes, particularly in females (**B**) [12].

Associated diseases

The development of other diseases associated with diabetes can occur during adolescence, and undoubtedly a sudden change in the stability of the diabetes requires attention. Specific diseases are associated with diabetes and these may lead to erratic and brittle control. Other autoimmune diseases are the most likely: antibodies to thyroid tissue have been reported in from 10% to as much as 50% of people with diabetes under the age of 25 years (**E**) [13] (see Chapter 11 for more details). Hypothyroidism or thyrotoxicosis are rarer (<5%), but these should be considered in any case of deteriorating control as should asymptomatic coeliac and Addisons diseases. Chronic infection (e.g. tuberculosis) is no longer associated with diabetes in many countries. However, all children with diabetes are open to other general childhood illnesses that should be considered, such as infection, anaemia and leukaemia. In addition, there are major behavioural changes and social and cultural influences in adolescence that also appear to affect the ability of young people to manage their diabetes successfully over time, leading to persistent high glycaemic levels. It is believed that these are the dominant factors in producing deterioration in glycaemia.

Psychological issues of adolescence and diabetes

Many studies show that, following on from well-established clinical education programmes, the understanding of diabetes information in children, young people and their parents is high (see Chapter 10). This suggests that the ability to translate the educational advice given by health professionals into their home management is not, for the vast majority, a lack of knowledge. Rather, evidence suggests that it is the desire and the want to take this information forward, which is the key to concordance with the diabetes regimens (**A**) [14]. It is not surprising, therefore, that many learn that insulin omission is a useful method of keeping weight down.

Insulin omission

Insulin deficiency producing erratic control with the possible scenario of, and subsequent brittle diabetes with, frequent episodes of diabetic ketocidosis (DKA) is most likely to be due to insulin omission. Manipulation and factitious insulin delivery have been seen in the most severe, psychologically disturbed patients. Several case reports have been published of hidden insulin, diluted insulin preparations, tampering with intravenous and intraperitoneal catheters. As mentioned, most of these have come to light with extensive hospital investigation (**E**) [13].

More recently, insulin omission has emerged as a common phenomenon, probably accounting for the vast majority of episodes of DKA in the older adolescents known to have diabetes. While clinicians have always suspected this, since the initial treatment of T1DM, direct evidence has only recently become available. Capillary blood glucose testing and glycated haemoglobin estimation in the 1980s firmly established the suboptimal control of many young people with diabetes (see above). It was appreciated that a lack of concordance with the prescribed therapy regimens (insulin and diet) may be the basis for such poor control and agreed with the developing literature on the psychological impact of this chronic disease (see below). As Steel so insightfully stated, '*There is a reluctance to believe that patients would deliberately cheat their doctor and, after all "she is such a nice girl she would never do anything like that"* ' (**E**) [15].

In our unit, Thompson described the differences between young people with DKA and the older, more established diabetes (**B**) [16]. No specific cause was established in the majority and they responded dramatically to simple fluid and insulin therapy. The often-quoted reason of infection as the cause of the DKA was not established. More specifically, we were able to show that in young people the reason for DKA was insulin omission. The DARTS/MEMO study allows for a direct measure of insulin prescription in the Tayside region. Using the community health index number, a six-figure unique identifier, we are able to measure individual encashment of prescriptions. We examined in 90 young people with T1DM (aged <25 yr) the insulin prescription rate over 1 year and compared the encashment rate with the prescribed insulin dose through the clinics (**B**) [17]. In the older subjects we found a failure to collect all of their prescribed insulin over 1 year in over 50% with on average 28% collecting less than one-third of their insulin. A low encashment of insulin was associated with a high admission rate for DKA and overall poor control (Figure 6.1). DKA and persisting poor control (HbA1c >11%) in our clinic is synonymous with a lack of concordance with prescribed insulin therapy (see below).

Insulin, weight and eating disorders

Diabetes, particularly for girls, is a battleground for the powerful effect that insulin has on fat metabolism and the culturally unacceptable body images of excessive weight gain in modern society. 'High doses' of insulin are frequently used to achieve as low blood glucose levels as possible. The effect on the glucose levels may be for many at the expense of extra carbohydrate intake and alteration in body fat distribution and mass. Data from the Hvidøre International Study Group (**B**) [4] confirm the 'excessive weight' of older girls and many of us have a group in our clinic with marked weight gain. For these girls this is a major problem.

At the same time it has been accepted that there is a relatively higher incidence of eating disorders (anorexia nervosa, bulimia and binge eating) in, particularly, girls with diabetes (**A**) [18]. With the realisation that eating disorders are common in young people, it is not surprising that this is increased in diabetes, with its emphasis on diet as a treatment modality. The combination of insulin omission and erratic eating habits is a powerful tool

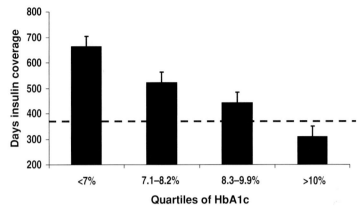

Figure 6.1 Lack of concordance in insulin encashment and influence on glycaemic control. Insulin omission in the middle teenage years is associated with poor HbA1c levels. (From Morris *et al.* [17] with permission.)

to reduce weight or keep weight steady at the expense of glycaemic control. For many this is acceptable but for some the erratic control of diabetes leads to a more brittle picture, with the risk of an episode of DKA.

Long-term consequences of diabetes

Concomitant with the poor glycaemic control is the concern for the development of the early signs of microvascular disease and changes in pathophysiology indicating an increased risk of future macrovascular disease. While the vast majority of older children and adolescents have no symptoms of vascular disease, most guidelines suggest that a screening programme should be introduced during this age range: guidelines produced by the National Institute for Clinical Excellence (NICE) (**E**) [19] and the International Society for Pediatric and Adolescent Diabetes (ISPAD) (**E**) [20] on balance suggest that screening for early biophysical markers of diabetic retinopathy and nephropathy, together with blood pressure screening, should start to be introduced systematically from the age of 12 years and be well established on an annual basis definitely by the age of 18 years (see Chapter 11).

Emotional and behavioural problems

The diagnosis of T1DM may be accompanied by a period of denial followed by gradual acceptance during which feelings of grief, stress and difficulty in coping are usually experienced. Whether the initial emotional response to diagnosis disappears, whether beneficial family dynamics exist (e.g. family cohesion), and how age at diagnosis affects children and young people and their families remains an issue and various elements of family adaptation to chronic illness (e.g. family system, adaptation to a stressful event, familial knowledge, skills and resources and use of coping strategies) determine the emotional and behavioural response in individuals (**E**) [21]. Children and young people with the least open and expressive families (as reported by children and young people and their mothers) demonstrated a greater deterioration in glycaemic control (as reported by mothers and children and young people). Males from less cohesive families and those with greater conflict showed a greater deterioration in HbA1c levels over 4 years compared with females **(B)** [22]. A 10-year follow-up study measuring the effect of diabetes on self-esteem in 57 children and young people with diabetes and 54 children and young people with acute illnesses **(B)** [23] showed that, when controlled for sex and socioeconomic status, there was no difference in self-esteem scores between the children and the young people with diabetes and the children and the young people with acute illnesses after 10 years. However, significant differences were reported in perceived competence, global self-worth and sociability. A Swiss study of 38 children and young people revealed that 24% of mothers and 22% of fathers had features of posttraumatic stress syndrome within 6 weeks of their children's diagnosis **(B)** [24].

The SIGN guideline reported that the following factors contributed to an increased risk of children and young people with T1DM developing psychological problems **(E)** [25]:
• avoidance of coping strategies
• increased responsibility given to the child
• family dysfunction
• non-effective communication between the family and the health professionals
• low socioeconomic status
• single-parent families
• maternal morbidity (particularly psychological morbidity).

Anxiety and depression

In 2000, the Office for National Statistics surveyed the prevalence of mental health problems in children and young people aged 5–15 years living in Great Britain: 5% had clinically significant conduct disorders and 4% suffered from emotional disorders (anxiety and depression) **(E)** [26]. In comparison, the prevalence of depression among adolescents with T1DM ranged from two to three times that of young people without diabetes **(E)** [27]. Correlates of depression in this population may include age, duration of diabetes and sex.

Psychological interventions

In 2004 Hampson *et al.* **(A)** [28] reported on the effects of educational and psychosocial interventions for adolescents with diabetes mellitus in a systematic review. Their findings are listed in Table 6.1. NICE recommended a series of approaches to behavioural support, listed in Table 6.2.

Social and cultural issues of adolescence and diabetes

Our group has systematically explored the wider issues of social and cultural factors that influence the delivery and response to health-care strategies for the young person with T1DM **(E)** [29]. Our observations have led us to the view that we should widen the debate about normative interpretations of adolescence by using the example of a 'culture-bound syndrome', as described by Hill and Fortenberry **(E)** [30], and to frame this debate within the context of diabetes care. We suggest that the concept of 'medicalisation of adolescence' brings into question the tendency in the NHS to talk about adolescence as if it were an age-based disorder that requires controlling alongside chronic illness and in this

Table 6.1 Effects of educational and psychosocial interventions for adolescents with T1DM

1 Educational and psychosocial interventions have small-to-medium beneficial effects on various diabetes management outcomes.
2 Well-designed trials of such interventions are needed in the UK. (No completed randomised controlled trials (RCTs) of educational or psychosocial interventions for adolescents with T1DM conducted in the UK were found.)
3 The evidence, arising primarily from studies in the USA, provides a starting point for the design of interventions in the UK.
4 Quantitative and narrative analysis of the evidence suggested that interventions are more likely to be effective if they demonstrate the inter-relatedness of the various aspects of diabetes management. The effectiveness of interventions should be evaluated by assessing outcomes that the intervention explicitly targets for change and at the appropriate point in time post-intervention to reflect the impact of the intervention.
5 Interventions need to be evaluated by well-designed studies, such as RCTs, including adequately powered patient-preference trials reporting results in such a way as to enable effect sizes to be calculated.
6 An important gap in the evidence is that there is no systematic understanding of whether interventions should be targeted (e.g. modified for different disease stages, different types of diabetes management problems or the different age groups subsumed by adolescence).
7 To reap economic returns, interventions need to show durable, favourable effects on behaviour and metabolic control, but there is a lack of cost-effective studies that fully address the resource implications of educational interventions for adolescents and long-term consequences.

From [28]. http://www.hta.nhsweb.nhs.uk/execsumm/summ510.htm

Table 6.2 Psychological support for the adolescent with diabetes recommendations from NICE

1 Diabetes care teams should be aware that poor psychosocial support has a negative impact on a variety of outcomes of T1DM in children and young people, including glycaemic control and self-esteem.
2 Children and young people with T1DM, especially young people using multiple-daily-injection regimens, should be offered structured behavioural intervention strategies because these may improve psychological well-being and glycaemic control.
3 Young people with T1DM should be offered specific support strategies, such as mentoring and self-monitoring of blood glucose levels supported by problem-solving, to improve their self-esteem and glycaemic control.
4 Families of children and young people with T1DM should be offered specific support strategies (such as behavioural family systems therapy) to reduce diabetes-related conflict between family members.
5 Children and young people with T1DM and their families should be offered timely and ongoing access to mental health professionals because they may experience psychological disturbances (such as anxiety, depression, behavioural and conduct disorders and family conflict) that can impact on the management of diabetes and well-being.
6 Diabetes care teams should have appropriate access to mental health professionals to support them in the assessment of psychological dysfunction and the delivery of psychosocial support.

From [19]. http://www.hta.nhsweb.nhs.uk/fullmono/mon510.pdf

way, also reveals the importance of seeing young people's lives in a broad context rather than purely through the filter of adolescence or diabetes. Relating to this is the idea that successful management of diabetes appears to relate not only to young people's strength of individuality, but also to the strength of their social support networks.

Conceptualisations of adolescence and diabetes

While puberty is viewed in many societies as a universal occurrence, the social positioning of adolescents, that is cultural beliefs about adolescents, is less easily defined (E, B) [30–32]. A number of societies choose to mark the transition from childhood to adulthood as a celebration and a public event involving formalised rites of passage (E) [33]. In the UK adolescence is more likely to be seen as an individual 'betwixt-and-between' affair, where young people must learn to work out, on a rather *ad hoc* and trial-and-error basis, the social roles of adulthood. Accordingly, this phase in the life cycle is typically defined in social and health policy terms as a problematic stage of adjustment, where normally developing young people start to confront parental boundaries and strive to become independent and autonomous decision-makers. In the diabetes arena this view understandably sets up the expectation that normal adolescents will behave badly by having 'poor control' of their diabetes and that 'good controllers' are somehow deficient in the normal qualities of social development and is illustrated in the following statement by a health professional, '*Adolescents with good control are abnormal; I would say, even a little bit worrying*' [34].

Yet, we also know that decisions about lifestyle made during adolescence may have an important bearing on the long-term health of the young person. The concept of patient-centred care, involvement and expertise (E) [35–38], as echoed in the Scottish Diabetes Framework (E) [39], involves both informing adult patients about the consequences of their risk-taking behaviour to their future health and relies on individuals playing an active role in safeguarding their own health. In the case of young people with T1DM, the concept of patient education, responsibility and expertise, however, seems infinitely more complex. This is because, on the one hand, health professionals are expected to acknowledge dominant western discourse about the normality of adolescent individualism and challenge to adult authority and on the other hand, they are increasingly pressurised to improve diabetes outcome in a group where greater independence appears to lead to a risk-taking lifestyle, such as the poor control of diabetes. Understandably, this leads many clinicians to strive merely to 'weather the storm of the teenage years' in the hope that as their patients get older they will develop a perception of their own vulnerability to complications, and thus improve their management of diabetes.

Adolescence as a culture-bound syndrome

As early as the 1920s, adolescence was perceived as a difficult phase of life in the West. The basis of this ideology is evident in the 'storm-and-stress' conceptualisations of the psychologist Hall in the early twentieth century (E) [40], along with other fashionable terms of the time, such as 'identity crisis', as explored in the work of Erikson (E) [41]. Despite protests in the 1950s about this style of framing youth culture by researchers such as Elkin and Westely, adolescence continued to be characterised as a phase of sexual frustration, social restrictions, difficulties in emancipation from the family and other authority relationships, in the form of conflict between the generations, and general risk taking (E) [42]. In fact, this view led Margaret Mead to Polynesia to discover whether adolescent Samoan girls were beset with the same developmental difficulties as Americans. Her conclusions were to begin to lead the way to rethinking the content of adolescence as being highly culture specific, rather than the result of characteristics that were universal to this age group (E) [43]. Nevertheless, adolescence today remains a twenty-first-century phenomenon associated with a disturbing and difficult development phase beleaguered with the problems of substance abuse, crime and sexually transmitted disease. As Hill and Fortenberry state, '*Adolescence per se is seen as the inevitable "risk" factor for these widespread problems as if the origins of these problems were innate to adolescents rather than a product of complex interactions of individual biology, personality, cultural preference, political expediency and social dysfunction. By creating adolescence as a development period defined by its problems, "adolescent health" becomes an oxymoron.*' (**E**) [30].

In the light of this view, adolescence appears to have been 'medicalised' into a condition that is inherently pathological and, in the case of adolescents with T1DM, adding to the impressions of health professionals that they are looking after patients with two conditions, diabetes and adolescence, which need controlling.

The concept of a culture-bound syndrome first appeared in medical literature in the 1950s (**E**) [42, 44] and continues to be drawn on (**E**) [45]. Our use of the term is based on Rittenbaugh's definition, which is described as '*a constellation of symptoms which has been categorised as a disease*' and which cannot be understood apart from a specific culture. Another example of a culturally specific syndrome might be obesity, where what is considered as a sign of beauty or health in one society may be seen in another as an epidemic (**E**) [46].

Action research

In diabetes literature, as described above, adolescence is described as a critical time for young people with diabetes as the result of puberty and the challenges of engaging with them to take responsibility for the management of their illness (**E, B**) [13, 47–51]. Co-currently, policy documents, in both diabetes and the care of the young (**E**) [39, 52], describe a new orientation in care delivery and a move in attention beyond developmental models that focus purely on how young people will turn out when they reach adulthood to those that validate the immediacy of their experiences of coping with a long-term illness. In social science literature, this reveals a change in ideology that shifts young people's position from 'social objects' of enquiry into active research agents with legitimate voices of their own (**E**) [53]. This, likewise, challenges beliefs about the commonality of youth culture and blanket prescriptions about what is needed in their best interests (**A, E**) [28, 51]. Our action research study drew on the theoretical and methodological frameworks of anthropology and psychology and generated a high-quality data set that allowed us to explore the above objectives in some detail. Our methods involved observing young people and health professionals in the clinic consultation and interviewing them separately in a place of their own choice to document issues that were of importance to both. The aim of this approach was to examine whether the rhetoric of patient-centred policy had been 'translated' into practice in the care of young people and, if not, to raise important questions about the lack of mechanisms in place to help health professionals 'action' patient-centred care for young people with diabetes (**E**) [29].

Results

A key issue about the delivery of care was the importance for young people of seeing their lives in a broad context rather than purely through the filter of diabetes, i.e. de-centring diabetes. While the design of our study enabled young people to talk about matters that were significant to them, the extent to which they were preoccupied by other issues and the centrality of these issues in their lives became increasingly apparent as fieldwork progressed. Many were facing a range of personal and familial challenges that were either prior or subsequent to having diabetes. These included issues around:

- sexuality
- schooling
- higher education (particularly the emphasis placed on assessments and exams)
- economic hardship and redundancy
- parental divorce
- peer friendships
- relationships with adults and the management of diabetes.

The inappropriateness of health professionals seeing diabetes as the central issue in their lives was something many spoke openly about and felt it was imposed upon them in a number of the clinics. In fact, many told us they had been unsure about taking part in the project for if it was merely about diabetes, then it was not seen as wholly relevant and would hold little meaning for them. This was particularly so for those who had had diabetes for a number of years and felt they had 'normalised' their situations by incorporating the illness into the normal complexities of lives.

The need to de-centre diabetes in a way that does not define it as the key life experience in a young person's life, which determines his or her subsequent life chances, is a theme pertained to in the Scottish Diabetes Framework (**E**) [39], but which appeared less well attended to in the narratives of some health professionals who felt they were struggling to cope with the rise in patient numbers and the constant changes in the NHS brought about by escalating performance assessments.

Issues relating to being an adolescent

Similarly, of importance to young people was the need for health professionals to see their lives in a broad context rather than purely through the 'filter' of adolescence, particularly, as it was associated with such negative connotations. As with diabetes, seeing adolescence as the central issue in their life and the cause of 'poor control' was a concept that few could identify with. Control was much more about issues related to coping with puberty and the pressure placed on them (by adults) to be independent and 'stand on their own two feet'. As such, notions of adolescence as an age-based disorder unintentionally drew attention away from other significant challenges in their lives. In relation to our data, there appeared to be a mismatch in understanding: health professionals, it seemed, were more inclined to see non-adherence as an inherent quality of adolescence and something they would grow out of, while young people were more likely to see themselves as master negotiators dealing with the challenges of a difficult illness in a life few felt they had any control over. Notions of independence, and the importance of it during adolescence, are related to a powerful ethos of individualism that seems to permeate Western discourse and influence medical attitudes towards young people (**E**) [54, 55]. An example of this is evident in a publication by the Royal College of Physicians and the British Paediatric Association that calls for health professionals to promote young people's accountability for disease management and not to 'mollycoddle' them (**E**) [56]. This raises important questions about the power of such discourse when evidence shows that early responsibility for diabetes management has been shown to increase poor glycaemic control and DKA (**A, E**) [57–59].

Social support networks

In fact, sharing diabetes management with supportive others, such as family, peers, teachers and employers, seemed of major importance to young people (**E**) [29]. Likewise, relationships with health professionals who related management issues to their specific needs were highly valued. However, many said that they were acutely aware of how preoccupied staff were with the lack of resources and the pressures to improve outcomes. Also, of importance, and in spite of having diabetes over many years, was how anxious many felt about attending clinic appointments. In particular, most feared learning about 'bad news' or 'feeling guilty' about a condition they felt they had little control over. Most, therefore, spoke about their preference for seeing staff that appreciated the efforts they made to come to clinic, reassuring them in the face of good or bad news, and 'warming them up' by framing the management of diabetes within the context of their daily routines and experiences. Continuity with the staff allowed them to problem-solve and build on their life experiences with diabetes and, in this way, increase their sense of control over a difficult condition. Solidarity with health professionals helped to promote a sense of claiming health-care relationships as a reciprocal process, suggestive of intimacy and familiarity between people.

Clinic non-attendance

Where the above features are missing, or inconsistently applied, such as being referred to inexperienced staff at clinic, the regimen of management and clinic attendance may become a trial for young people. Non-attendance is therefore often a sign of a one-way process, expressing low self-esteem, anger, disillusionment and resolve. This suggests that the task of sustaining diabetes management over many years is challenging for young people and that disadvantaged relationships with staff may begin to outweigh the efforts that young people make towards rigorous management of diabetes. Of importance then is how health professionals manage the inherent power relations embedded in medical encounters; moreover, how, despite the best intentions, adult knowledge may be prioritised over the young persons. It is clear that young people are receptive to supportive relationships during adolescence and appear to be major agents in thinking about these relationships and how their meanings and practices are shaped.

It therefore appears that the outcome of Western views of adolescence, in relation to a chronic disorder such as diabetes, is the stereotyping of adolescence as an age-based disorder. This, as Hill and Fortenberry argue and our study suggests, draws attention away from the important bases of youth morbidity and mortality in the form of racism, poverty, unemployment and inadequate education. The conceptualisation of adolescence as a disease or an epidemic that needs control and prevention merely contributes to a misconception about the essence of adolescence, and with it their experiences and needs. It is our hope that consideration of these issues (Table 6.3) may help to reshape care strategies for this age group and lead to its necessary part in care delivery reform and the research agenda setting.

Table 6.3 Young people's priorities for care delivery

1 The need to *de-centre diabetes* and see their lives in a broad context rather than purely through the filter of diabetes, i.e. by acknowledging the range of personal and familial challenges they face.
2 The need to *de-centre diabetes* in a way that does not define it as the key life experience that defines them and determines their subsequent life chances.
3 The need to *de-centre adolescence* and see their lives in a broad context rather than purely through the filter of adolescence; i.e. notions of adolescence as an age-based disorder draw attention away from other significant challenges in their lives.
4 The need to *de-centre adolescence* and reconsider the pressure on this age group to manage diabetes independently, which may increases its sense of isolation, low self-esteem, anger, disillusionment and resolve.
5 The need to *recognise* the significance of young people's social support networks in managing diabetes; i.e. inclusion of family, friends, mentors, teachers and employers may help to reduce a sense of isolation.
6 The need to *recognise* the importance of continuity with supportive health professionals that recognise young people's specific needs, i.e. framing diabetes management in the context of the other significance challenges in their lives.
7 The need to recognise that reciprocity between young people and health professionals helps to promote diabetes ownership, suggestive of intimacy and familiarity between people.

Transition of care from the paediatric to the adult service

The commonest age of diagnosis of T1DM is during childhood, with 10 years being the current average in the UK (**E**) [19]. Consequently, as they move through puberty and adolescence, they have to cope not only with the issues of their society and culture surrounding their position as adolescents, but also with the practical issues of managing their diabetes (see above). As they move from the children's health service into the adult health-care system, it is accepted that young people with T1DM have specific health needs relating to these physical and sociocultural changes of adolescence.

Offering a special service for adolescents with T1DM

NICE, through the National Collaborating Centre for Women's and Children's Health, systematically reviewed and published the evidence of effective transition of care as part of the guidelines for the UK on the management of T1DM in children and young (**E**) [19].

Effectiveness of young adult clinics

In the UK a number of centres across the country transfer young people into special transition clinics rather than transfer them directly from paediatric to the general adult diabetes clinics (**E**) [60]. NICE found no studies that examined the clinical or cost-effectiveness of transition clinics. However, there are some studies that have compared the differences between various outcomes between children's and adult clinics. A survey investigating the transfer of young people from children's to adult clinics in the Oxford region showed that age of transfer ranged from 13.3 to 22.4 years (mean age 17.9 yr) (**B**) [61]. A similar range occurs currently in Scotland (SSGCYD, personal data). The rate at which clinic attendance occurred at least every 6 months dropped from 98% at 2 years before transfer to 61% at 2 years after transfer. A letter of transfer was identified in the clinical records for 86%

of the young people, and the attendance rate at the first appointment in the new clinic was 79%.

Another study from the UK National Children's Bureau examined young people's knowledge of adult clinics before transfer, preparation for transfer and how young people felt about the move (**E**) [62]. Young people who were attending an adolescent or transition clinic seemed to have little knowledge about the clinic they would be going to in the future. Of the young people attending adult clinics, 35% had discussed the change beforehand, 16% reported having had a choice about the move, 84% felt they were ready to move and 40% felt they were well prepared by staff for the move. However, 79% were not pleased to move.

A Canadian survey examined the experience of young people with T1DM during the period of transfer from paediatric to adult care (**B**) [63]. The mean age at transfer was 18.5 years, and this was lower than the age of transfer suggested by the patients (18.8 yr): 21% of patients felt that they should have been transferred earlier, whereas 65% felt that they should have been transferred later. After transfer, 13% had no regular contact with adult-care services, 3% had contact with a family physician and the remainder had contact with an endocrinologist or a diabetes clinic. Thirty-three per cent of patients felt they had a problem with the transition from paediatric to adult care. Twenty-seven per cent experienced a delay of more than 6 months between their last visit to the paediatric clinic and their first visit to the adult clinic. (In 17% of patients this delay was greater than 1 yr.)

A Finnish study examined glycaemic control in young people 1 year before and 1 year after they were transferred from a paediatric clinic to an adult clinic (**B**) [64], with the mean age of transfer 17.5 years and the mean HbA1 level improving from 1 year before transfer to 1 year after transfer (11.2% vs 9.9%).

Where to and when to transfer?

An Australian survey of young people with T1DM found that patients wished to be treated in a range of care places: 72% public hospital, 43% private specialist and 14% general practitioner only (**B**) [65]. Also, they had differing views on the age of transfer: 6% felt that transfer should occur before the age of 17 years, 49% felt that transfer should occur between the ages of 17 and 20 years and 45% felt that transfer should occur at any age up to 25 years.

A UK survey of young people in Exeter showed that the average age of transfer was 15.9 years (range 12–20 yr), and 27% offered some reason for transfer of care (**B**) [66]. The patients thought that it would be more helpful to visit the young adults' clinic before transfer than for a nurse or physician from the young adults' clinic to visit the paediatric clinic. The young people thought that the staff in the paediatric clinic assigned more importance to school progress and family relations than did staff in the young adults' clinic but less importance to exercise, avoidance of complications and blood glucose. The paediatric and young adults' clinic staff did not differ in their assignment of importance to diet, insulin management or privacy.

In preparation of the guideline, NICE organised a young people's consultation day, where it was found that some parents suggested that age of transfer of young people with T1DM from paediatric to adult services should be standardised and that clinics should be jointly run by paediatric and adult services to provide continuity of care, whereas other parents thought that young people with T1DM should be involved in the decision about

Table 6.4 Recommendations for the transition of care in adolescents with T1DM

1 Young people with T1DM should be encouraged to attend clinics on a regular basis (three or four times per year) because regular attendance is associated with good glycaemic control.
2 Young people with T1DM should be allowed sufficient time to familiarise themselves with the practicalities of the transition from paediatric to adult services because this has been shown to improve clinic attendance.
3 Specific local protocols should be agreed for transferring young people with T1DM from paediatric to adult services.
4 The age of transfer to the adult service should depend on the individual's physical development and emotional maturity, and local circumstances.
5 Transition from the paediatric service should occur at a time of relative stability in the individual's health and should be coordinated with other life transitions.
6 Paediatric diabetes care teams should organise age-banded clinics for young people and young adults jointly with their adult specialty colleagues.
7 Young people with T1DM who are preparing for transition to adult services should be informed that some aspects of diabetes care will change at transition. The main changes relate to targets for short-term glycaemic control and screening for complications.

From [19]. http://www.hta.nhsweb.nhs.uk/fullmono/mon510.pdf

when transfer should occur. Young people with T1DM appear to like age-banded clinics, in both the paediatric and adult services.

How to transfer

The UK National Service Framework for Diabetes states that transfer of young people with diabetes from paediatric services to adult services often occurs at a sensitive time in relation to the young person's diabetes and personal life (**E**) [67]. The cultural change that occurs at transition is found to be unacceptable by many young people, and young people's attendance rates at adult clinics are often low. Sensitive and skilled care at transition can assist in achieving good diabetes management, with a consequent avoidance of complications. A multidisciplinary approach is particularly effective for young people at transition. Young people with T1DM who are preparing for transition to adult services should be informed that some aspects of diabetes management will change at transition.

NICE drew attention to some points that had been recommended in the adult guidelines that had a different emphasis in the children's and young person's guideline. Of particular note was:

• the increasing emphasis on screening for not only microvascular but also macrovascular disease
• the emphasis on tight glycaemic control with pre- and postprandial blood glucose targets of 4–7 mmol/L and less than 9 mmol/L, respectively.

Recommendations for transition

NICE summed up its recommendations for transition of care in seven points (see Table 6.4). The recommendations are broad and assume that each individual young adult will receive a personalised-care package from a multidisciplinary team, experienced in the issues of teenagers in their respective cultural setting.

A recent review (**B**) [68] of provision of services for children and adolescents with diabetes in the UK did not specifically assess the transition process, but did show continuing improvements in organisational structure of services for older children. NICE recommended that paediatric diabetes care teams should organise age-banded clinics for adolescents and young adults jointly with their adult colleagues: 71% of hospitals clinics surveyed in 2005 ($n = 119$) have age-stratified clinics of which 63% have an adolescent clinic and 48% of the centres have joint clinics with adult colleagues. This is a marked change since the previous surveys in the previous 15 years.

From the limited evidence base the recommendations were weighted based on the NICE criteria. NICE strongly suggested that further research is needed to investigate young people's experiences of transition from paediatric to adult services for people with T1DM.

Forming a transition service

Undoubtedly, teenagers are a special group that requires a different clinical service compared with young children. Several issues, however, should be considered in establishing a transition service:
• Perhaps, most importantly, the children's team needs to communicate with and be comfortable working closely with the adult team.
• Both must share a philosophy, as well as an understanding of the social positioning in their culture of adolescence.
• The transition clinic should be serviced by both teams, to their mutual convenience.
• Agreement should be made on the culturally designed and influenced:
  – venue
  – age range
  – position of parents and peers
  – clinical standards and care strategies.
• The service should have easy access to psychological support.
• Education programmes should include advice and direction on the management of diabetes and various lifestyle issues:
  – alcohol
  – smoking cessation
  – avoidance of recreational drugs
  – pre-pregnancy planning and contraception
  – work and diabetes
  – extreme sports and diabetes.
The limited evidence for the UK suggests that transition clinics should start around 18 years of age (following on from age-banded clinics in the paediatric service), facilitate the participation of family and peers and encourage an intensive approach to insulin therapy, accompanied by formalised and frequent screening for micro- and macrovascular complications.

Post transition

A dilemma is arising with the management of patients who were managed as children with T1DM in the paediatric service and who were then transferred through a successful transition service. Most groups recommend the end of transition to be around 22–25 years of age, usually coinciding with the finishing of tertiary education. This raises the question of who provides the service for older people with T1DM. Should they be retained into a special T1DM service or be managed by their general practitioner or family physician? If the latter, should these health professionals be designated as diabetes specialists?

In reality, certainly in the UK, a considerable number of these young adults 'disappear' from the health service. This 'lost tribe of T1DM' then re-emerges with the clinical declaration of micro- and macrovascular disease. The adult diabetes service is often unable to cope with additional workload against the background explosion of T2DM. A way forward could be to develop specialised family practitioners, trained in T1DM management, and/or to consider a dedicated specialist service for T1DM, which could offer continuity across the age range.

Summary

A matching of priorities and goals between young people with T1DM and health professionals appears to be a significant factor in producing good clinical outcome.

This chapter suggests several themes that interfere with the process of matching priorities and goals.

Despite differences in organisation and resources in the diabetes centres studied, these themes appeared constant.

References

1 Greene SA. Factors influencing glycemic control in young people with type 1 diabetes in Scotland: a population-based study (DIABAUD2). *Diabetes Care* 2001; **24**: 239–44.

2 Diabetes Control and Complications Trial Research Group. The effect of intensive treatment of diabetes on the development and progression of long-term complications in insulin-dependent diabetes mellitus. The Diabetes Control and Complications Trial Research Group. *N Engl J Med* 1993; **329**: 977–86.

3 Mortensen HB, Marinelli K, Norgaard K *et al.* A nation-wide cross-sectional study of urinary albumin excretion rate, arterial blood pressure and blood glucose control in Danish children with type 1 diabetes mellitus. Danish Study Group of Diabetes in Childhood. *Diabet Med* 1990; **7**: 887–97.

4 Mortensen HB, Hougaard P. Comparison of metabolic control in a cross-sectional study of 2,873 children and adolescents with IDDM from 18 countries. The Hvidore Study Group on Childhood Diabetes. *Diabetes Care* 1997; **20**: 714–20.

5 Rosilio M, Cotton JB, Wieliczko MC *et al.* Factors associated with glycemic control: a cross-sectional nationwide study in 2,579 French children with type 1 diabetes. The French Pediatric Diabetes Group. *Diabetes Care* 1998; **21**: 1146–53.

6 Scottish Study Group for the Care of the Young with Diabetes. A longitudinal observational study of insulin therapy and glycaemic control in Scottish children with type 1 diabetes: DIABAUD 3. *Diabet Med* 2006; **23**: 1216–21.

7 Hindmarsh PC, Matthews DR, Di Silvio L *et al.* Relation between height velocity and fasting insulin concentrations. *Arch Dis Child* 1988; **63**: 665–66.

8 Dunger DB, Cheetham TD, Holly JM *et al.* Does recombinant insulin-like growth factor I have a role in the treatment of insulin-dependent diabetes mellitus during adolescence? *Acta Paediatr Suppl* 1993; **388**: 49–52.

9 Green F, Khan F, Kennedy G *et al.* Syndrome X and endothelial function in children. *Diabet Med* 1999; **16**(suppl 1): 49–52.

10 White EM, Wilson AC, Greene SA *et al.* Body mass index centile charts to assess fatness of British children. *Arch Dis Child* 1995; **72**: 38–41.

11 Pinhas-Hamiel O, Zeitler P. Type 2 diabetes in adolescents, no longer rare. *Pediatr Rev* 1998; **19**: 434–5.

12 Gregory JW, Wilson AC, Greene SA. Body fat and overweight among children and adolescents with diabetes mellitus. *Diabet Med* 1992; **9**: 344–8.

13 Greene SA. Diabetes in childhood and adolescence. In: Pickup J, Williams G, eds. *Textbook of Diabetes*. Blackwell, Oxford, 1997.

14 Franklin VL, Waller A, Pagliari C *et al*. A randomized controlled trial of Sweet Talk, a text-messaging system to support young people with diabetes. *Diabet Med* 2006; **23**: 1332–8.

15 Steel JM. 'Such a nice girl'. *Lancet* 1994; **344**: 765–6.

16 Thompson CJ, Cummings F, Chalmers J *et al*. Abnormal insulin treatment behaviour: a major cause of ketoacidosis in the young adult. *Diabet Med* 1995; **12**: 429–32.

17 Morris AD, Boyle DI, McMahon AD *et al*. Adherence to insulin treatment, glycaemic control, and ketoacidosis in insulin-dependent diabetes mellitus. The DARTS/MEMO Collaboration. Diabetes Audit and Research in Tayside Scotland. Medicines Monitoring Unit. *Lancet* 1997; **350**: 1505–10.

18 Jones JM, Lawson ML, Daneman D *et al*. Eating disorders in adolescent females with and without type 1 diabetes: cross sectional study. *BMJ* 2000; **320**: 1563–6.

19 NICE Type 1 Diabetes in Children and Young People: Full Guideline, 2004. Available at: http://www.nice.org.uk/page.aspx?o=CG015childfullguideline

20 ISPAD. *ISPAD Consensus Guidelines for the Management of Type 1 Diabetes Mellitus in Children and Adolescents*. Medical Forum International, Zeist, Netherlands, 2000.

21 Clawson JA. A child with chronic illness and the process of family adaptation. *J Pediatr Nurs* 1996; **11**: 52–61.

22 Jacobson AM, Hauser ST, Lavori P *et al*. Family environment and glycemic control: a four-year prospective study of children and adolescents with insulin-dependent diabetes mellitus. *Psychosom Med* 1994; **56**: 401–9.

23 Jacobson AM, Hauser ST, Willett JB *et al*. Psychological adjustment to IDDM: 10-year follow-up of an onset cohort of child and adolescent patients. *Diabetes Care* 1997; **20**: 811–18.

24 Landolt MA, Ribi K, Laimbacher J *et al*. Posttraumatic stress disorder in parents of children with newly diagnosed type 1 diabetes. *J Pediatr Psychol* 2002; **27**: 647–52.

25 Scottish Intercollegiate Guidelines Network. *SIGN 50: A Guideline Developer's Handbook*. Scottish Intercollegiate Guidelines Network, Edinburgh, 2001.

26 Meltzer H, Gatward R, Goodman R *et al*. *The Mental Health of Children and Adolescents in Great Britain*. Summary Report. Office of National Statistics, London, 2000.

27 Grey M, Whittemore R, Tamborlane W. Depression in type 1 diabetes in children: natural history and correlates. *J Psychosom Res* 2002; **53**: 907–11.

28 Hampson SE, Skinner TC, Hart J *et al*. Effects of educational and psychosocial interventions for adolescents with diabetes mellitus: a systematic review. *Health Technol Assess* 2001; **5**: 1–79.

29 Greene A, Skinner C, Greene S. *Quality Care in Young People with Type 1 Diabetes*. Diabetes UK, London, 2003.

30 Hill RF, Fortenberry JD. Adolescence as a culture-bound syndrome. *Soc Sci Med* 1992; **35**: 73–80.

31 Mayall B. *Children, Health and the Social Order*. Buckingham: Open University Press, 1996.

32 Young B, Dixon-Woods M, Windridge KC *et al*. Managing communication with young people who have a potentially life threatening chronic illness: qualitative study of patients and parents. *BMJ* 2003; **326**: 305.

33 van Gennep A. *The Rites of Passage: A Classic Study of Cultural Celebrations*. Chicago: University of Chicago Press, 1961.

34 Greene A. Health carers' and young peoples' conceptualisations of chronic illness: an anthropological interpretation of diabetes mellitus. Unpublished PhD thesis, 2000.

35 Department of Health. *The Expert Patient: A New Approach to Chronic Disease Management for the 21st Century*. Department of Health, London, 2001.

36 Department of Health Patient and Public Involvement. Available at: http://www.dh.gov.uk/PolicyAndGuidance/OrganisationPolicy/PatientAndPublicInvolvement/fs/en

37 Detmer DE, Singleton PD, MacLeod A *et al*. *The Informed Patient: Study Report*. Cambridge University Press, Cambridge, 2003.

38 Patient Information Forum. Patient Information Forum: Better Communication, Better Health. Available at: http://www.pifonline.org.uk/mod_sys/site_search.asp

39 Scottish Executive. Scottish Diabetes Framework: Action Plan. Available at: http://www.scotland.gov.uk/Publications/2006/06/12111211/0

40 Hall GS. *Adolescence: Its Psychology and Its Relations to Psychology, Anthropology, Sociology, Sex, Crime, Religion and Education.* New York: Appleton, 1904.

41 Erikson E. *Childhood and Society.* New York: Norton, 1950.

42 Yap PM. Mental diseases peculiar to certain culture: a survey of comparative psychiatry. *J Ment Sci* 1951; **97**: 313–27.

43 Mead M. *Coming of Age in Samoa: A Psychological Study of Primitive Youth for Western Civilisation.* New York: Dell, 1968.

44 Yap PM. Koro – a culture bound depersonalization syndrome. *Br J Psychiatry* 1965; **111**: 43–50.

45 Helman CG. Heart disease and the cultural construction of time: the type A behaviour pattern as a Western culture-bound syndrome. *Soc Sci Med* 1987; **25**: 969–79.

46 Ritenbaugh C. Obesity as a culture-bound syndrome. *Cult Med Psychiatry* 1982; **6**: 347–64.

47 Grey M, Boland EA, Davidson M *et al.* Short-term effects of coping skills training as adjunct to intensive therapy in adolescents. *Diabetes Care* 1998; **21**: 902–8.

48 Ingersoll GM, Orr DP, Herrold AJ *et al.* Cognitive maturity and self-management among adolescents with insulin-dependent diabetes mellitus. *J Pediatr* 1986; **108**: 620–3.

49 Meldman LS. Diabetes as experienced by adolescents. *Adolescence* 1987; **22**: 433–4.

50 Olsen R, Sutton J. More hassle, more alone: adolescents with diabetes and the role of formal and informal support. *Child Care Health Dev* 1998; **24**: 31–9.

51 Skinner C, Petzing J, Johnston C. Peer support and metabolic control in adolescence. *J Diab Nurs* 1999; **3**: 140–4.

52 Department of Health. *National Service Framework for Children, Young People and Maternity Services: Core Standards.* Department of Health, London, 2004.

53 Greene A. The caring relationship: chronic adolescent illness in Scotland. *Proceedings of the British Scientific Association* Glasgow, 2001.

54 Brannen J, Dodd K, Oakley A, Storey P. *Young People, Health and Family Life.* Buckingham: Open University Press, 1995.

55 Williams C. Alert assistants in managing chronic disease: the case of mothers and teenage sons. *Sociol Health Illn* 2000; **22**: 254–72.

56 Royal College of Physicians. Alcohol and the young. Report of a joint working party of the Royal College of Physicians and the British Paediatric Association. Royal College of Physicians, London, 1995.

57 Burroughs TE, Harris MA, Pontious SL *et al.* Research on social support in adolescents with IDDM: a critical review. *Diabetes Educ* 1997; **23**: 438–48.

58 Drotar D. Relating parent and family functioning to the psychological adjustment of children with chronic health conditions: what have we learned? What do we need to know? *J Pediatr Psychol* 1997; **22**: 149–65.

59 Snoek F, Skinner TC. *Psychology in Diabetes Care.* Chichester: John Wiley & Sons, 2000.

60 Rawlins MD. NICE work – providing guidance to the British National Health Service. *N Engl J Med* 2004; 351: 1383–5.

61 Jefferson IG, Swift PG, Skinner TC *et al.* Diabetes services in the UK: third national survey confirms continuing deficiencies. *Arch Dis Child* 2003; **88**: 53–6.

62 Datta J. *Moving up with Diabetes: The Transition from Paediatric to Adult Care.* National Children's Bureau, London, 2003.

63 Pacaud D, McConnell B, Huot C *et al.* Transition from pediatric care to adult care for insulin-dependent diabetes patients. *Can J Diabet Care* 1996; **20**: 14–20.

64 Salmi J, Huupponen T, Oksa H *et al.* Metabolic control in adolescent insulin-dependent diabetics referred from pediatric to adult clinic. *Ann Clin Res* 1986; **18**: 84–7.

65 Court JM. Issues of transition to adult care. *J Paediatr Child Health* 1993; **29**(suppl 1): S53–5.

66 Eiser C, Flynn M, Green E *et al.* Coming of age with diabetes: patients' views of a clinic for under-25 year olds. *Diabet Med* 1993; **10**: 285–9.

67 Diabetes NSF Implementation Group. National Service Framework for Diabetes: Delivery Strategy. Available at: http://www.dh.gov.uk/prod_consum_dh/groups/dh_digitalassets/@dh/@en/documents/digitalasset/dh_4032823.pdf

68 Edge JA, Swift PG, Anderson W *et al.* Diabetes services in the UK: fourth national survey: are we meeting NSF standards and NICE guidelines? *Arch Dis Child* 2005; **90**: 1005–9.

CHAPTER 7

Management of special situations in diabetes

Fergus J. Cameron & Jeremy Allgrove

> *The first precept was never to accept a thing as true until I knew it as such without a single doubt.*
>
> —Rene Descartes, '*Le Discours de la Methode*', 1637
> French mathematician and philosopher (1596–1650)

Good control of diabetes depends on a balance between insulin given in suitable doses, the maintenance of a healthy diet and participation in adequate amounts of exercise. However, even excellent control can be disrupted by a variety of intercurrent problems, such as illness, the need for surgery, travel and holidays. This chapter aims to present the evidence, such as it is, for how to address these issues as and when they arise.

Illness

Fergus Cameron

Despite some *in vitro* evidence of altered immune function in diabetes (**B**) [1–3], children and adolescents with well-controlled diabetes do not appear to be at greater risk of infectious disease than their peers (**C**) [4]. However, they are not immune to infection either and intercurrent illnesses are largely unavoidable.

Intercurrent illnesses can be divided into three categories according to their impact upon glycaemia:
• those illnesses that elevate blood glucose levels
• those illnesses that lower blood glucose levels
• those illnesses that have no impact upon blood glucose levels.

Examples of the first category include viral and bacterial infections associated with significant pyrexia and malaise, and examples of the second category include vomiting and diarrhoeal illnesses. Illnesses that have no impact upon glycaemia include trivial or mild viral infections. Ketogenesis is associated with impaired insulin action due to either low circulating insulin levels (e.g. following a dose reduction in order to deal with hypoglycaemia) or impaired insulin bioactivity (e.g. with increased counter-regulatory hormone secretion during significant pyrexia). Frequently, elevations in blood glucose and ketones may precede the overt signs and symptoms of the underlying illness (**E**) [5].

Generic principles of management include treating the underlying illness and ensuring adequate rest and hydration. The main aims of diabetes-specific therapy are to avoid

Table 7.1 Extra insulin doses required during sick-day management

Blood glucose (mmol/L)	Urinary ketones	Blood ketones (mmol/L)	Extra rapid-acting insulin requirement
< 15	Nil	< 1.0	Nil
> 15	Nil	< 1.0	Increase scheduled dose by 5%
> 15	Trace/small	1.0–1.4	Give extra insulin every 2–4 h (5–10% of the total daily dose)
> 15	Moderate/large	> 1.5	Give extra insulin every 2–4 h (10–20% of the total daily dose)

Adapted from [7].

Table 7.2 Minidose glucagon rescue doses

Age (yr)	Glucagon dose (μg)	Glucagon dose if drawn up in an insulin syringe (units)
< 2	20	2
2–15	10 per year of age	1 per year of age
> 15	150	15

diabetic ketoacidosis and hypoglycaemia. Glycaemia and ketosis are usually unstable, and frequent (1–2 hourly) monitoring of blood glucose levels and ketones is therefore critical. Measurement of blood β-hydroxybutyrate levels has significant advantages over measuring urinary acetoacetate levels (**B**) [6].

Illnesses that result in hyperglycaemia and ketosis require increased insulin doses. The ways in which this can be done will depend upon the underlying insulin-replacement regimen and the degree of hyperglycaemia/ketosis. Glycaemia and ketosis thresholds for dose changes will vary from centre to centre. The Australasian guidelines for patients receiving intermittent subcutaneous insulin injections are summarised in Table 7.1 (**E**) [7].

Patients who are receiving continuous subcutaneous insulin infusion (or insulin-pump) therapy require a different regimen. In the absence of ketones a correctional bolus should be given (e.g. calculated using the '100 rule' (**E**) [8]). If this fails to correct the blood glucose levels and/or ketones develop then pump failure should be presumed and the pump should be disconnected and a subcutaneous injection of insulin given. In this context there may be no active insulin 'on board' and an increased insulin dose may need to be given.

Illnesses that result in hypoglycaemia can be dealt with in various ways. Initially, patients should be given 'hypo' foods or fluids if possible. If vomiting renders this option impracticable, then glucagon can be given either in the standard way if the patient is unconscious or alternatively using the 'Minidose glucagon rescue' protocol (Table 7.2) (**B**) [9]. If hypoglycaemia persists then insulin doses may need to be reduced by 20–50%. It is critical that insulin not be ceased altogether, as this will trigger lipolysis and ketogenesis. It is also important to remind patients to check for ketones even if their blood glucose is not elevated in this situation.

Critical to the success of any of these above-mentioned strategies is the requirement of frequent blood glucose and ketone testing and ongoing contact with a suitable member of the diabetes care team. When these ambulatory strategies are unsuccessful, prompt hospital admission is usually required.

Travel

Young people and adolescents travel frequently for recreational, sporting and educational reasons. Fear of diabetes-related problems, however, can deter many young diabetic people from pursuing such activities (**B**) [10]. Travel can present challenges for diabetes management with the following aspects of a planned trip needing to be considered:
- the length of the planned trip
- the medical resources of the planned destination country (countries)
- the climate of the planned destination countries
- planned activities
- foods available in destination countries
- change in time zones between the place of origin and the place of destination
- likelihood of infectious illness
- health/travel insurance needs.

Generally speaking, travel that involves either changing time zones (east–west travel by plane), physical activity or travel to countries of differing health resources for extended periods of time (e.g. a 2–3-week, high-altitude trekking holiday in a third-world country) is more likely to have an impact upon diabetes control than that of a more simple and less adventurous trip (**E, C**) [11, 12]. Several weeks prior to departure a plan for insulin adjustment during the trip should be negotiated with the diabetes care team. This will vary according to what the usual insulin regime is (twice daily, multiple daily injections or pump therapy), time zone change, duration of flight and any stopovers. Plans should include contingencies for unscheduled events, such as missed flight connections, etc.

The young persons or their families should inform themselves as to the medical system of the country of destination and idiosyncratic needs for immunisations, travel insurance, etc. Letters of introduction and explanation of the need to carry diabetes equipment are usually required for security services, customs and overseas health providers. Plans should be discussed for how to deal with unexpected illnesses, etc.

Medical supplies (insulin, glucagon, test strips, batteries, needles, etc.) should be carried as hand luggage in an insulated container during travel. Adequate supplies should be taken for the duration of the trip, with some extra in case of loss or destruction. Allowances should be made for extremes in climate, which may affect insulin storage, electronic function of blood glucose meters/pumps, etc. (**B**) [13], and how needles/lancets will be disposed of appropriately. Young people with diabetes should not rely on meal services during flights/cruises/bus trips and should carry their own supply of 'hypo' foods to treat any hypoglycaemia. Blood glucose monitoring will need to be more frequent during travel, particularly in the first 24 hours after arrival if active or if eating unfamiliar foods. The usual guidelines for insulin adjustment with activities or sick days should apply. Non-urgent advice can sometimes be provided by the diabetes care team in the country of origin, using either e-mail or phone contact.

Exercise

There is conflicting evidence as to underlying fitness levels in children and adolescents with type 1 diabetes mellitus (T1DM) (**B**) [14, 15] and the frequency with which they undertake exercise. Different studies have indicated that children and adolescents with T1DM undertake more, less and the same amounts of exercise as their non-diabetic peers (**B**) [16–18].

Most diabetes care centres encourage regular exercise amongst their patients. Whilst the cardiovascular and psychosocial benefits of exercise are recognised (**C**) [19, 20], there appear to be inconsistent data as to the metabolic benefits of exercise in the context of T1DM and the risks of marked fluctuations in glycaemia. In general terms, the glycaemic impact of exercise will depend upon the type and frequency of the exercise (**C**) [21], as well as the mode and type of insulin delivery.

The impact of exercise upon overall glycaemic control is unclear. The FinnDiane Study of 1030 adults with T1DM showed that leisure-based exercise had no impact upon HbA1c levels in men but was associated with increased HbA1c levels in women (**A**) [22]. In another study of 91 adolescents with T1DM, regular exercise was associated with better glycaemic control, with the improvement correlating with duration of exercise (measured in minutes per week) (**B**) [16].

Repeated episodes of prolonged exercise of both low and moderate intensities appear to cause some degree of hypoglycaemia unawareness through blunted counter-regulatory hormone responses (**C**) [23]. Whilst intercurrent/short-term hypoglycaemia during exercise is avoidable using supplemental carbohydrate ingestion (**C, B**) [24–26], it appears that longer (>60 min duration) exercise is best managed by a 20–30% reduction in insulin dose (**B**) [27]. A study of 50 adolescents undergoing exercise on a treadmill in the afternoon showed that prolonged, moderate, aerobic exercise resulted in a mean fall of blood glucose of 2.6 mmol/L (47 mg/dL) by 45 minutes after completion of the exercise (**C**) [28]. Eighty-three per cent of subjects experienced a fall in blood glucose of ≥25% of their baseline value with hypoglycaemia occurring frequently if the baseline blood glucose value was <6.6 mmol/L (120 mg/dL) (**C**) [28]. These changes occurred despite significant increases in both growth hormone and norepinephrine during the exercise protocol. The same group reported that later-onset nocturnal hypoglycaemia occurred significantly more frequently when compared with a non-exercise afternoon (**C**) [29]. A study of 10 exercising children and adolescents who were receiving insulin-pump therapy had no greater intercurrent hypoglycaemia incidence whether pumps were continued at 50% of the usual basal rate or suspended. However, later-onset hypoglycaemia was more likely in those children who did not totally suspend their insulin-pump therapy leading the investigators to recommend that this practice be adopted (**C**) [30]. There is some evidence that subcutaneous absorption of the long-acting insulin analogue glargine may not be affected by exercise (**C**) [30, 31]. It should also be recognised that perturbations in electrolytes such as potassium can also occur after intense exercise if hypoinsulinaemia is present (**B**) [32].

Consensus guidelines (**E**) [7, 33, 34] have suggested that an extra 15 grams of carbohydrate be ingested for every 30 minutes of planned moderate-to-intense physical activity. In addition, if blood glucose levels are <7 mmol/L then 'hypo' foods/fluids should be taken. The DIRECNET (Diabetes Research in Children Network) Study Group's findings; however; indicate that 15 grams of carbohydrate was not enough reliably to treat hypoglycaemia during four sequential 15-minute moderate exercise sessions (**C**) [28]. Guidelines recommend that exercise should be avoided if significant hyperglycaemia or ketones are present. However, mild hyperglycaemia (12.4 ± 2.1 mmol/L) under clamp conditions does not appear to influence exercise capacity or intracellular glucose oxidation (**C**) [35].

Increasing body mass index throughout puberty and adolescence is a problem in T1DM, particularly for females (**B**) [36]. Significant obesity leading to metabolic syndrome in the FinnDiane Study was present in 33% of 18–30-year olds with T1DM (**B**) [37]. Metabolic syndrome in this cohort was found to be independently associated with a 3.75-fold risk of developing diabetic nephropathy (**B**) [37]. Therefore, regardless of any potential benefits upon glycaemic control, physical fitness and associated weight control are desirable amongst diabetic adolescents. Managing diabetes with exercise and sporting activities does present some challenges but these can be largely overcome through an understanding of glucose/exercise physiology, planning, 'trial-and-error' approaches and by being flexible in choice of insulin regimen (**E**) [38].

Surgery

Diabetes management during elective and emergency surgery requires both medical and nursing expertise. Most guideline statements therefore recommend that such surgery should be undertaken in hospitals with dedicated paediatric and diabetes facilities (**E**) [7, 33, 34].

Ideally, patients should be as metabolically stable as possible prior to any surgery and if ketoacidosis is present then surgery should be delayed if at all possible whilst this is corrected. If the underlying diabetes control is poor and the surgery is elective, then pre-operative optimisation of glycaemic control should be attempted, sometimes requiring inpatient diabetes care. Most guidelines recommend that patients undergoing elective surgery be placed at the beginning of the surgical list, preferably in the morning. Intravenous dextrose and hourly testing of blood glucose are common to most protocols. Perioperative insulin regimens vary between centres and between patients according to their underlying insulin-replacement strategy and time of surgery. Strategies have been published, which rely either on intermittent subcutaneous insulin or alternatively on intravenous insulin (**E**) [7, 39]. There has been one published trial comparing these two options in children and adolescents undergoing surgery (**C**) [40]. This study found that insulin requirements increased by up to 66.6% in the perioperative period and that glycaemia was most stable using intravenous insulin delivery. It is noteworthy that this trial used regular and intermediate-acting insulin and pre-dated the newer analogue insulins.

Perioperative glycaemic management for patients using insulin pumps is relatively straightforward for minor surgical procedures. Basal infusion rates should allow for maintenance of euglycaemia in the context of fasting and hence these usually do not require adjustment. Given that patients are fasting, meal boluses are omitted until oral intake is re-established. Patients need to be frequently monitored however (blood glucose/ketones every 1–2 h, whilst conscious and blood glucose every 20–30 min whilst anaesthetised). Major surgical procedures will require the use of intravenous insulin and dextrose as mentioned above.

Alcohol consumption

It is a fact of life that, despite prohibition of alcohol consumption under various age limits, alcohol is readily accessible and is consumed by adolescents (**C**) [41, 42]. This is concerning not only because of the unknown effects of alcohol on still-developing neurocognition, but also because of the patterns and context of alcohol consumption in this age group. Adolescents are more likely to engage in binge drinking (E) [43], mix alcohol consumption with other recreational drugs [44] (see below) and associate alcohol consumption with risk-taking behaviours, such as unprotected sexual activity, violence and distinctly adolescent activities including 'train surfing', 'car joyriding' or graffiti writing in hazardous environments (E, C) [45–47]. There is some evidence that patients with T1DM consume alcohol to a similar extent to the general population (B) [48].

In the context of T1DM there is a theoretical risk of hypoglycaemia associated with alcohol consumption due to reduced hepatic gluconeogenesis and depletion of hepatic glycogen stores (E) [49]. In practice though, alcohol can have a variety of effects most of which are context dependent. There have been several small studies in adults with T1DM that have shown late-onset hypoglycaemia or no glycaemic effect at all (C, B) [50–52]. In a study of 26 adult patients with either T1DM or insulin-requiring T2DM, 1g/kg of alcohol with a meal caused no hypoglycaemia (C) [50]. Two recent studies have used continuous glucose-sensing technology to study this issue further. In a controlled ambulant setting in adults, 0.85 g/kg of vodka resulted in more reported symptomatic hypoglycaemia and a mean 1.2 mmol/L lower interstitial tissue glucose than placebo (C) [53]. In a non-controlled ambulant setting in adolescents, however, social consumption of alcohol was associated with increased glycaemic lability but no increase in hypoglycaemia (B) [54]. These differences have been postulated to be due to alcohol type, associated beverages (particularly, premixed sweetened alcoholic drinks), intercurrent activity and food ingestion [54]. In an analysis of 141 adult patients presenting with severe hypoglycaemia and insulin-dependent diabetes (including T1DM, T2DM and secondary diabetes), alcohol was present in blood samples of 17% of the patients (E) [55]. Other studies have reported comparable rates of 6 and 19% (C, E) [56, 57]. It should be stressed that literature in this field deals overwhelmingly with adults, the study by Ismail et al. (B) [54] being the only study investigating adolescents.

In adults there appear to be interdependent and additive effects of alcohol consumption and hypoglycaemia upon cognitive function (B) [58, 59]. In addition, alcohol consumption appears to be associated with reduced adherence to insulin in adolescents (E) [60] and in adults (B) [61]. However, there is some limited evidence that alcohol consumption lessens over time in adult patients with either T1DM or T2DM [62].

Given that alcohol consumption is inevitable for most young patients with T1DM, it appears that the most pragmatic approach to adopt is that of harm minimisation. Patients need to be informed of the risks of alcohol consumption in a non-judgemental fashion and taught techniques (such as eating a substantial meal with or before alcohol, avoid binge drinking, using 'diet' or non-sugar mixers and checking blood glucose levels after drinking) to decrease the risk of marked glycaemic fluctuations.

Recreational drug use

Whilst recreational drug use is common amongst adolescents, generally (E) [63], there has been little research into recreational drug usage amongst adolescents with T1DM. In one study of diabetic British adolescents and young adults, 29% admitted to using recreational drugs, with 68% of these using them habitually more often than once per month (E) [64]. Worryingly, 72% of respondents were unaware of what impact such drug usage had upon glycaemic control. The adverse effects of recreational drug use in adolescents with diabetes are in some respects the same as those for their non-diabetic peers. In the context of T1DM, however, there are additional risks summarised as:

- potential interactions between drug effects and body metabolism
- confusion between hypoglycaemia and an altered sensorium for other reasons
- longer term effects of drugs upon motivation to maintain diabetes control.

Multiple recreational drugs are often taken simultaneously, further confusing the overall glycaemic outcome (**E**) [65]. Ketamine and alcohol, either individually or in combination, can trigger and exacerbate ketoacidosis (**E**) [65]. In a prospective study of diabetic Danish adult patients experiencing severe hypoglycaemia, marijuana and amphetamines were identified in 5% and amphetamines in 1% of patients, respectively, with 4% of patients having both alcohol and an illicit drug present on screening (**E**) [55].

The context of recreational drug taking will also have a significant impact upon glycaemia (e.g. increased caloric intake with cannabis, associated rave dancing/frenzied activity with 'Ecstasy' or methamphetamine and vomiting with alcohol bingeing). Thus the short-term effects upon glycaemia are not only drug dependent but also context dependent, and it is hard to be dogmatic when counselling adolescents about generic harm-minimisation strategies. One overarching strategy is to recommend having a decent meal before going out for a night's social activity and checking blood glucose levels as often as possible during the night, particularly before going to bed. The credibility of any advice from medical experts will depend upon an up-to-date knowledge of recreational drug-taking mores/activities and a non-judgemental, realistic approach.

Immunisation advice

It is recommended that children and adolescents with T1DM be routinely immunised according to their regional immunisation schedules (**E**) [7]. The value of optional, additional immunisations, such as influenza and pneumococcal vaccines, in adolescents is still unclear. However, T1DM should not be seen as a contraindication in this group. Similarly, immunisations for travel should be undertaken as for the non-diabetic population.

Fasting and feasting

Jeremy Allgrove

Many religions include, as part of their beliefs, periods of fasting that are often ended by feasting. These have been well reviewed by Green (**E**) [66]. Thus, in the Christian faith, Lent is a time of relative abstinence, although it is not usually accompanied by any prolonged fasting. The Jewish faith includes two periods during the year, Yom Kippur and Tisha B'Av, when adolescents and adults are required to fast for a full 24-hour period. Children, pregnant women and those who are unwell are exempt.

In the Muslim faith, Ramadan lasts for a full 30-day period. During this 'holy month of Islam', it is an obligatory duty for all healthy adolescents and adult Muslims to fast during daylight hours. Prepubertal children and sick patients are exempted by 'the holy Q'uran' from fasting during Ramadan. Strict fasting involves eating and drinking nothing between dawn and dusk, a period that can vary from 11 to 19 hours depending on latitude and the time of the year. Therefore, diabetic patients are theoretically at high risk of developing acute complications, particularly hypoglycaemia and/or ketoacidosis, during fasting. Despite this, many diabetic patients, including some children and many adolescents, insist on fasting regardless of medical advice.

There has been one small observational study in children and adolescents using 'conventional' twice daily soluble insulin with isophane insulins (**C**) [67]. Most other studies have been in adults, mainly in T2DM, although one study (**B**) [68] in patients with T1DM, including a few adolescents, showed that the incidence and frequency of hypoglycaemia were lower in those patients taking insulin lispro instead of soluble insulin as the short-acting component of a basal-bolus insulin regimen.

However, since the introduction of basal-bolus insulin regimens, it has been suggested that fasting during Ramadan might be less likely to result in hypoglycaemia than with more conventional twice-daily-insulin regimens and it has been recommended (**E**) [69] that patients wishing to fast should be on a multiple-daily-dose regimen using either once daily insulin glargine or twice daily insulin detemir as the basal insulin. One study in adults with T1DM showed that the use of insulin glargine was safe and maintained reasonable insulin levels in plasma over the period of the fast (**C**) [70]. No such studies have been conducted in children.

Fasting during the day influences the control of diabetes because of changes in meal times, the type of food eaten and daily lifestyle (**E**) [69]. Several previous studies have made recommendations for treatment of adults with diabetes (both T1DM and T2DM) wishing to fast during Ramadan (**E**) [71, 72] but no similar recommendations for children or adolescents have been made and no observations made on children using basal-bolus insulin regimens. Our own preliminary unpublished studies have suggested that it is possible for adolescents with diabetes to fast successfully during Ramadan if they are on a basal-bolus regimen but that they should consider reducing the dose of basal insulin to prevent hypoglycaemia in the late afternoon but may need to use larger doses of rapid-acting insulin to compensate for the greater rise in blood glucose that occurs at times of breaking the fast during the hours of darkness (**E**).

The episodes of feasting that follow periods of fasting may need to be treated with increased doses of short- or rapid-acting insulin to compensate for the increased calorie intake at these times, particularly as these calories are often largely obtained from carbohydrate. In this respect, those patients who are on a basal-bolus or insulin-pump regimen are likely to find it easier to deal with than those who are taking twice daily insulin.

It is important to be sensitive to strongly held religious views and, rather than being dogmatic about not fasting, to try to adapt the insulin regimen to the person's way of life rather than vice versa (**E**) [73].

References

1 Delamaire M, Maugendre D, Moreno M *et al.* Impaired leucocyte functions in diabetic patients. *Diabet Med* 1997; **14**: 29–34.

2 Gallacher SJ, Thomson G, Fraser WD *et al.* Neutrophil bactericidal function in diabetes mellitus: evidence for association with blood glucose control. *Diabet Med* 1995; **12**: 916–20.

3 Mowat A, Baum J. Chemotaxis of polymorphonuclear leukocytes from patients with diabetes mellitus. *N Engl J Med* 1971; **284**: 621–7.

4 Liberatore RdRJ, Barbosa S, Alkimin M *et al.* Is immunity in diabetic patients influencing the susceptibility to infections? Immunoglobulins, complement and phagocytic function in children and adolescents with type 1 diabetes mellitus. *Pediatr Diabetes* 2005; **6**: 206–12.

5 Schade DS, Eaton RP. Metabolic and clinical significance of ketosis. *Spec Top Endocrinol Metab* 1982; **4**: 1–27.

6 Laffel LMB, Wentzell K, Loughlin C *et al.* Sick day management using blood 3-hydroxybutyrate 3-OHB compared with urine ketone monitoring reduces hospital visits in young people with T1DM: a randomized clinical trial. *Diabet Med* 2006; **23**: 278–84.

7 NHMRC. *The Australian Clinical Practice Guidelines on the Management of Type 1 Diabetes in Children and Adolescents 2005.* Available at: http://www.nhmrc.gov.au/publications/synopses/cp102syn.htm

8 Walsh J, Roberts R. *Pumping Insulin: Everything You Need for Success with an Insulin Pump.* Torrey Pines, San Diego, CA, 2000.

9 Haymond MW, Schreiner B. Mini-dose glucagon rescue for hypoglycemia in children with type 1 diabetes. *Diabetes Care* 2001; **24**: 643–5.

10 Nordfeldt S, Ludvigsson J. Fear and other disturbances of severe hypoglycaemia in children and adolescents with type 1 diabetes mellitus. *J Pediatr Endocrinol Metab* 2005; **18**: 83–91.

11 Brubaker P. Adventure travel and type 1 diabetes: the complicating effects of high altitude. *Diabetes Care* 2005; **28**: 2563–72.

12 Driessen SO, Cobelens FG, Ligthelm RJ. Travel-related morbidity in travelers with insulin-dependent diabetes mellitus. *J Travel Med* 1999; **6**: 12–15.

13 Fink K, Christensen D, Ellsworth A. Effect of high altitude on blood glucose meter performance. *Diabetes Technol Ther* 2002; **4**: 627–35.

14 Heyman E, Briard D, Gratas D *et al.* Normal physical working capacity in prepubertal children with type 1 diabetes compared with healthy controls. *Acta Paediatr* 2005; **94**: 1389–94.

15 Komatsu W, Gabbay M, Castro M *et al.* Aerobic exercise capacity in normal adolescents and those with type 1 diabetes mellitus. *Pediatr Diabetes* 2005; **6**: 145–9.

16 Bernardini A, Vanelli M, Chiari G *et al.* Adherence to physical activity in young people with type 1 diabetes. *Acta Biomed Ateneo Parmense* 2004; **75**: 153–7.

17 Massin MM, Lebrethon MC, Rocour D *et al.* Patterns of physical activity determined by heart rate monitoring among diabetic children. *Arch Dis Child* 2005; **90**: 1223–6.

18 Särnblad S, Ekelund U, Aman J. Physical activity and energy intake in adolescent girls with type 1 diabetes. *Diabet Med* 2005; **22**: 893–9.

19 Mosher PE, Nash MS, Perry AC *et al.* Aerobic circuit exercise training: effect on adolescents with well-controlled insulin-dependent diabetes mellitus. *Arch Phys Med Rehabil* 1998; **79**: 652–7.

20 Roberts L, Jones T, Fournier P. Exercise training and glycemic control in adolescents with poorly controlled type 1 diabetes mellitus. *J Pediatr Endocrinol Metab* 2002; **15**: 621–7.

21 Guelfi K, Jones T, Fournier P. The decline in blood glucose levels is less with intermittent high-intensity compared with moderate exercise in individuals with type 1 diabetes. *Diabetes Care* 2005; **28**: 1289–94.

22 Wadén J, Tikkanen H, Forsblom C *et al.* Leisure time physical activity is associated with poor glycemic control in type 1 diabetic women: the FinnDiane study. *Diabetes Care* 2005; **28**: 777–82.

23 Sandoval D, Guy D, Richardson M *et al.* Effects of low and moderate antecedent exercise on counter-regulatory responses to subsequent hypoglycemia in type 1 diabetes. *Diabetes* 2004; **53**: 1798–1806.

24 Dubé M, Weisnagel SJ, Prud'homme D *et al.* Exercise and newer insulins: how much glucose supplement to avoid hypoglycemia? *Med Sci Sports Exerc* 2005; **37**: 1276–82.

25 Francescato M, Geat M, Fusi S *et al.* Carbohydrate requirement and insulin concentration during moderate exercise in type 1 diabetic patients. *Metabolism* 2004; **53**: 1126–30.

26 Perrone C, Laitano O, Meyer F. Effect of carbohydrate ingestion on the glycemic response of type 1 diabetic adolescents during exercise. *Diabetes Care* 2005; **28**: 2537–8.

27 Grimm JJ, Ybarra J, Berné C *et al.* A new table for prevention of hypoglycaemia during physical activity in type 1 diabetic patients. *Diabetes Metab* 2004; **30**: 465–70.

28 Tansey M, Tsalikian E, Beck R *et al.* The effects of aerobic exercise on glucose and counterregulatory hormone concentrations in children with type 1 diabetes. *Diabetes Care* 2006; **29**: 20–5.

29 Tsalikian E, Mauras N, Beck R *et al.* Impact of exercise on overnight glycemic control in children with type 1 diabetes mellitus. *J Pediatr* 2005; **147**: 528–34.

30 Admon G, Weinstein Y, Falk B *et al.* Exercise with and without an insulin pump among children and adolescents with type 1 diabetes mellitus. *Pediatrics* 2005; **116**: e348.

31 Peter R, Luzio S, Dunseath G *et al.* Effects of exercise on the absorption of insulin glargine in patients with type 1 diabetes. *Diabetes Care* 2005; **28**: 560–5.

32 Harmer A, Ruell P, McKenna M *et al.* Effects of sprint training on extrarenal potassium regulation with intense exercise in type 1 diabetes. *J Appl Physiol* 2006; **100**: 26–34.

33 NICE. *Type 1 Diabetes in Children and Young People: Full Guideline*, 2004. Available at: http://www.nice.org.uk/page.aspx?o=CG015childfullguideline

34 ADA. Standards of medical care in diabetes. *Diabetes Care* 2006; **29**: S4–42.

35 Stettler C, Jenni S, Allemann S *et al.* Exercise capacity in subjects with type 1 diabetes mellitus in eu- and hyperglycaemia. *Diabetes Metab Res Rev* 2006; **22**: 300–6.

36 Dabadghao P, Vidmar S, Cameron FJ. Deteriorating diabetic control through adolescence – do the origins lie in childhood? *Diabet Med* 2001; **18**: 889–94.

37 Thorn L, Forsblom C, Fagerudd J *et al.* Metabolic syndrome in type 1 diabetes: association with diabetic nephropathy and glycemic control the FinnDiane study. *Diabetes Care* 2005; **28**: 2019–24.

38 Lisle D, Trojian T. Managing the athlete with type 1 diabetes. *Curr Sports Med Rep* 2006; **5**: 93–8.

39 ISPAD. *Consensus Guidelines for the Management of Type 1 Diabetes Mellitus in Children and Adolescents.* Medical Forum International, Zeist, Netherlands, 2000.

40 Kaufman FR, Devgan S, Roe TF *et al.* Perioperative management with prolonged intravenous insulin infusion versus subcutaneous insulin in children with type I diabetes mellitus. *J Diabetes Complications* 1996; **10**: 6–11.

41 Carballo J, Oquendo M, Giner L *et al.* Prevalence of alcohol misuse among adolescents and young adults evaluated in a primary care setting. *Int J Adolesc Med Health* 2006; **18**: 197–202.

42 Chisholm D, Kelleher K. Admission to acute care hospitals for adolescent substance abuse: a national descriptive analysis. *Subst Abuse Treat Prev Policy* 2006; **1**: 17.

43 Bonomo Y. Adolescent alcohol problems: whose responsibility is it anyway? *Med J Aust* 2005; **183**: 430–2.

44 Baumann M, Spitz E, Predine R *et al.* Do male and female adolescents differ in the effect of individual and family characteristics on their use of psychotropic drugs? *Eur J Pediatr* 2007; **166**(1): 29–35.

45 Eaton D, Kann L, Kinchen S *et al.* Youth risk behavior surveillance – United States 2005. *MMWR CDC Surveill Summ* 2006; **55**: 1–108.

46 Marshall C, Boyd KT, Moran CG. Injuries related to car crime: the joy-riding epidemic. *Injury* 1996; **27**: 79–80.

47 Strauch H, Wirth I, Geserick G. Fatal accidents due to train surfing in Berlin. *Forensic Sci Int* 1998; **94**: 119–27.

48 Ingberg CM, Palmér M, Aman J *et al.* Social consequences of insulin-dependent diabetes mellitus are limited: a population-based comparison of young adult patients vs healthy controls. *Diabet Med* 1996; **13**: 729–33.

49 Plougmann S, Hejlesen O, Turner B *et al.* The effect of alcohol on blood glucose in type 1 diabetes: metabolic modelling and integration in a decision support system. *Int J Med Inform* 2003; **70**: 337–44.

50 Koivisto VA, Tulokas S, Toivonen M *et al.* Alcohol with a meal has no adverse effects on postprandial glucose homeostasis in diabetic patients. *Diabetes Care* 1993; **16**: 1612–14.

51 Moriarty KT, Maggs DG, Macdonald IA *et al.* Does ethanol cause hypoglycaemia in overnight fasted patients with type 1 diabetes? *Diabet Med* 1993; **10**: 61–5.

52 Turner BC, Jenkins E, Kerr D *et al.* The effect of evening alcohol consumption on next-morning glucose control in type 1 diabetes. *Diabetes Care* 2001; **24**: 1888–93.

53 Richardson T, Weiss M, Thomas P *et al.* Day after the night before: influence of evening alcohol on risk of hypoglycemia in patients with type 1 diabetes. *Diabetes Care* 2005; **28**: 1801–2.

54 Ismail D, Gebert R, Vuillermin P *et al.* Social consumption of alcohol in adolescents with type 1 diabetes is associated with increased glucose lability, but not hypoglycaemia. *Diabet Med* 2006; **23**: 830–33.

55 Pedersen-Bjergaard U, Reubsaet J, Nielsen S *et al.* Psychoactive drugs, alcohol, and severe hypoglycemia in insulin-treated diabetes: analysis of 141 cases. *Am J Med* 2005; **118**: 307–10.

56 Hart SP, Frier BM. Causes, management and morbidity of acute hypoglycaemia in adults requiring hospital admission. *Q J Med* 1998; **91**: 505–10.

57 Potter J, Clarke P, Gale EA *et al.* Insulin-induced hypoglycaemia in an accident and emergency department: the tip of an iceberg? *BMJ* 1982; **285**: 1180–2.

58 Cheyne EH, Sherwin RS, Lunt MJ *et al.* Influence of alcohol on cognitive performance during mild hypoglycaemia; implications for type 1 diabetes. *Diabet Med* 2004; **21**: 230–7.

59 Kerr D, Macdonald IA, Heller SR *et al.* Alcohol causes hypoglycaemic unawareness in healthy volunteers and patients with type 1 insulin-dependent diabetes. *Diabetologia* 1990; **33**: 216–21.

60 Kyngas HA, Kroll T, Duffy ME. Compliance in adolescents with chronic diseases: a review. *J Adolesc Health* 2000; **26**: 379–88.

61 Ahmed AT, Karter AJ, Liu J. Alcohol consumption is inversely associated with adherence to diabetes self-care behaviours. *Diabet Med* 2006; **23**: 795–802.

62 Gallagher A, Connolly V, Kelly WF. Alcohol consumption in patients with diabetes mellitus. *Diabet Med* 2001; **18**: 72–3.

63 Greene J, Ahrendt D, Stafford E. Adolescent abuse of other drugs. *Adolesc Med Clin* 2006; **17**: 283–318.

64 Ng RSH, Darko DA, Hillson RM. Street drug use among young patients with type 1 diabetes in the UK. *Diabet Med* 2004; **21**: 295–6.

65 Lee P, Nicoll AJ, McDonough M *et al*. Substance abuse in young patients with type 1 diabetes: easily neglected in complex medical management. *Intern Med J* 2005; **35**: 359–61.

66 Green V. Understanding different religions when caring for diabetes patients. *Br J Nurs* 2004; **13**: 658–62.

67 Salman H, Abdallah MA, Abanamy MA *et al*. Ramadan fasting in diabetic children in Riyadh. *Diabet Med* 1992; **9**: 583–4.

68 Kadiri A, Al-Nakhi A, El-Ghazali S *et al*. Treatment of type 1 diabetes with insulin lispro during Ramadan. *Diabetes Metab* 2001; **27**: 482–6.

69 Al-Arouj M, Bouguerra R, Buse J *et al*. Recommendations for management of diabetes during Ramadan. *Diabetes Care* 2005; **28**: 2305–11.

70 Mucha GT, Merkel S, Thomas W *et al*. Fasting and insulin glargine in individuals with type 1 diabetes. *Diabetes Care* 2004; **27**: 1209–10.

71 Omar MA, Motala AA. Fasting in Ramadan and the diabetic patient. *Diabetes Care* 1997; **20**: 1925–6.

72 Pinar R. Management of people with diabetes during Ramadan. *Br J Nurs* 2002; **11**: 1300–3.

73 Burden M. Culturally sensitive care: managing diabetes during Ramadan. *Br J Community Nurs* 2001; **6**: 581–5.

CHAPTER 8

Dietary management: optimising diabetes outcomes

Sheridan Waldron

> *He that takes medicine and neglects diet, wastes the skill of the physician.*
> —Chinese proverb

Introduction

Diet is integral to successful diabetes care for young people with type 1 diabetes mellitus (T1DM), and yet dietary education methods remain controversial and poorly evaluated. Dietary education is primarily concerned with glycaemic control with limited evidence regarding the effect of diet on serum lipids, cardiovascular outcomes, the incidence of hypoglycaemia, weight management, education models, adherence to dietary recommendations and psychosocial interventions.

Successful self-management education for young people with diabetes can result in optimum glycaemic control, prevention of hypoglycaemia and a reduction in micro- and macrovascular complications. When used in combination with other components of diabetes care, effective dietary intervention can contribute to improving clinical and metabolic outcomes through attention to:

- motivation
- behaviour-management approaches
- tailoring information to the individual
- individualised diet history
- altering insulin dosages for varying food intake
- intensive insulin therapy
- regular dietary advice
- education (**A, B, E**) [1–3].

Effective methods of education need to be found to optimise diabetes outcomes for children and young people (**E**) [4–6] whilst maintaining quality of life (**E, B**) [4, 7].

Aims of dietary management

Expert consensus exists over the aims of dietary management in childhood (**E**) [3, 6, 8–11] to:

- provide sufficient and appropriate energy intake and nutrients for optimal growth, development and good health

- encourage healthy, lifelong eating habits whilst preserving and maintaining social, cultural and psychological well-being and respecting the individual's wishes and willingness to change
- achieve a balance between food intake, metabolic requirements, energy expenditure and insulin profiles/levels to attain optimum glycaemic control without excessive hypoglycaemia
- achieve and maintain an appropriate body mass index (BMI) and waist circumference. This includes the strong recommendation for children and young people to undertake regular physical activity
- prevent and treat acute complications of diabetes, such as hypoglycaemia, hyperglycaemic crises, illness and exercise-related problems
- reduce the risk of microvascular complications through optimising glycaemic control
- modify nutrient intake and lifestyle as appropriate for the prevention and treatment of the chronic complications of diabetes, obesity, dyslipidaemia, cardiovascular disease, hypertension and nephropathy.

Growth, development, nutrients and energy balance

Dietary habits and food preferences form early in childhood (**E**) [5] and therefore good habits need to be established from the start of diabetes. Dietary recommendations are based on achieving optimal growth, development and health for all children and adults (**E**) [12]. In addition, young people with diabetes are at a higher risk of diabetic complications that can be delayed or prevented by dietary intervention. Therefore, to optimise outcomes, an individualised approach for each child is essential to combine:
- the eating pattern
- appetite
- food preferences
- lifestyle
- personal wishes of the child/young person as to the most appropriate insulin regimen. Care should be in the context of the families' culture, ethnicity and traditions.

Children's growth rate is continually changing but the phases of particularly rapid growth are in infancy and puberty. Growth rapidly increases the nutritional requirements of children. However, after these rapid phases of growth, or cessation of growth, failure to reduce energy intake will lead to obesity. Adjusting dietary intake during these continually changing metabolic demands is central to the dietary management of childhood diabetes and requires ongoing regular review.

Growth potential may not be fulfilled when glycaemic control is poor, as glycosuria can cause significant urinary energy loss, while insufficient insulin treatment can cause inadequate anabolism. Energy requirements, carbohydrate intake and insulin doses increase throughout childhood and rise markedly during puberty. Adolescents and parents need to be reassured that increasing carbohydrate intake is both normal and essential at this time and will not jeopardise overall metabolic control. Parents often compensate for the increased appetite of puberty by increasing inappropriate non-carbohydrate foods that are high in fat and/or protein.

Total daily energy intake should be distributed as follows:
- protein 10–15% decreasing with age
- fat 30–35%:
  - <10% saturated fat+trans fatty acids
  - <10% polyunsaturated fat
  - >10% monounsaturated fat (MUFA; up to 20% total energy)
  - $n - 3$ fatty acids (cis configuration): 0.15 g/d
- carbohydrate 50–55%:
  - based on non-starch polysaccharide (fibre) containing foods such as whole-grain cereals, fruits and vegetables
  - moderate sucrose intake (up to 10% total energy)

Protein (10–15% of total daily energy)

Animal sources of protein are associated with higher fat intake, especially saturated fat, and therefore should not be consumed in large amounts. Intake decreases during childhood from approximately 2 g/kg/d in early infancy to 1 g/kg/d for a 10-year old and from 0.8 to 0.9 g/kg/d in later adolescence (**E**) [12, 13]. Protein can be used for growth only if sufficient total energy is available.

When persistent microalbuminuria or established nephropathy occurs, excessive protein intake may be detrimental; protein intake at the lower end of the recommended range should be considered (**E**) [14]. Modifications to protein intake in adolescence should not be allowed to interfere with normal growth.

Lean sources of animal protein, including lean cuts of meat and fat-reduced dairy products, are also recommended. Sources of vegetable protein such as beans, legumes and lentils should be encouraged.

Dietary fat (30–35% total daily energy)

Fat is necessary in children's diets to provide energy, fat-soluble vitamins and essential fatty acids for normal growth and development. Some countries, e.g. Canada, recommend that from the age of 2 years to the end of linear growth there should be a transition from the high-fat diet of infancy (approximately 50% of total energy) to adult recommendations (<30% of energy as fat and <10% of energy as saturated fat) (**E**) [15]. During this transition, energy and nutrient intake should be sufficient to achieve normal growth and development. The Canadian Paediatric Society and Health, Canada, believe there is insufficient evidence to support lowering fat intake to adult levels during childhood to prevent chronic diseases of adulthood.

Other countries recommend that children should follow adult guidelines from >5 years (**E**) [6, 8–12]. Up to the age of 5 years it is expected that the proportion of energy derived from dietary fats will fall from about 50%, as supplied by breast-feeding or infant formula, to those recommended for adults. This change should not occur before 2 years of age. In practice, this means that the change from whole-fat milk to semi-skimmed or even skimmed milk should be delayed until the age of 2. Below this age, a high energy density of foods is important and, in addition, if low-fat foods are given to toddlers, there can be associated rapid gastric emptying and diarrhoea.

A key goal for all people is to decrease total fat intake, with particular attention given to decreasing saturated and trans fatty acids. Daily fat intake should be ≤30% of total energy requirements, comprised of ≤10% saturated fat due to its effect on cholesterol and low-density (LDL) levels, ≤10% polyunsaturated fat, with the remainder coming from MUFA due to its effect on cholesterol and low-density lipoprotein (LDL) levels. High MUFA intakes have several potential metabolic advantages, including improving insulin sensitivity and glycaemic control and possibly reducing atheroma (**E**) [16]. A major benefit of a higher MUFA diet is palatability and aiding compliance to an otherwise low-fat diet.

Unsaturated fatty acids of the $n - 3$ variety found in oily fish and certain vegetable oils may be particularly beneficial (**A**) [17, 18]. Advice for children is to eat oily fish once to twice weekly in amounts of 80–120 g (**E**) [19]. The use of plant sterol and stanol esters (in margarine and dairy products) may be considered for children of 5 years and older if total and/or LDL cholesterol is elevated (**B**) [20, 21].

Carbohydrate (50–55% total daily energy)

There is international agreement that carbohydrate should not be restricted, as it may have deleterious effects on growth. The energy distribution of 50–55% is based on requirements for healthy children/adolescents (**E**) [11]. If carbohydrate intake provides only 45% energy then carbohydrate and MUFA together should provide 60–70% energy (**E**) [9].

Evidence suggests that children with diabetes achieve between 44 and 55% of their total energy intake from carbohydrate (**A, C, E**) [22–25]. Practical suggestions may be useful to encourage larger amounts of carbohydrate to prevent excess protein and fat intakes and to encourage healthy sources of carbohydrate foods, such as whole-grain breads and cereals, fruits, vegetables and low-fat dairy products.

Sucrose (<10% total daily energy)

Sucrose does not increase glycaemia more than isocaloric amounts of starch (**A**) [26]. The recommendation of 10% total energy is the same as for the general population (**E**) [3, 11]. Sucrose can be substituted for other carbohydrate sources in moderation without causing hyperglycaemia or, if added, should be appropriately covered with insulin (**E**) [8]. Sucrose-sweetened drinks may cause hyperglycaemia and large amounts should be avoided. Also, sucrose-rich foods are often energy dense with poor nutritional value, so care must be taken to ensure a balanced diet.

Non-starch polysaccharide (fibre)

Non-starch polysaccharides may be classified into two broad categories – soluble (including gums, gels and pectin) and insoluble (including cellulose and lignin). Soluble fibre can benefit both glycaemic control and lipid metabolism, reducing fasting and postprandial glucose values. An improvement in insulin sensitivity is postulated as the mechanism by which soluble fibre can improve fasting hyperglycaemia. Studies support the benefit of increasing soluble fibre (**A, B, E**) [27–29].

Intakes are recommended to the level suggested for the general population. A range of fibre intakes have been reported in children with diabetes (**A, B**) [23, 30–32]. Some children find it more difficult than others to achieve desired targets. Emphasis needs to be placed on increasing fibre intake along with particular emphasis on increasing fruit and vegetable intake [33]. Fibre intake should be increased slowly to prevent abdominal discomfort and should be accompanied by an increase in fluid intake.

Vitamins and antioxidant nutrients

Foods naturally rich in dietary antioxidants (tocopherols, carotenoids, vitamin C and possibly, flavanoids) should be strongly encouraged. Highly reactive oxygen-free radicals are increasingly implicated in the pathogenesis of atherosclerosis. Foods rich in antioxidants, such as fresh fruit and vegetables, should be encouraged. Five portions of fruit and vegetables are recommended [33], and this may provide a means of protecting against long-term cardiovascular disease in populations at increased risk.

Scientific evidence on the benefits of vitamins and dietary antioxidants is still evolving, and further research is required in children before firm recommendations can be made. In the meantime, it is appropriate to achieve at least the recommended values for dietary vitamins (E) [12] and promote foods that naturally contain significant quantities of dietary antioxidants (E) [34]. Current evidence does not support the routine use of dietary supplementation with vitamins or minerals.

Salt

Salt intake is in general too high and in Western countries it is difficult to decrease, as it is added to many processed foods. Only 20% of intake is added at the table and in cooking. Reducing processed and manufactured foods is essential and practical advice is to develop cooking skills with a lower salt intake. Reduction is recommended to the general adult population. In most European countries this constitutes a reduction of 50%, to less than 6 g of salt daily (E) [14].

Alcohol

Alcohol has no place in the normal nutrition of young people with or without diabetes, and in many countries alcohol ingestion in children and young people is either illegal or age restricted and culturally unacceptable. However, adolescents do experience and experiment with alcoholic drinks, and the effect of alcohol on their diabetes requires discussion. It is important to explain the risks of alcohol-induced hypoglycaemia and stress the dangers of nocturnal hypoglycaemia induced by inhibition of gluconeogenesis and glycogenolysis. The benefits of taking complex carbohydrates before, during and after drinking alcohol to reduce the risk of hypoglycaemia need to be explained, and it may also be necessary to adjust the insulin dose particularly if rigorous exercise is performed before or after drinking. Practical education is needed on the alcohol content of different drinks (see Chapter 7 for a fuller discussion of this).

Weight management

At diagnosis, appetite and energy intake are often high to restore the preceding catabolic weight loss. Energy intake should be reduced when appropriate weight is restored (E) [11].

Children and young people with diabetes are heavier at all ages when compared with healthy controls (E) [35]. The reason for this is not clear but may result from intensive insulin therapy (A, B, E) [35–38]. In addition, female adolescents with diabetes are particularly at risk of being overweight (B, E) [35, 39, 40] and lower physical activity levels may also contribute (B) [41].

Achieving ideal body weight in T1DM is essential, as being overweight or obese predisposes individuals to insulin resistance and dyslipidaemia, which are linked to increased risk of cardiovascular disease. Weight should be regularly monitored in the child with diabetes and appropriate weight-management advice should be provided. Targeting females would also seem appropriate, not only because of their higher risk of being overweight but also because of the higher relative mortality rate from cardiovascular disease compared with males with diabetes (**A**) [42]. However, it is important to approach weight management with sensitivity and care, as females with diabetes appear to be at a higher risk of dysfunctional eating behaviour and eating disorders than their peers without diabetes (**A, E**) [43, 44].

Promoting a healthy weight should include eating habits, lifestyle and physical activity advice from diagnosis and should be part of the holistic care to promote cardiovascular health and prevent obesity. Successful weight management is difficult in this group of children, and carefully organised trials of lifestyle management and interventions are required.

Practical management

• In puberty, energy intake and nutritional demands increase substantially along with significant increases in insulin dosage
• Careful attention given to monitoring total energy and lifestyle activity is essential to prevent weight increase in the developing child: plot the growth curve, BMI (SDS/Z score) (**B**) [45, 46] and possibly waist circumference (**B**) [47] every 3 months (**B**) [46]. Currently, there are no international reference ranges for waist circumference in children younger than 16 years. Target reference values for young people aged 16 years and older are <80 cm for women and <94 cm for men (**E**) [48]
• The insulin (amount and type) should be adapted where possible to the child's eating pattern and appetite. Having a child eat consistently without an appetite or withholding food in an effort to control blood glucose should be discouraged, as this may impact adversely on weight gain and development (**E**) [9]
• Consistent advice should be given in the prevention and treatment of hypoglycaemia by all team members
• Review of the insulin regimen should be done to minimise hypoglycaemia and the need for large snacks
• Emphasis on food quantity, portion size and fat and sugar intake is essential (**E**) [11]
• Psychological counselling should be considered for severely obese and young people with disordered eating/eating disorders (**E**) [50].

The influence of diet on glycaemic control

Effective dietary management plays a key role in optimising glycaemic control (**A**) [36, 51]. The Diabetes Control and Complications Trial (DCCT) also highlighted the expanded role of the dietitian in achieving these targets (**A**) [1, 2].

The DCCT (**A**) [1] used many methods to achieve target HbA1c levels, including meal planning, exchange systems, carbohydrate counting and weighing and measuring foods. In the trial it appears that the particular method of dietary education was less important than diet behaviours, factors that were associated with a statistically significant reduction in HbA1c levels were:

- Adherence to the agreed meal plan
- Adjusting food and insulin in response to hyperglycaemia
- Appropriate treatment of hypoglycaemia
- Consumption of agreed snacks within the meal plan.

The DCCT also showed that intensive nutrition education, not necessarily carbohydrate assessment, with frequent blood glucose monitoring in conjunction with adjustment of insulin doses on a meal-to-meal and day-to-day basis, improved glycaemic control. This requires motivation, recording blood glucose results and altering insulin doses according to experience and often using an insulin-adjustment algorithm.

There are still persistent differences amongst international centres in glycaemic control and hypoglycaemia in children and adolescents with T1DM (**B**) [52], and the influence of diet behaviours between these centres still requires further research. Initial findings of international comparisons between centres have shown some diet behaviours and lifestyle activities to be associated with poorer glycaemic control (**B**) [53]. These include:

- consumption of unhealthy food choices
- skipping breakfast
- bingeing
- increased television watching.

Also, Danne *et al.* (**B**) [52] found lower severe hypoglycaemic events in centres with HbA1c values below the grand mean of the study. The authors suggested that the reason may be better education programmes and management from the onset of the disease. Thus differing attitudes of the diabetes team and/or differing degrees of patient empowerment may represent a major factor underlying differences between centres (**B**) [52, 54].

Education

Education provides the child, parent and carer with the knowledge and skills needed to perform diabetes self-care, manage critical events and make lifestyle changes to manage the condition successfully [10]. Major factors that will affect the content of an educational package include age, maturity, sex, ethnic/cultural background, the psychosocial infrastructure and support available and the level of educational attainment of the child and family. Consequently, education should be varied, with a range of methods and delivery styles that adhere to child learning principles [55]. Education opportunities include individual consultations, play sessions, structured patient education, activity weekends and holidays. These should be appropriate to the needs of the family and staged at a pace with which the family is comfortable (**E**) [4, 56]. As families become more confident with managing diabetes, education may become more complex, and as children grow and take more responsibility, regular re-education is essential. Education is most effective when integrated into routine care, parents are involved and self-efficacy is promoted (**E**) [10].

Structured patient education

There is a distinct lack of well-designed education programmes in children's diabetes (**E**) [4, 5]. Although many centres have educational programmes for young people, few if any are structured, assess outcomes, are based on theoretical principles, use formal curricula or provide training for educators (**E**) [4, 5]. Therefore, the value of these programmes is uncertain. Guidance from the Diabetes National Service Framework (**E**) [57], and the National Institute for Clinical Excellence (**E**) [6], Department of Health and Diabetes UK,

(**E**) [5] support the delivery of structured education that is designed to meet the needs and learning styles of the population and is delivered by appropriately trained staff.

Recent structured patient-education programmes for children have been developed (**B, E**) [56, 58, 59], drawing on the long-established, successful, adult education programmes (**E**) [60, 61] and the more recent dose adjustment for normal eating (DAFNE) programme (**B**) [62]. These programmes are intensive, skill-based education with estimation of carbohydrate content of food (using 10–15-g carbohydrate portions), adjusting insulin and intensive blood glucose monitoring. Pilot studies have been performed in young people in the UK and Germany respectively (**B, E**) [56, 58], with promising results in improvements in quality of life. These approaches have many benefits, although they require extensive nutrition education. Young people enjoy the freedom of eating a wider variety of foods and the flexibility of a less rigid meal pattern, sensitive to the varying daily energy expenditure of childhood and addressing postprandial glycaemic excursions, all of which are inadequately managed by conventional therapy.

Education tools

Dietary education tools need to be selected carefully for each child and family to achieve maximum understanding and compliance. Food pyramid (Figure 8.1) and food plate (Figure 8.2) models are useful in providing basic nutritional information and healthy eating concepts. They also visually illustrate carbohydrate in relation to other food components and are attractive visual aids for children.

Carbohydrate assessment

Expert consensus agrees that the *total* carbohydrate intake from a meal or snack is a relatively reliable predictor of postprandial blood glucose (**A, E**) [9, 65]. Many methods of counting or estimating carbohydrate intake are used in paediatric practice, e.g. qualitative approach, portions/servings, carbohydrate exchanges, intensive nutritional management with estimation of carbohydrate effects and low glycaemic index (GI) (**B**) [66, 67]. There is no consensus in favour of one particular method and some methods are better suited to particular children and families. The necessity to achieve optimum glycaemic control and the introduction of insulin analogues into the clinical care of children have increased the use of carbohydrate quantification, particularly for children and adolescents on intensive insulin therapy (**E**) [3, 8, 11].

The impact of the *type* of carbohydrate on postprandial glucose levels has continued to be an area of debate. However, a recent analysis (**B**) [68] of the randomised controlled trials that have examined the efficacy of the GI on overall blood glucose control indicates that the use of this technique can provide an additional benefit over that observed when total carbohydrate is considered alone. The American Diabetes Association accepts that both the amount and the type of carbohydrate are important in the management of diabetes (**A, E**) [9, 69].

Carbohydrate counting

Historically, carbohydrate was counted in order to achieve regular carbohydrate intake, with great attention given to precise quantities at meals and snacks (**E**) [70]. This method was inaccurate and was likely to underestimate the true carbohydrate requirement. It is also likely that this method caused a restriction of carbohydrate and an attendant increase in fat to meet energy requirements (**B**) [63]. Changing one nutrient (e.g. carbohydrate)

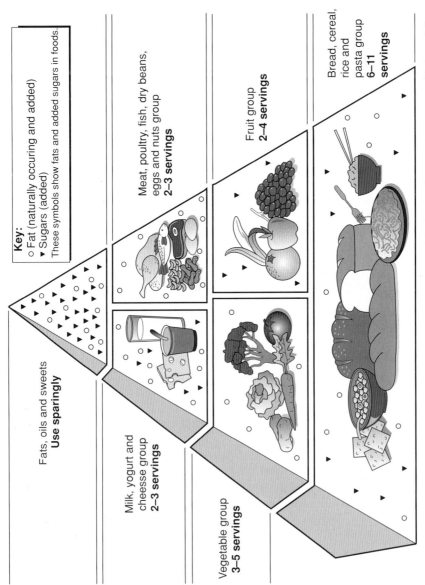

Key:
○ Fat (naturally occuring and added)
▶ Sugars (added)
These symbols show fats and added sugars in foods.

Fats, oils and sweets
Use sparingly

Meat, poultry, fish, dry beans, eggs and nuts group
2–3 servings

Fruit group
2–4 servings

Bread, cereal, rice and pasta group
6–11 servings

Milk, yogurt and cheese group
2–3 servings

Vegetable group
3–5 servings

Figure 8.1 Illustration of the 'food pyramid' demonstrating the principal food types that constitute a normal balanced diet. (Reproduced from http://teamnutrition.usda.gov/resources/mpk_close.pdf, with permission.)

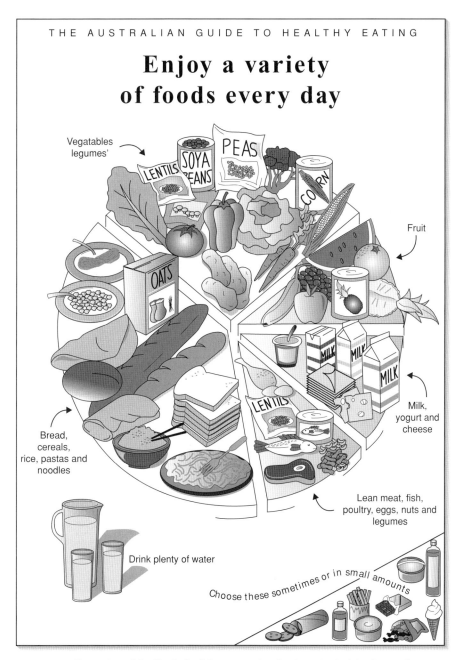

THE AUSTRALIAN GUIDE TO HEALTHY EATING

Enjoy a variety of foods every day

Vegatables legumes'

Fruit

Bread, cereals, rice, pastas and noodles

Milk, yogurt and cheese

Lean meat, fish, poultry, eggs, nuts and legumes

Drink plenty of water

Choose these sometimes or in small amounts

Figure 8.2 Illustration of the 'food plate' demonstrating the five principal food types that constitute a normal balanced diet [64]. (© Commonwealth of Australia, reproduced with permission.)

is likely to have a detrimental effect upon another nutrient (e.g. fat), which may in turn affect other diabetes outcomes (i.e. cardiovascular risk factors). Restricting carbohydrate also makes no allowances for diversity of energy expenditure [71] and growth. There is a danger that such dietary prescriptions can lead to carbohydrate constraint as the child is growing, restricting growth and creating abnormal eating practices that are detrimental to normal family functioning [72]. Children and families find it difficult to follow a restrictive carbohydrate plan, and rigid approaches to diabetes management may contribute to disordered eating behaviour (**E, C**) [44, 73]. These findings illustrate the importance of evaluating macronutrient intake following dietary education.

Modern carbohydrate counting

Carbohydrate counting received renewed interest when it was used as one of the four methods in the DCCT (**A**) [36]. Modern carbohydrate counting is a meal-planning approach that focuses on improving glycaemic control while allowing maximum flexibility of food choices. This system is used in conjunction with self-management education for insulin dose adjustments.

A stepwise learning approach to carbohydrate counting has been identified by the American Dietetic Association and the American Diabetes Association [74].

Level 1: consistent carbohydrate intake. This level introduces the concept of carbohydrate as the food component that raises blood glucose. A consistent intake of carbohydrate is encouraged, using exchange or portion lists of measured quantities of food that contain all types of sugars and starches. This level allows a greater variety of carbohydrate foods (based on knowledge of the GI) than was previously accepted. With regular carbohydrate intake and blood glucose monitoring results, it is possible for a dietitian (if permitted by regulatory body and within scope of practice), nurse or doctor to advise on appropriate baseline insulin doses.

Level 2: pattern management principles. This level is an intermediate step in which patients continue to eat regular carbohydrate, use a consistent baseline insulin dose and frequently monitor blood glucose levels. They learn to recognise patterns of blood glucose response to carbohydrate intake modified by insulin and exercise. With this understanding, they learn to make their own adjustments to insulin doses or alter carbohydrate intake or timing of exercise to achieve blood glucose goals. Alterations to baseline insulin doses should be made in response to a pattern of blood glucose results over a few days, not in response to a single high or low level.

Levels 1 and 2 may assist in achieving better adherence to recommendations and improved blood glucose control, even for those young people not on intensive insulin regimens (**B**) [54]. Twice-daily-insulin regimes of short- and long-acting insulin require day-to-day consistency in carbohydrate intake (often as 'snacks') to prevent hypoglycaemia during periods of hyperinsulinaemia (**E**) [75]. Particular attention should be paid to the energy profile of snacks to prevent excessive weight gain, and low-fat choices should be encouraged.

Level 3: carbohydrate to insulin ratios. This level of self-management education for carbohydrate counting is appropriate for people on multiple-dose-insulin or insulin-pump therapy. It requires a solid understanding of the first two levels and motivation in order to be able to monitor blood glucose levels closely. Once the appropriate baseline insulin doses have been established on a regular intake of carbohydrate, an insulin-to-carbohydrate ratio can be calculated (e.g. 1 unit rapid-acting insulin to 10 g carbohydrate). With the determined insulin-to-carbohydrate ratio, it allows the adjustment of the premeal insulin according to the estimated carbohydrate content of the meal or snack. This provides greater dietary flexibility than a traditional exchange diet and helps reduce the frequency of hypoglycaemia as well as postprandial hyperglycaemia after large meals.

Extensive patient education materials are available in most countries to help people estimate the carbohydrate content of foods. Considerable time is spent educating patients on how to read and interpret food labels, assess the carbohydrate content of the snack/meal and understand the nutrient content of foods in order to make healthy choices. Most national diabetes associations also produce useful literature on how to read food labels.

Use of the full carbohydrate-counting system at Level 3 requires intensive self-management education and an ongoing support from an experienced multidisciplinary diabetes team and motivated patients. This type of structured patient education programme has been shown to improve dietary freedom and quality of life in adults with T1DM (**E**) [62]. It is at present being evaluated in young people by several centres (**E, B**) [56, 58].

Further advantages of multiple-daily-injection regimes include more flexible meal times and the decreased need for between meal snacks. It is also possible to give the rapid-acting insulin after the meal if the quantity of the carbohydrate is not known. This is especially useful in younger children.

Glycaemic index and glycaemic load

GI is the measure of the change in blood glucose following ingestion of carbohydrate-containing foods. The type of carbohydrate is best described by its GI. Foods are ranked according to their immediate effect on blood glucose levels; the higher the GI number, the greater the glycaemic impact. Extensive GI tables are available [76].
• Low-GI carbohydrate foods (GI <55) may assist with postprandial hyperglycaemia when they are chosen to replace higher GI foods (GI >70)
• Examples of low-GI food sources include whole-grain breads, pasta, temperate fruits and dairy products.

The GI ranking of a food does not take into account the effect of portion size of the food. The glycaemic load (GL) of a food is the product of the GI of the food and the amount of carbohydrate in the serving. The addition of the GL of individual foods will give the GL of the whole meal.
• GL is another method to predict the postprandial blood glucose response, which also takes into account the portion size and the GI of the food (**A, E**) [68, 77].

Further evaluation of the practical application of the use of GI and GL diets in children is required. However, a recent study in children showed a statistically significant reduction in HbA1c levels after they were taught to follow a low-GI diet (**A**) [78]. Other advantages of this method are that it is easy for children and families to implement by including low-GI foods at every meal and snack without having to adhere to defined quantities of carbohydrate.

Cardiovascular considerations

Evidence confirms the increased incidence of cardiovascular disease in people with early onset T1DM compared with the general population (**A**) [79]. This establishes high HbA1c as an independent risk factor in the development of premature atherosclerosis and increased cardiovascular events.

High serum cholesterol and LDL-C are important predictors of cardiovascular disease in people with T1DM, and higher levels have been documented in children with T1DM (**E, B**) [80, 81]. The association between dietary intake, glycaemic control and cardiovascular risk in young people with T1DM still needs further investigation in prospective studies. Virtanen *et al.* (**B**) [81] found lower total cholesterol and triglycerides values in young T1DM subjects who had better glycaemic control. The authors concluded that serum total cholesterol and low-density cholesterol could be lowered by improving their metabolic control and decreasing their saturated fatty acid intake. Other authors have shown (**B**) [82] that even a modest increase in MUFA in adolescents with T1DM seemed to improve insulin sensitivity. Forsander *et al.* [22] found that children with poor glycaemic control consumed more fat, and an association was found between saturated fat and insulin dose. Similar findings of better glycaemic control and healthier food habits were found by Lodefalk and Aman (**B**) [30].

However, there have been no longitudinal studies in children and young people with diabetes to prove that a reduction in dietary fat, saturated fat and trans fatty acids will reduce either serum cholesterol, LDL-C or cardiovascular disease. However, it would seem prudent to promote all dietary factors that are cardioprotective, recommended in the ISPAD consensus guidelines to reduce CV risk (**E**) [10], e.g. optimum weight, reduction in total fat, promote the ideal fatty acid profile, aim for vitamin and antioxidant daily intake, increase soluble fibre.

Do children achieve dietary guidelines?

The dietary habits of children across the world are changing rapidly; in general these changes include poor-quality, energy-dense, low-nutrient foods [83, 84], contributing to the increase in childhood obesity. It is against this background that young people with diabetes strive to make dietary change. International dietary comparisons [23] show variation in adherence to dietary recommendations (**E**) [10]. Some authors report good adherence (**E**) [23, 31], whilst other authors report poorer adherence, i.e. a higher intake of fat (**C, B**) [24, 32, 54, 85] and lower intake of fibre (**E, B**) [31, 54]. This indicates that certain dietary recommendations may be more difficult to achieve than others, with the likelihood that the indigenous diet has a major impact on food choices. Evidence is inconclusive in relation to dietary compliance during adolescence. Some authors report a deterioration in dietary quality as the child moves into adolescence, seeing rises in saturated fat (**B**) [86, 87] and general diabetes mismanagement, e.g. missed meals and snacks (**B**) [88]. However, some authors [30, 89–91] report that the food habits of young people with T1DM were mainly healthier than those of control subjects.

Psychological difficulties, dysfunctional eating behaviour and eating disorders

Care and education should include acknowledging developmental and psychosocial factors [92, 93] for, although diabetes is not inevitably associated with psychological difficulties, it may result in additional psychosocial vulnerabilities, e.g. eating problems and depression [43, 94]. It is known that psychological issues such as behaviour disorders and depression are greater in young children with diabetes, and this in turn is associated with poor metabolic control (**B**) [95].

Disordered eating behaviour has long been recognised in young people with T1DM [44, 73]. It has become increasingly recognised that adolescents may manipulate their insulin dose and/or diet because of weight and shape concerns in ways that may not be immediately or easily identified as symptoms of an eating disorder (**B**) [96]. Recent evidence shows that the incidence of eating disorders in adolescent girls with diabetes is higher than that in the non-diabetic population, and its incidence is increasing (**A**) [43].

In association with eating disorders, the omission of insulin is a well-described tactic in attempts at weight loss in overweight, insulin-treated patients (**B**) [39, 97]. Individuals with eating disorders have higher HbA1c levels and an earlier age of onset of diabetic complications; one study reported that eating disorders were associated with a threefold increase in the risk of diabetic retinopathy (**A**) [43]. This early onset of diabetic complications is more of a concern when accompanied by ineffective treatment for the eating disorder (**B**) [98]. The disordered eating patterns are also an indication of mental health problems, requiring psychological support (**B**) [99].

It is not only adolescent girls that are vulnerable but there are some indications that binge eating and misuse of insulin is also common in adolescent boys. Evidence from the Young Diabetes Conference in 1987 indicated that 71% of young people with T1DM admit to 'binge' eating, which is often associated with feelings of extreme guilt [100].

Classical approaches to eating-disorder diagnosis and management need to be modified to incorporate the specific demands of diabetes regimens (**B**) [99]. Clinicians need to take into account potential insulin omission, glycaemic control, dietary dissatisfaction or manipulation, body dissatisfaction and family functioning, as well as hospital attendance history.

There are clear, evidence-based guidelines for the management of eating disorders (**E**) [50]. These recommend a range of psychotherapeutic approaches for the treatment of anorexia and bulimia. Motivational enhancement therapy has recently been suggested as a clinically effective approach in the treatment of adolescents with abnormal eating behaviours [101]. Solution-focused therapy has also been used to encourage young people to focus on positive skills in order to take control of the eating disorder and diabetes; it also empowers families to participate in the day-to-day management of diabetes.

The treatment of severe malnutrition related to an eating disorder associated with diabetes should be substantially the same as for eating disorder unrelated to diabetes. Nasogastric tube feeding should be instituted for significant malnutrition where the young person is unable or refuses to take the required calorie intake.

Behavioural approaches in diabetes education

The management of diabetes in young children is recognised as requiring a multidisciplinary team approach, and parents are in need of understanding and non-judgemental support from all health-care professionals [102]. Paediatric dietitians should be trained in communication to promote listening and the ability to respond and manage developing psychopathology in the child and necessary early referrals to mental health specialists. The inclusion of behavioural approaches, such as empowerment, cognitive behavioural therapy and motivational interviewing to patient education, provides an alternative model of patient care (**E**) [103]. It has also been shown that exploring problem-solving skills through experiential learning leads to greater self-efficacy and improved dietary outcomes (E) [104]. There is some evidence that these behavioural interventions are effective for adolescents with T1DM (A, E) [105, 106]. Dietary goal-setting is also a very useful technique to measure dietary interventions [89]. Education and/or counselling should be regularly reviewed to meet the constantly changing needs and requirements of the developing child, parents and carers.

Summary

The nutritional care of children with diabetes is complex. It involves not only the child but also the family and multiple carers. It requires a deep understanding of the relationship between treatment regimens and constantly changing physiological requirements, including growth, fluctuations in appetite associated with changes in growth velocity, varying nutritional requirements and sporadic episodes of physical activity. In addition, diabetes management is set within the current context of frequently dysfunctional family dynamics, deteriorating national dietary characteristics, issues of non-compliance, peer pressure, emerging independence and the ultimate aim of maintaining quality of life. However, evidence suggests that it is possible to improve diabetes outcomes through meticulous attention to nutritional management and an individualised approach. This requires a clear focus on the dietetic targets in relation to glycaemic control and reduction in cardiovascular risk. The fundamental premise of successful dietary outcomes is the development of a trusting relationship between the health professional, the child and the family/carer, which will facilitate behaviour change during the challenges and turbulence of childhood and adolescent development.

References

1 Delahanty LM, Halford BN. The role of diet behaviors in achieving improved glycemic control in intensively treated patients in the Diabetes Control and Complications Trial. *Diabetes Care* 1993; **16**: 1453–8.

2 Delahanty LM. Clinical significance of medical nutrition therapy in achieving diabetes outcomes and the importance of the process. *J Am Diet Assoc* 1998; **98**: 28–30.

3 Wolever T, Gougeon R, Freeze C *et al*. Clinical practice guidelines for the prevention and management of diabetes in Canada. Chapter 9: Nutrition Therapy. *Can J Diabet* 2003; **27**(suppl 2): S27–31.

4 Making Every Young Person with Diabetes Matter: Report of the Children and Young People with Diabetes Working Group. Department of Health, 2007. Available at: http://www.dh.gov.uk/en/Publicationsandstatistics/Publications/PublicationsPolicyAndGuidance/DH_073674

5 Department of Health. *Structured Patient Education in Diabetes: Report from the Patient Education Working Group*. Available at: http://www.diabetes.nhs.uk/downloads/structured_patient_education_diabetes_report.pdf

6 NICE. *Type 1 Diabetes in Children and Young People: Full Guideline*, 2004. Available at: http://www.nice.org.uk/page.aspx?o=CG015childfullguideline

7 Hoey H, Aanstoot HJ, Chiarelli F *et al*. Good metabolic control is associated with better quality of life in 2,101 adolescents with type 1 diabetes. *Diabetes Care* 2001; **24**: 1923–8.

8 American Diabetes Association. Nutrition principles and recommendations in diabetes. *Diabetes Care* 2004; **27**(suppl 1): S36–46.

9 Franz MJ, Bantle JP, Beebe CA *et al*. Evidence-based nutrition principles and recommendations for the treatment and prevention of diabetes and related complications. *Diabetes Care* 2003; **26**(suppl 1): S51–61.

10 Swift PGF. ISPAD Clinical Practice Consensus Guidelines 2006–2007. Diabetes Education. *Pediatric Diabetes* 2007; **8**: 103–109.

11 NHMRC. *The Australian Clinical Practice Guidelines on the Management of Type 1 Diabetes in Children and Adolescents*, 2005. Available at: http://www.nhmrc.gov.au/publications/synopses/cp102syn.htm

12 Department of Health. Dietary reference values for food energy and nutrients for the United Kingdom. Report of the Panel on Dietary Reference Values of the Committee on Medical Aspects of Food Policy. *Rep Health Soc Subj (Lond)* 1991; **41**: 1–210.

13 Dewey KG, Beaton G, Fjeld C *et al*. Protein requirements of infants and children. *Eur J Clin Nutr* 1996; **50**(suppl 1): S119–147.

14 Mann JI, De L, I, Hermansen K *et al*. Evidence-based nutritional approaches to the treatment and prevention of diabetes mellitus. *Nutr Metab Cardiovasc Dis* 2004; **14**: 373–94.

15 Canadian Paediatric Society (Joint Working Group). Nutrition recommendations update: dietary fat and children. Report of the Joint Working Group of the Canadian Paediatric Society (CPS) and Health, Canada, 2004. Available at: http://www.cps.ca/english/statements/n/n94-01.htm.

16 Ha TK, Lean ME. Recommendations for the nutritional management of patients with diabetes mellitus. *Eur J Clin Nutr* 1998; **52**: 467–81.

17 Friedberg CE, Janssen MJ, Heine RJ *et al*. Fish oil and glycemic control in diabetes: a meta-analysis. *Diabetes Care* 1998; **21**: 494–500.

18 Hooper L, Thompson RL, Harrison RA *et al*. Risks and benefits of omega 3 fats for mortality, cardio-vascular disease, and cancer: systematic review. *BMJ* 2006; **332**: 752–60.

19 de Deckere EA, Korver O, Verschuren PM *et al*. Health aspects of fish and $n-3$ polyunsaturated fatty acids from plant and marine origin. *Eur J Clin Nutr* 1998; **52**: 749–53.

20 Amundsen AL, Ntanios F, Put N *et al*. Long-term compliance and changes in plasma lipids, plant sterols and carotenoids in children and parents with FH consuming plant sterol ester-enriched spread. *Eur J Clin Nutr* 2004; **58**: 1612–20.

21 Ketomaki AM, Gylling H, Antikainen M *et al*. Red cell and plasma plant sterols are related during consumption of plant stanol and sterol ester spreads in children with hypercholesterolemia. *J Pediatr* 2003; **142**: 524–31.

22 Forsander G, Malmodin B, Eklind C *et al*. Relationship between dietary intake in children with diabetes mellitus type 1, their management at diagnosis, social factors, anthropometry and glycaemic control. *Scand J Nutr* 2003; **47**: 75–84.

23 Virtanen SM, Virta-Autio P, Rasanen L *et al*. Changes in food habits in families with a newly diagnosed child with type 1 diabetes mellitus. *J Pediatr Endocrinol Metab* 2001; **14**(suppl 1): 627–36.

24 Waldron S, Swift PG. Can children in the UK achieve the ISPAD nutritional guidelines? *J Pediatr Endocrinol Metab* 2000; **13**(suppl 4): 53.

25 Waldron S. PhD Thesis *The Evaluation of a Low Fat Dietary Intervention in Children with Diabetes*. Leicester University, Leicester, UK, 2004.

26 Rickard KA, Loghmani ES, Cleveland JL *et al*. Lower glycemic response to sucrose in the diets of children with type 1 diabetes. *J Pediatr* 1998; **133**: 429–34.

27 Magrath G, Hartland BV. Dietary recommendations for children and adolescents with diabetes: an implementation paper. British Diabetic Association's Professional Advisory Committee. *Diabet Med* 1993; **10**: 874–85.

28 Pereira MA, O'Reilly E, Augustsson K *et al*. Dietary fiber and risk of coronary heart disease: a pooled analysis of cohort studies. *Arch Intern Med* 2004; **164**: 370–6.

29 Toeller M, Buyken AE, Heitkamp G *et al*. Fiber intake, serum cholesterol levels, and cardiovascular disease in European individuals with type 1 diabetes. EURODIAB IDDM Complications Study Group. *Diabetes Care* 1999; **22**(suppl 2): B21–8.

30 Lodefalk M, Aman J. Food habits, energy and nutrient intake in adolescents with type 1 diabetes mellitus. *Diabet Med* 2006; **23**: 1225–32.

31 Pinelli L, Mormile R, Gonfiantini E *et al*. Recommended dietary allowances (RDA) in the dietary management of children and adolescents with IDDM: an unfeasible target or an achievable cornerstone? *J Pediatr Endocrinol Metab* 1998; **11**(suppl 2): 335–46.

32 Schober E, Langergraber B, Rupprecht G *et al*. Dietary intake of Austrian diabetic children 10 to 14 years of age. *J Pediatr Gastroenterol Nutr* 1999; **29**: 144–7.

33 *Eating 5 a day is easy*. Available at: http://www.5aday.nhs.uk

34 World Health Organization. *Diet, Nutrition and the Prevention of Chronic Diseases.* Technical Report Series 916. Geneva, Switzerland, 2003. Available at: http://whqlibdoc.who.int/trs/WHO_TRS_916.pdf

35 Mortensen HB, Robertson KJ, Aanstoot HJ *et al.* Insulin management and metabolic control of type 1 diabetes mellitus in childhood and adolescence in 18 countries. Hvidore Study Group on Childhood Diabetes. *Diabet Med* 1998; **15**: 752–9.

36 The effect of intensive treatment of diabetes on the development and progression of long-term complications in insulin-dependent diabetes mellitus. The Diabetes Control and Complications Trial Research Group. *N Engl J Med* 1993; **329**: 977–86.

37 Danne T, Kordonouri O, Enders I *et al.* Factors influencing height and weight development in children with diabetes. Results of the Berlin Retinopathy Study. *Diabetes Care* 1997; **20**: 281–5.

38 Holl RW, Grabert M, Sorgo W *et al.* Contributions of age, gender and insulin administration to weight gain in subjects with IDDM. *Diabetologia* 1998; **41**: 542–7.

39 Bryden KS, Neil A, Mayou RA *et al.* Eating habits, body weight, and insulin misuse: a longitudinal study of teenagers and young adults with type 1 diabetes. *Diabetes Care* 1999; **22**: 1956–60.

40 Domargard A, Sarnblad S, Kroon M *et al.* Increased prevalence of overweight in adolescent girls with type 1 diabetes mellitus. *Acta Paediatr* 1999; **88**: 1223–8.

41 Sarnblad S, Ekelund U, Aman J. Physical activity and energy intake in adolescent girls with type 1 diabetes. *Diabet Med* 2005; **22**: 893–9.

42 Laing SP, Swerdlow AJ, Slater SD *et al.* Mortality from heart disease in a cohort of 23,000 patients with insulin-treated diabetes. *Diabetologia* 2003; **46**: 760–5.

43 Jones JM, Lawson ML, Daneman D *et al.* Eating disorders in adolescent females with and without type 1 diabetes: cross sectional study. *BMJ* 2000; **320**: 1563–6.

44 Rodin GM, Daneman D. Eating disorders and IDDM: a problematic association. *Diabetes Care* 1992; **15**: 1402–12.

45 Cole TJ, Freeman JV, Preece MA. Body mass index reference curves for the UK, 1990. *Arch Dis Child* 1995; **73**: 25–9.

46 Cole TJ, Bellizzi MC, Flegal KM *et al.* Establishing a standard definition for child overweight and obesity worldwide: international survey. *BMJ* 2000; **320**: 1240–3.

47 Fernandez JR, Redden DT, Pietrobelli A *et al.* Waist circumference percentiles in nationally representative samples of African-American, European-American, and Mexican-American children and adolescents. *J Pediatr* 2004; **145**: 439–44.

48 World Health Organization. *Obesity: Preventing and Managing the Global Epidemic. Report on a WHO Consultation Technical Report Series, No 894.* Available at: http://www.who.int/bookorders/anglais/detart1.jsp?sesslan=1&codlan=1&codcol=10&codcch=894

49 Chanoine JP, Hampl S, Jensen C *et al.* Effect of orlistat on weight and body composition in obese adolescents: a randomized controlled trial. *JAMA* 2005; **293**: 2873–83.

50 National Collaborating Centre for Mental Health. *Eating Disorders Guidelines: Core Interventions in the Treatment and Management of Anorexia Nervosa, Bulimia Nervosa and Related Eating Disorders.* Available at: http://www.bps.org.uk/publications/core/eating/eating_home.cfm?&redirectCount=0

51 Effect of intensive diabetes treatment on the development and progression of long-term complications in adolescents with insulin-dependent diabetes mellitus: Diabetes Control and Complications Trial. Diabetes Control and Complications Trial Research Group. *J Pediatr* 1994; **125**: 177–88.

52 Danne T, Mortensen HB, Hougaard P *et al.* Persistent differences among centers over 3 years in glycemic control and hypoglycemia in a study of 3,805 children and adolescents with type 1 diabetes from the Hvidore Study Group. *Diabetes Care* 2001; **24**: 1342–7.

53 Daneman D, Swift PGF, De Beaufort C *et al.* Do differences in nutritional intake, eating habits and lifestyle in adolescents influence glycaemic outcome and explain the differences between international centers? *Pediatr Diabetes* 2006; **7**(suppl 5): 65.

54 Dorchy H, Bourguet K. Nutritional intake of Belgian diabetic children. *Diabetes Care* 1997; **20**: 1046–7.

55 Kyriacou C. *Essential Teaching Skills*, 2nd edn. Nelson Thomas Ltd., Cheltenham, UK, 1998.

56 Knowles J, Waller H, Eiser C *et al.* The development of an innovative education curriculum for 11–16 yr old children with type 1 diabetes mellitus (T1DM). *Pediatr Diabetes* 2006; **7**: 322–8.

57 Department of Health. *National Service Framework for Diabetes: Delivery Strategy.* Available at: http://www.dh.gov.uk/en/Publicationsandstatistics/Publications/PublicationsPolicyAndGuidance/DH_4003246

58 von Sengbusch S, Muller-Godeffroy E, Hager S *et al.* Mobile diabetes education and care: intervention for children and young people with type 1 diabetes in rural areas of northern Germany. *Diabet Med* 2006; **23**: 122–7.

59 Waller H, Eiser C, Heller S *et al.* Implementing a new paediatric structured education programme. *J Diabet Nurs* 2005; **9**: 332–8.

60 Berger M, Muhlhauser I. Implementation of intensified insulin therapy: a European perspective. *Diabet Med* 1995; **12**: 201–8.

61 Pieber TR, Brunner GA, Schnedl WJ *et al.* Evaluation of a structured outpatient group education program for intensive insulin therapy. *Diabetes Care* 1995; **18**: 625–30.

62 DAFNE Study Group. Training in flexible, intensive insulin management to enable dietary freedom in people with type 1 diabetes: dose adjustment for normal eating (DAFNE) randomised controlled trial. *BMJ* 2002; **325**: 746.

63 Price KJ, Lang JD, Eiser C *et al.* Prescribed versus unrestricted carbohydrate diets in children with type 1 diabetes. *Diabet Med* 1993; **10**: 962–7.

64 Australian Government Department of Health and Ageing. *Australian Guide to Healthy Eating – What is the National Food Selection Guide?* 2001. Available at: www.health.gov.au/internet/wcms/ Publishing.nsf/ Content/health-pubhlth-strateg-food-guide-index.htm

65 Wolever TM, Bolognesi C. Source and amount of carbohydrate affect postprandial glucose and insulin in normal subjects. *J Nutr* 1996; **126**: 2798–806.

66 Hanas R. *Type 1 Diabetes in Children, Adolescents and Young Adults: How to Become an Expert in Your Own Diabetes*, 2nd edn. London: Class, 2004.

67 Waldron S, Swift PG, Raymond NT *et al.* A survey of the dietary management of children's diabetes. *Diabet Med* 1997; **14**: 698–702.

68 Brand-Miller J, Hayne S, Petocz P *et al.* Low-glycemic index diets in the management of diabetes: a meta-analysis of randomized controlled trials. *Diabetes Care* 2003; **26**: 2261–7.

69 Sheard NF, Clark NG, Brand-Miller JC *et al.* Dietary carbohydrate (amount and type) in the prevention and management of diabetes: a statement by the American Diabetes Association. *Diabetes Care* 2004; **27**: 2266–71.

70 Lawrence RD. *The Diabetic Life: Its Control by Diet and Insulin. A Concise Practical Manual for Practitioners and Patients*, 16th edn. Churchill, London, 1927.

71 Swift PG. Flexible carbohydrate. *Diabet Med* 1997; **14**: 187–8.

72 Swift PGF, Waldron S, Glass C. A child with diabetes: distress, discrepancies and dietetic debate. *Pract Pediatr* 1995; **12**: 59–62.

73 Steele JM, Young RJ, Lloyd GG *et al.* Abnormal eating attitudes in young insulin-dependent diabetics. *Br J Psychiatr* 1989; **155**: 515–21.

74 Gillespie SJ, Kulkarni KD, Daly AE. Using carbohydrate counting in diabetes clinical practice. *J Am Diet Assoc* 1998; **98**: 897–905.

75 Wolever TM, Hamad S, Chiasson JL *et al.* Day-to-day consistency in amount and source of carbohydrate associated with improved blood glucose control in type 1 diabetes. *J Am Coll Nutr* 1999; **18**: 242–7.

76 Foster-Powell K, Holt SH, Brand-Miller JC. International table of glycemic index and glycemic load values: 2002. *Am J Clin Nutr* 2002; **76**: 5–56.

77 Colombani PC. Glycemic index and load-dynamic dietary guidelines in the context of diseases. *Physiol Behav* 2004; **83**: 603–10.

78 Gilbertson HR, Brand-Miller JC, Thorburn AW *et al.* The effect of flexible low glycemic index dietary advice versus measured carbohydrate exchange diets on glycemic control in children with type 1 diabetes. *Diabetes Care* 2001; **24**: 1137–43.

79 Nathan DM, Lachin J, Cleary P *et al.* Intensive diabetes therapy and carotid intima-media thickness in type 1 diabetes mellitus. *N Engl J Med* 2003; **348**: 2294–303.

80 Dorchy H. Dietary management for children and adolescents with diabetes mellitus: personal experience and recommendations. *J Pediatr Endocrinol Metab* 2003; **16**: 131–48.

81 Virtanen SM, Rasanen L, Virtanen M *et al.* Associations of serum lipids with metabolic control and diet in young subjects with insulin-dependent diabetes mellitus in Finland. *Eur J Clin Nutr* 1993; **47**: 141–9.

82 Donaghue KC, Pena MM, Chan AK *et al.* Beneficial effects of increasing monounsaturated fat intake in adolescents with type 1 diabetes. *Diabetes Res Clin Pract* 2000; **48**: 193–9.

83 *EU Platform on diet, Physical Activity and Health. Synopsis. Commitments 2006.* Available at: http://ec.europa.eu/health/ph_determinants/life_style/nutrition/platform/docs/synopsis_commitments2006_en.pdf

84 Rolls BJ. The supersizing of America: portion size and the obesity epidemic. *Nutr Today* 2003; **38**: 42–53.

85 Kalk WJ, Kruger M, Slabbert A *et al.* Fat, protein and carbohydrate content of diets of white insulin-dependent diabetic adolescents and young adults. *S Afr Med J* 1992; **81**: 399–402.

86 Pietilainen KH, Virtanen SM, Rissanen A *et al.* Diet, obesity, and metabolic control in girls with insulin dependent diabetes mellitus. *Arch Dis Child* 1995; **73**: 398–402.

87 Virtanen SM, Rasanen L, Tumme R *et al.* A follow-up study of the diet of Finnish diabetic adolescents. *Acta Paediatr* 1992; **81**: 153–7.

88 Weissberg-Benchell J, Glasgow AM, Tynan WD *et al.* Adolescent diabetes management and mismanagement. *Diabetes Care* 1995; **18**: 77–82.

89 Waldron S, Swift PGF, Kurinczuk J *et al.* Goal setting as a tool for focused dietary management of UK children with type 1 diabetes. *Pediatr Diabetes* 2004; **5**(suppl I): 26.

90 Waldron S, Swift PGF. Positive food choices in children and adolescents with type 1 diabetes. *J Pediatr Endocrinol Metab* 2003; **16**(suppl 4): 941.

91 Waldron S, Morgan G, Swift P; Trent Paediatric Diabetes Interest Group. Prospective audit of the food intake of children and adolescents. International Society for Pediatric and Adolescent Diabetes Annual Meeting, Cambridge, UK., *Pedaitr Diab* 2006; 7(suppl 5): 41–2.

92 Datta J. *Moving up with Diabetes: The Transition from Paediatric to Adult Care.* National Children's Bureau, London, 2003.

93 Eiser C. *Growing up with a Chronic Disease: The Impact on Children and Their Families.* Jessica Kingsley Publishers, London, 1993.

94 Doherty Y, Dovey-Pearce G. Understanding the developmental and psychological needs of young people with diabetes. *Pract Diabetes Int* 2005; **22**: 59–64.

95 Northam EA, Matthews LK, Anderson PJ *et al.* Psychiatric morbidity and health outcome in type 1 diabetes – perspectives from a prospective longitudinal study. *Diabet Med* 2005; **22**: 152–7.

96 Fairburn CG, Peveler RC, Davies B *et al.* Eating disorders in young adults with insulin dependent diabetes mellitus: a controlled study. *BMJ* 1991; **303**: 17–20.

97 Takii M, Komaki G, Uchigata Y *et al.* Differences between bulimia nervosa and binge-eating disorder in females with type 1 diabetes: the important role of insulin omission. *J Psychosom Res* 1999; **47**: 221–31.

98 Peveler RC, Bryden KS, Neil HA *et al.* The relationship of disordered eating habits and attitudes to clinical outcomes in young adult females with type 1 diabetes. *Diabetes Care* 2005; **28**: 84–8.

99 Olmsted MP, Daneman D, Rydall AC *et al.* The effects of psychoeducation on disturbed eating attitudes and behavior in young women with type 1 diabetes mellitus. *Int J Eat Disord* 2002; **32**: 230–9.

100 Newton RW, Connacher A, Morris AD *et al.* Dilemmas and directions in the care of the diabetic teenager: the Arnold Bloom Lecture 1999. *Pract Diabetes Int* 2000; **17**: 15–20.

101 Nielsen S, Molbak AG. Eating disorder and type 1 diabetes: overview and summing-up. *Eur Eat Disord Rev* 1998; **6**: 4–26.

102 Anderson B, Bracket J. Diabetes during childhood. In: Snoek FJ, Skinner TC, eds. *Psychology in Diabetes Care.* John Wiley & Sons, Winchester, 2000.

103 Anderson RM, Funnell MM, Hernandez CA. Choosing and using theories in diabetes education research. *Diabetes Educ* 2005; **31**: 513–18, -20.

104 Turan B, Osar Z, Molzan TJ *et al.* The role of coping with disease in adherence to treatment regimen and disease control in type 1 and insulin treated type 2 diabetes mellitus. *Diabetes Metab* 2002; **28**: 186–93.

105 Hampson SE, Skinner TC, Hart J *et al.* Behavioral interventions for adolescents with type 1 diabetes: how effective are they? *Diabetes Care* 2000; **23**: 1416–22.

106 Meetoo D. Clinical skills: empowering people with diabetes to minimize complications. *Br J Nurs* 2004; **13**: 644–51.

CHAPTER 9

Education in childhood diabetes

Peter G.F. Swift

The important thing is not to stop questioning. Curiosity has its own reason for existing. One cannot help but be in awe when one contemplates the mysteries of eternity, of life, of the marvellous structure of reality. It is enough if one tries merely to comprehend a little of this mystery every day.
 —Albert Einstein, US (German-born) physicist (1879–1955)

Education is what survives when what has been learned has been forgotten.
 —BF Skinner (after Einstein), American psychologist (1904–1990)

Introduction

Historically, treatment of disease has been prescribed by doctors. Although this prescriptive process of treatment may have applied to diabetes when insulin was first discovered, it was soon realised that type 1 diabetes mellitus (T1DM) required far more than just insulin (**E**) [1]. Numerous enlightened physicians, paediatricians and other health-care professionals (HCPs) realised that managing T1DM demands a much more holistic, patient-centred, non-didactic management approach (**E**) [2–4].

In 1922 insulin was, as it is now, a miraculous life saver but, particularly in children and young adults, it changed diabetes from a rapidly fatal disease into a chronic disorder with serious long-term complications. As time has progressed it has become more apparent that diabetes requires constant, lifelong attention to complex details of treatment to keep it under consistently good control. It also intrudes into the normal lives of affected individuals and their carers. Not surprisingly, therefore, diabetes is now seen as a condition requiring serious lifestyle management to deal with it successfully. This conclusion applies to T1DM in children and probably even more to the emerging problem in paediatric practice of T2DM most commonly associated with obesity and a family history of T2DM (**E**) [5].

There is a philosophical debate as to the most effective methods of patient education based on the strong evidence that a large proportion of patients do not comply or adhere to treatment schedules (**E**) [6]. This debate has been mainly conducted around adult diabetes and particularly with regard to T2DM but, of course, in the adolescent age group, non-adherence is well recognised (**B**) [7]. The debate then focuses upon the most effective methods of preventing or managing such non-adherence.

Education is always quoted as being the key to successful management and outcomes but what diabetes education is required and what style of education is most effective? The traditional medical model as described above is often criticised for its lack of empathy, its didactic nature, its judgemental approach fostering conflict and tension and, of course, engendering a feeling of frustration in the physician because of the lack of effectiveness (**E**) [2, 6, 8]. Do these criticisms apply to paediatric care; and is the alternative of empowerment education, based on counselling psychology, the way forward for childhood diabetes?

What is diabetes education?

A suggested definition is:

'*The process of providing the person with the knowledge and skills needed to perform diabetes self-care, manage crises and to make lifestyle changes to successfully manage the disease*' [8].

This definition incorporates several important features (**E**):
• Education should involve not only acquisition of knowledge but also development of practical skills.
• Practical skills that enable the performance of self-care procedures.
• Self-care involves change in lifestyle (essential for diabetes management).

Until relatively recent times, education in both adults and children has utilised general common-sense guidelines without an evidence base, often in an unstructured *ad hoc* manner, generally without much thought as to whether or not the educational process is likely to be successful. A lack of, or inadequate, education may result in poor outcomes both for glycaemic control (**A**) [9] and in levels of patient satisfaction, quality of life and a higher risk of complications (**A**) [10, 11]. Inadequate education may be in part also responsible for the fact that alterations in insulin regimens *per se*, even using newer insulin regimens, have not resulted in better glycaemic outcomes (**B**) [12].

We should ask whether the two landmark studies the Diabetes Control and Complications Trial (DCCT) (**A**) [10, 11] in T1DM and the UK Prospective Diabetes Study (UKPDS) [13] in T2DM provide evidence for education in improving diabetes management and outcomes. Both of these studies were constructed to compare the relationship of different levels of glycaemia with the development and progression of vascular and neurological complications. The DCCT unequivocally showed that sustained and lower levels of glycaemia (as reflected in lower HbA1c) were associated with significantly lower risks of vascular complications. These results have been emphasised more recently by the follow-up EDIC (Epidemiology of Diabetes Interventions and Complications) studies showing the longer term benefits of earlier better glycaemic control (**A**) [14, 15]. The UKPDS showed that better blood glucose control reduced the risk of vascular eye and kidney disease by around a quarter and better blood pressure control also significantly reduced diabetes-related deaths, strokes and visual deterioration [16]. But the question remains as to whether the better outcomes were the result of treatment schedules or altered behaviour or a combination of both and whether increased education was the critical factor.

There is no doubt from the DCCT experience that the participants, especially in the adolescent age group (**A**) [11], were a very special group of people who were difficult to recruit, and the intensively treated group received an enormous amount of (very expensive) support, over a long period of time [17]. After the DCCT was completed and the level of education and support diminished, the participants demonstrated a deterioration in glycaemic control [14]. Although there are no publications from the UKPDS on the role of education, summaries of its findings highlight the fact that more educational staff (for better blood pressure control) and 'ensuring a good understanding of targets for blood glucose and blood pressure' were important, using 'culturally appropriate education' (**E**) [18]. The DCCT illustrates very clearly the value of more frequent contact with patients, continuing education and unconditional consistent psychosocial support and advice. But, as neither trial was designed to have directly comparable control groups, it is impossible to dissect out the effect size of different parts of the intervention.

This chapter will further explore the evidence base for using education to improve the clinical practice of diabetes care in children, adolescents and young adults. Evidence-based practice in medicine is usually expected to involve controlled trials and interventions, but in diabetes care of young people, appropriately conducted qualitative research may be equally instructive in demonstrating the effectiveness of different educational approaches. Have they been performed and are they available for analysis?

What does the literature say about different modes of education and educational interventions?

Diabetes outcomes in young people have frequently been disappointing but variable between countries, and so guidelines to improve the quality of management have proliferated. In childhood diabetes there are numerous national guidelines, all of them identifying education as an essential component of management (**E**) [19–22]. The only global guidelines for children and adolescents put education '*at the centre of clinical management... providing not only a knowledge base but also, when delivered in a style which is patient-centred and appropriate for the age and maturity of the young person and the culture of the family, it becomes the vehicle for optimal self-management, the key to success*' [23]. This publication has no scientific references and no evidence gradings but its advice is based on worldwide consensus by experts in the field (**E**). It has been widely quoted and translated into 10 different languages. In contrast to other guidelines it has a separate chapter on diabetes education.

The four major-referenced and evidence-graded national guidelines for childhood diabetes also strongly recommend the theoretical importance of education but only one of them devotes much space to an analysis of the evidence (**E**) [21].

In a broader context, the Diabetes Education Study Group (DESG), founded in 1979 by JP Assal, was established with the aim of '*realising the importance of patient education as a therapeutic measure*'. The group has published many practical documents to assist in the development of successful educational techniques, including its *Basic Curriculum for Health Professionals* on diabetes therapeutic education (**E**) [24]. This publication contains many useful referenced recommendations.

The term 'therapeutic patient education', the words often used by DESG, has been usurped by other titles, such as structured patient education (SPE) and diabetes self-management education (DSME) (**E**) [25]. Diabetes UK has recently published, jointly with the UK Department of Health, a guidance booklet on SPE and notes that a structured education programme should be based on four clear criteria (**E**) [26]. It should:
• have a structured, agreed, written curriculum
• use trained educators
• be quality assured
• be audited.

These criteria are also highlighted in the DSME document (**E**) [25] and a guidance document from National Institute for Clinical Excellence UK (**E**) [27], and putting them into practice it has been recommended that:

• structured education should be available to all people with diabetes at the time of initial diagnosis, or when it is appropriate for them, and then as required on an ongoing basis, based on a formal, regular individual assessment of need (**E**)

• education should be provided by an appropriately trained interdisciplinary team – the team should have a sound understanding of the principles governing teaching and learning (**E**)

• interdisciplinary teams providing education should include, as a minimum, a diabetes specialist nurse and a dietitian (**E**)

• sessions should be held in a location accessible to individuals and families, whether in the community or the inpatient centre (**E**)

• educational programmes should use a variety of teaching techniques, adapted wherever possible to meet the different needs, personal choices, learning styles of both the young people with diabetes and the parents and local models of care (**E**).

What is the evidence that SPE is effective in T1DM? Most of the evidence comes from adult work (see [27] which unfortunately does not include references). However, the document quotes studies that are small in number and the only randomised controlled trial (RCT) of an education intervention alone did not show a significant difference in glycaemic control (**C**) [28]. Other controlled trials in both adults and young people have tested the effects of intensified insulin therapy or self-monitoring of blood glucose but included strong educational elements (**B, C**) [29–32] with variable results. Not surprisingly, the educational element itself did not always have a significant effect on glycaemia but had an additional impact when used alongside a new technology or skill. Another widely quoted study, and the only UK intervention at that time, the Dose Adjustment for Normal Eating (DAFNE) study in adults, did not meet the inclusion criteria, as there was a concurrent 'control' group for only 6 months after which this group attended a delayed DAFNE training course. The study reported significant differences in glycaemic control between the intervention group and the delayed intervention group at 6 months, a significant but less impressive lowering of HbA1c at 12 months and improved quality of life (**B**) [33].

A systematic review of educational and psychosocial interventions in adolescents was published by Hampson *et al.* in 2001 (**A**) [34]. This was the first time such a database had been constructed. The studies analysed revealed numerous methodological weaknesses, including inadequate descriptions of the skills and reasoning behind interventions, and outcome measures were often unclear and seemed to change during analysis. No data had been published about the longer term effectiveness of the interventions. Of 62 studies, 25 were RCTs, none performed in the UK. Conclusions drawn from this review included (**A**):

• educational and psychosocial interventions having small-to-medium beneficial effects on:
  – psychosocial outcomes (effect size 0.37)
  – glycated haemoglobin (effect size 0.33–0.08 excluding outliers)
• interventions most likely to be effective if they demonstrate the interrelatedness of various aspects of diabetes management

• an important gap in the evidence where the interventions should be targeted, e.g. age of patient, duration of diabetes and type of management problem
• the need of more carefully constructed research, which is also able to show longer term effects and provide estimates of cost-effectiveness.

Many of these conclusions were also reached in a further review of the intervention literature in paediatrics (**B**) [35]. This review investigated the results of predominantly behavioural or psychosocial interventions (1985–2003) that might put it outside the scope of this chapter on education but it highlights the overlap between the two areas of intervention that are inextricably connected (see also Chapter 10). Most of the more effective interventions discussed at length were the same ones discussed by Hampson *et al.* (**A**) [34].

Six research groups were highlighted that initiated diabetes-related interventions, using control groups. One group taught communication and problem-solving skills around diabetes (**C**) [36], while another group, working with recently diagnosed children, compared:
• supportive counselling focusing on psychosocial adjustment and family cooperation around diabetes care
• advanced teaching on self-blood-glucose monitoring to problem-solve and adjust insulins
• standard care (**A**) [37].

The group from the Joslin clinic evolved a series of studies based on trained teamworkers, using clear written protocols and psychoeducational materials to deliver sessions designed to enhance not only diabetes skills but also family cooperation and conflict reduction (**B, A**) [38–40]. Others have used group coping skills training used specifically around intensified insulin regimens utilising cognitive behavioural principles (**C**) [41]. Some have focused on problem-solving around diabetes self-care and stress reduction (**B**) [42] or others on stress-management training (**C**) [43]. The outcomes of these studies were of variable effectiveness but, in general, show improvements in psychosocial measures, with little effect on glycaemic control. All the aforementioned studies focused attention on modifications of diabetes management, whereas Wysocki *et al.* have tested the efficacy of a generic (not diabetes-related) intervention in families and adolescents with diabetes (**A**) [44, 45]. This structured behavioural family systems therapy is used to enhance communication within families, improve problem-solving and aid conflict resolution. In controlled studies the intervention groups showed improvements in parent–adolescent relations and reduction in family conflicts and diabetes-related conflicts, sustained to 12 months. There was no impact on glycaemic control. The authors of this review (**A**) [35] make some important comments that echo some of those made by Hampson *et al.* [34]:
• These highlighted controlled interventions appear to provide us with evidence that interventions which were directed by good theoretically based methodologies had greatest impact. They tend to be driven by cognitive behavioural techniques to enhance education, family cohesion, problem-solving, coping, communication, stress reduction and conflict resolution.
• The quality of many other studies is questionable with low participation rates, poorly defined theoretical constructs to interventions, selection bias and many studies have no control or comparison groups.
• Wysocki's group perhaps gives a clue that the interventions do not necessarily have to be diabetes specific [44, 45]. This must, however, be a guarded conclusion, as the positive

results of most of these interventions appear to apply mainly to psychosocial outcomes rather than improvements in glycaemic control.

Recently, the systematic review by Hampson *et al.* has been updated by analysing a further 168 papers (1999–2005) of which 24 were psychoeducational interventions and 13 were RCTs (**A**) [46]. The review noted that the quality of studies had improved, demonstrating greater clarity in the methodology of intervention used. This, as reported by Northam *et al.* (**B**) [35], was most often of a behavioural therapeutic nature, sometimes using cognitive behaviour therapy (**C**) [41, 47] or motivational interviewing (**C**) [48]. Studies that enhance both psychosocial support and education utilising modern technology (continuous glucose monitoring (**C**) [49], text messaging (**C**) [50], telephone contacts, telemedicine (**C**) [51] were discussed, including the first UK-based RCT (**A**) [52] involving negotiated telephone support that showed a significant improvement in self-efficacy but not in HbA1c. The interesting conclusion from that study was that the frequency and duration of telephone contact seemed to be of more importance than the (educational) content of the conversation.

Accepting that the outcomes of routine or conventional clinical care remain suboptimal, the overall summary and conclusions of this further systematic review (**A**) [46] are of considerable interest, indicating that:
• education appears to be most effective when integrated into routine care, e.g. added contacts, teamwork intervention, behavioural therapy, involvement of parents and when adolescent self-efficacy is promoted
• education alone has only a modest effect on outcomes unless linked to intensive insulin management or behavioural interventions (although studies comparing similar levels of intervention in more conventional therapy have not been tested in an RCT)
• it is likely that several modalities of interventions, by different motivated interventionists in a variety of settings, might show positive effects with certain targeted groups of individuals.

The review concludes by stating that *'there are no adequately powered, randomised, multicentre trials examining the feasibility, effectiveness and consistency of delivering psychoeducational interventions in paediatric populations'*.

Of particular interest to paediatricians should be:
• the teamwork approach of Anderson *et al.* to make more effective use of staff to increase the frequency and duration of contacts (**C**) [38–40]
• the use of new technologies to improve self-efficacy, interest and motivation (**C, A**) [50–52]
• the establishment of clear goals and targets
• the involvement and maintenance of parental support (**A**) [44, 45].

Winkley *et al.* (**A**) [53] have recently looked at psychological interventions in T1DM, comparing adult studies with those in children and adolescents. Many of the studies analysed were again those reviewed by Hampson *et al.* [34] and Northam *et al.* [35]. Not surprisingly, therefore, this further review provides evidence that psychological interventions can modestly improve glycaemic control in children and adolescents, but not in adults. The psychological effect size (-0.46) is greater than the impact on glycaemic control (effect size -0.35, equivalent to reduction in HbA1c of nearly 0.5%). The authors comment that previous reviewers have not always distinguished between educational and psychological interventions, between T1DM and T2DM, nor even between children and adults. They state that *'educational interventions use didactic and enhanced* *learning methods to improve self management by reducing identifiable gaps in knowledge, whereas psychological therapies use the alliance between patient and therapist, in which the patient's problems are understood in terms of emotions, cognitions and behaviours'*. Whether the reasoning behind these comments might have influenced the identification, grading or even the analysis of the review is open to debate. Educationists might contest words such as didactic, although it has been one of the criticisms levelled at medical teaching.

All the interventions summarised so far have been in T1DM and in young people. Deakin *et al.* (**A**) [54] have concluded an important study in adults with T2DM that involved a carefully planned, structured educational package for the intervention group that was compared with a control group. The study deserves analysis because it illustrates the difficulties of carrying out purely educational interventions. At 14 months the intervention group showed improvements in HbA1c (−0.6%), body mass index, waist circumference, total cholesterol, need for medication, nutritional intake, knowledge, self-management skills and satisfaction with treatment. In an accompanying editorial, Skinner (**E**) [55] argues that this was a well-conducted study of an educational intervention with blinding at randomisation and at final analysis with strictly specified outcome measures and a control group which also had increased contact time with HCPs. He contrasts these excellent features with the previously cited DAFNE intervention in adult T1DM (**B**) [33] that did not have a true control group and whose results showed that the advantages of the primary outcome group at 6 months regressed by 12 months. He also questioned the effect of group work as compared with individual therapy. '*Without a psychologically equivalent placebo, we have no means of knowing that the effects of these group programmes is no more than the impact of intensive contact with highly motivated, charismatic and enthusiastic educators, and the well documented therapeutic effects of groups through increased affiliation, social support and social comparison*'. Skinner concludes that the study '*provides further compelling evidence that when enthusiastic and motivated healthcare professionals invest more time with patients in a structured way to help them manage their diabetes, we see improved biomedical outcomes*'. Clearly, even though it is extraordinarily difficult, we have to apply the same critical scientific principles to self-management education as we do to pharmacological research.

Can primarily educational interventions in 61-year-old adults with T2DM be applied to children and adolescents with either type of diabetes? Although a major problem with paediatric research in diabetes is the underpowering of studies due to the lack of large numbers, the answer is probably affirmative in view of the carefully structured controlled studies described previously (**C**) [37–40, 44, 45]. Moreover if research interventions are targeted [35] or large multicentre studies are carefully designed, requiring substantial resourcing [56], there may be a possibility of carrying out an adequately powered, randomised, multicentre trial, examining '*the feasibility, effectiveness and consistency of delivering psycho-educational interventions in paediatric populations*' (**A**) [46].

In summary, psychoeducational interventions that have been used to improve the clinical care of young people have been very thoroughly analysed in recent years. Virtually all the controlled studies have been performed in the USA and it may be that this biases the selection of individuals, the style of intervention and the very need for interventions that have a stronger psychological/behavioural element than more purely educational. Reviewing evidence in the literature seems to allow some general conclusions that might perhaps help to shape future research and clinical practice guidelines:

1 Purely educational interventions produce modest benefits to young people with diabetes (**A**) [34, 46].

2 Interventions are most often a combination of educational and psychosocial elements (**C**) [41], (**A**) [34, 46, 53].

3 Psychoeducational interventions produce greater benefits in psychological domains than glycaemic control (**A**) [53].

4 Psychoeducational interventions should be based on clear theoretical principles (**A**) [34], (**B**) [35].

5 Interventions are best adapted to or added onto routine clinical care especially as an adjunct to intensive insulin management (**C**) [29, 31, 32, 41, 49].

6 The success of interventions might not be a result of the educational package itself but in part be accounted for by greater frequency and/or duration of contact (**B**) [33, 46], (**A**) [52].

7 Highly motivated, enthusiastic, charismatic interventionists may strongly influence results (**C**) [29, 31, 33, 41, 49], (**B**) [46, 54], (**E**) [55].

8 Parental or family involvement is important because most successful interventions involve behavioural elements (**A, B**) [37–40, 44, 45].

9 The educational and behavioural domains that appear to be most frequently used are related to:
- problem-solving (**A, C**) [36, 37, 44, 45]
- communication skills (**C**) [36]
- conflict resolution (**B, A**) [37–40, 44, 45]
- coping skills training including stress management (**C, B**) [41–43, 47]
- motivational interviewing (**C**) [48]
- enhancement of self-efficacy (**A**) [52]
- empowerment (**E**) [2].

How should education for young people be implemented?

Authors who have studied educational methods and have understood the unsatisfactory outcomes and lack of compliance/adherence, which is so common in medicine generally, and diabetes in particular, are very critical of the medical model (**E**) [2, 3, 57, 58]. Despite attempts by medical schools to teach students, the principles of holistic patient-centred medicine, personal observations and those of many others indicate that many medical students and junior doctors maintain the didactic, prescriptive practices of their forebears. The usual excuse is that there is no time to invest in 'proper' education or guidance. Recent focus groups with adolescents in the UK confirm that doctors often give out the wrong signals (**E**) [21] and are the least convincing teachers in the health-care team (personal communication and (**E**) [59]). So, what can be done to enable medical (and other health care) professionals to improve their success in diabetes education?

First and foremost, HCPs need to understand that, although meta-analyses and reviews consistently demonstrate that knowledge is predictive of better self-care and glycaemic control (**E**) [60], the association is weak. The acquisition of knowledge is unlikely by itself to alter behaviour significantly to improve diabetes control, especially in those who find diabetes difficult to manage. There seems, therefore, a need to train HCPs in the principles of education and teaching sufficient to effect and maintain behaviour change (**E**) [57–59].

Table 9.1 Principles and practice of education in children

1 Motivation
     The learner needs to and/or have a desire to learn
2 Context
     Where is the learner now?
     Where does the leaner want to be later?
3 Environment
     Learner centred, comfortable and trusting
     Enjoyable/entertaining/interesting/'open'
4 Significance
     Meaningful, important, links or joins up
     Reward or gain
5 Concepts
     Simple to complex in gentle steps (*short attention span*)
6 Activity
     Constantly interactive
     Practical (*fitting into real life*)
7 Reinforcement
     Repetition, review and summarise
8 Reassess, evaluate and audit
9 Move forward, continuing education

Table 9.2 Qualities looked for by OFSTED (**E**)

1 Lessons should be purposeful with high expectations conveyed
2 Learners should be given some opportunities to organise their own work
     [*guard against overdirection by teachers*]
3 Lessons should elicit and sustain learner's interest and be perceived by
   pupils to be relevant and challenging
4 The work should be well matched to learner's abilities and learning
   needs
5 Learner's language should be developed and extended
     [*teachers' questioning skills play a part here*]
6 A variety of learning activities should be employed
7 Good order and control should be largely based on skilful management
   of learner's involvement in the lesson and mutual respect

Adapted from [59].

HCPs should consider what children need when they are being taught. Table 9.1 is adapted from texts on teaching practice and discussions with teachers and young people. The evidence base for this is then the experience of the educational establishment (**E**).

Similarly, the HCPs who are teaching need to understand how lessons are to be formulated and in the UK the schools inspectorate (Office for Standards in Education, OFSTED; see [59]) has introduced qualities that they expect in the planning of lessons. These are shown in Table 9.2 and may be adapted to improve standards in teaching in the medical scene.

Modern teachers are also advised to develop some sort of agreement or contract with the learners in order to emphasise the two-way flow of responsibilities required in successful education.

Of necessity, diabetes education is very different from school education in that it must involve as many of the relatives and carers who will be involved in helping the child to manage the disease as confidently as possible. This added responsibility for carers as well as patient puts a different and sometimes troublesome perspective on paediatric diabetes education.

How should these principles be put into practice in diabetes care? The ISPAD Consensus Guidelines, 2000 (**E**) [23], introduced the following universal principles for childhood diabetes (quoted also in [20–22]):

• Children and adolescents, their parents and other care providers should all have easy access to and be included in the educational process.

• Diabetes education should be delivered by HCPs with a clear understanding of the special and changing needs of young people and their families as they grow through the different stages of life.

• Diabetes education needs to be adaptable and personalised so that it is appropriate to each individual's age, stage of diabetes, maturity and lifestyle, culturally sensitive and at a pace to suit individual and family needs.

• The priorities for HCPs in diabetes education may not match those of the child and family. Thus diabetes education should be based on a thorough assessment of the person's attitudes, beliefs, learning style, ability and readiness to learn existing knowledge and goals.

• Educators (doctors, nurses, dietitians and other health care providers) should have access to continuing specialised training in diabetes education and educational methods.

• Diabetes education needs to be a continuous process and repeated for it to be effective.

Levels of diabetes education

Level 1 – at diagnosis

The education programme for young people necessarily divides itself into two time scales. The first is at the time of diagnosis, a time when there may be enormous anxiety, fear, anger, guilt and misunderstandings about the new diagnosis. The child may have become exceedingly ill in diabetic ketoacidosis or in contrast shown few symptoms and appeared well despite the devastating diagnosis. There is of course no documented evidence that missing out various parts of the following curriculum has particular consequences, but common sense suggests that education at this time needs to follow a carefully planned but flexible schedule, be empathetic but informative and, over a period of time, either inside or outside the hospital environment, needs to impart both 'survival skills' and most of the list below (Table 9.3) (**E**). The content of this teaching programme is extensive and, in contrast to most other diseases, is a uniquely complex combination of emergency knowledge base, immediately applicable practical skills, lifestyle changes and short- to long-term educational principles of self-care, monitoring and readjustments.

Level 2 – continuing education

Soon after the family has adjusted to the new diagnosis, there is a need to follow a continuing and continuous process of further education (see Table 9.4), without which the young person and family may drift away from satisfactory glycaemic control (**B**) [61, 62]. This is

Table 9.3 Primary (Level 1) education: at diagnosis – survival skills

1	Explanation of how the diagnosis has been made and reasons for symptoms
2	Simple explanation of the uncertain cause of diabetes. No cause for blame
3	The need for immediate insulin and how it will work
4	What is glucose? Normal blood glucose levels and glucose targets
5	Practical skills Insulin injections Blood and/or urine testing and reasons for monitoring
6	Basic dietetic advice
7	Simple explanation of hypoglycaemia
8	Diabetes during illnesses. Advice not to omit insulin
9	Diabetes at home or at school including the effects of exercise
10	Identity cards, necklets, bracelets and other equipment
11	Membership of a diabetes association and other available support services
12	Psychological adjustment to the diagnosis
13	Details of emergency telephone contacts

Adapted from [23].

Table 9.4 Secondary (Level 2) continuing educational curriculum

1	Pathophysiology, epidemiology, classification and metabolism
2	Insulin secretion, action and physiology
3	Insulin injections, types, absorption, action profiles, variability and adjustments
4	Nutrition: Food plans Qualitative and quantitative advice on intake of carbohydrate, fat, proteins and fibre Coping with special events and eating out Growth and weight gain, 'diabetic foods', sweeteners and drinks (see Chapter 8)
5	Monitoring, including glycated haemoglobin and clear (agreed) targets of control
6	Hypoglycaemia and its prevention, recognition and management including glucagon
7	Intercurrent illness, hyperglycaemia, ketosis and prevention of ketoacidosis
8	Problem-solving and adjustments to treatment
9	Micro- and macrovascular complications and their prevention; the need for regular assessment
10	Exercise, holiday planning and travel, including educational holidays and camps
11	Smoking, alcohol and drugs
12	School, college, employment and driving vehicles
13	Sexuality, contraception, pregnancy and childbirth

Adapted from [23].

also the educational phase when, without frequent and positive support, diabetes has the potential to be devastatingly destructive both physically and psychologically.

Once again it can be seen that this list of contents is very complex and, for HCP educators to be successful, there needs to be a high level of commitment, motivation, expertise and experience. Such a resource is not always available as surveys have shown, with poorer outcomes, where expertise is unavailable (**E**) [63].

Earlier in the chapter, attention was drawn to interventions to improve clinical care and outcomes. Little mention was made about the fundamental differences between the education of adults, adolescents and children. This differentiation between age groups, the levels of maturity and understanding, differing cultures, beliefs and attitudes are all part of the challenge of paediatric diabetes. Moreover, the essential ingredient of childhood, its ever-changing circumstances associated with growth, maturity and position in society, means that diabetes educators at both the clinical and the researcher level have to adapt to these changing perspectives. It is also important to know that the impact and burden of diabetes may be viewed from different perspectives by adolescents, parents and HCPs (**B**) [64]. Although parents might be satisfied with the attention given to them, focus groups of adolescents have criticised HCPs for talking to parents and not to the patient (**E**) [21].

Other texts describe the educational requirements of different age groups (**E**) [20, 22, 23]. Practical experience makes it obvious that continuing or specific re-education courses are essential for older children who have been diagnosed as young children.

Barriers to education and their consequences

The education of children is very different from adults and it should be helpful that school children are already within an educational system, with teachers and learning being part of their usual daily lives. Most of the children being taught the practicalities of diabetes care assimilate the information with extraordinary speed. Unfortunately, however, a proportion of young people do not enjoy school or education, and some have adverse experiences. Diabetes teaching usually takes place alongside parents (and perhaps siblings) which for some people enhances the experience but for others it may seriously interfere and inhibit successful learning. When the family is under significant stress, or parents exhibit little motivation in learning or are in conflict, this is likely to have a negative effect on diabetes education and care in the young person (**E, B, C**) [65–67]. Educators will see here the challenging opportunities of involving both child and parent equally and synergistically. The enormous variability of educational ability and maturity has also to be taken into consideration such that the HCP has to assess the learning capabilities and concentration span of individuals (see Table 9.1). There have been no studies which have compared the use of individual education as against group education (**A**) [34]. Both modes of education can be successful in the correct settings.

Most young people are most attracted to education if it is fun. It is also much more engaging if the learning process is grounded in practical activity and perhaps role-play. The Chinese proverb of '*give a man a fish and he will not go hungry today; teach a man to fish and he will not go hungry for the rest of his life*' (**E**) [65] can be considered, in more academic terms, like the Miller pyramid of competence that starts with 'knowing' but ends with 'doing' [68]. In childhood education, doing something successfully is very important in breeding confidence and self-efficacy.

It is commonly argued, and there is abundant evidence to prove it, that non-compliance or non-adherence is common in childhood and adolescence (**B**) [7]. However, it has been suggested that these terms are counter-productive, especially as non-compliance may result from behavioural or communication difficulties and insufficient or poorly delivered education. The relationships developed between HCPs, children and parents must therefore involve an educational process that empowers the young person towards self-care and autonomy (**E**) [2, 60] with the unconditional support of parents.

Total 'compliance' may be construed as a pathological state. HCPs should not be perfectionistic but should expect all patients to stray from recommended paths during some phases of diabetes care (**E**) [2].

So, is there evidence that changes in educational input (or other interventions) can promote positive patterns of behaviour to help in the successful management of diabetes? The research on cognitive behavioural approaches to education and training in conflict resolution would seem to add support to the notion of preventing further deterioration in behaviour (**A**) [37, 44, 45]. Perhaps we should screen our clinic population to pick out those at greatest risk or showing early signs of adverse behaviour (**B**) [35] and intervene early with evidence-based interventions (**A, B**) [36–40, 44, 45]. The alternative strategy is that clinic staff are trained to use mental-health skills (**B, A**) [38–40] in identifying behavioural problems and either utilise those skills in managing the problems or enlist the help of mental-health experts (**A**) [44, 45]. It would seem clear from these approaches that services for children with diabetes benefit from the assistance of mental-health experts, either to initiate behaviourally based interventions or to educate or train other HCPs in behavioural techniques or to provide clinical management for young people and families when required. Unfortunately, such expertise is not readily available in most clinics (**E**) [63].

Is there evidence on how education should be implemented?

It has been argued that the three overriding aims of diabetes management are the best possible glycaemic control, without excessive hypoglycaemia and with optimal quality of life. There is evidence from many countries that the quality of glycaemic control in young people falls far short of the optimum expected by HCPs (**A**) [69]. There is also no doubt that some centres achieve far better levels of glycaemic control than others, with lower levels of hypoglycaemia and also with some evidence that quality of life is at least equal and may be better (**A, B**) [64, 70].

The question is how do these centres achieve such superior results and is this due to higher and more successful levels of education? If education is the key element in this mechanism, what are the secrets of success, and can they be reproduced elsewhere?

This author, having had first-hand knowledge of the Hvidøre Study Group (HSG) since its inception in 1994, has developed bias as to reasons for the success of certain groups, but is there evidence emerging from these and other successful groups which might be transferable to help other centres? There are numerous non-randomised studies reported of improvements in glycaemic control with fewer hypoglycaemic episodes and improvements in quality of life after changes to treatment regimens, such as multiple-daily-injection therapy or pump therapy (**A, B, C, E**) [29, 49, 71, 72]. Having accepted that there is a great deal of evidence to suggest that the insulin regimen itself is not a major factor influencing glycaemic control (**A**) [12], we must assume that these results are associated with an intervention effect (**E**) [73], albeit usually associated with increased education from enthusiastic educators (**E, A**) [71, 72].

Two major centres in Europe have reported on their successful management of diabetes in terms of excellent glycaemic control and low rates of hypoglycaemia (**C, B**) [49, 74]. These two centres have very different approaches to the insulin regimens but their reports, and those of others, once again emphasise the point that it is not the regime *per se* that makes a difference but the ways in which these regimens are put into practice. Indeed, one of the centres compared those children on twice daily insulin with those on basal bolus and found no differences in outcome. One centre reports seeing patients in clinic on average six to nine times per year with 70-minute consultations, the other four times per year but with other contacts by nurse educators and other points of contact outside the clinic. Both centres have a lead clinician who is a full-time paediatric diabetologist and both have frequent diabetic clinics. After every clinic all the patients are discussed with all the team. There is emphasis in their reports of the overriding importance of education, psychosocial support, attending to family dynamics, problem-based education, self-management with nutritional and insulin adjustments. Both departments have the support of psychologist and social worker to discuss and manage the difficulties experienced by a proportion of their patients.

Some other centres in the HSC also have consistently excellent results. One of these centres has been the subject of comparison with a centre achieving significantly poorer glycaemic control (HbA1c 7.6 vs 9.1%). A qualitative study was carried out by medical anthropologists looking at differences between the centres which might have influenced their discordant results (C) [74]. The results suggested that the centre with the lower HbA1c was working in a cultural environment which was more egalitarian, family centred, more constantly supportive and empowering (especially to adolescents), had a more consistent family dietary education and the service offered was diabetes dedicated. In contrast, the culture of the other centre was individualistic with less family support and it medicalised the adolescent, assuming the adolescent to be non-adherent but expected to take over management at a younger age. The service was not dedicated to diabetes (there were multiple other paediatric responsibilities), had fewer clinics and was less patient centred and empowering. The researchers suggested that cultural factors, independent of clinical practice, appear to determine a variety of social behaviours resulting in a low level of motivation and higher degrees of non-adherence. It is of interest that the author from one of the successful European centres analysed above also suggests that perhaps his results are '*not exportable without adjustment to the local way of life*' (E) [75]. This view would seem to be validated by comments from other centres in the HSG that have consistently excellent results and yet have an almost entirely hospital (non-community)-based treatment and virtually all the education is performed by physicians and not nurse educators (personal communication). This seems to bear out the commentary referred to above about the success of interventions being dependent not so much on the intervention but the interventionist – the personal charisma and style of the educator who implements the education or the intervention.

In 2005, the HSG completed a further study to examine the factors that might be responsible for the differences in glycaemic outcomes between centres. The results have not been completely analysed but it is already apparent that education and service provision factors that influence glycaemic control are target setting insulin and nutritional adjustments, 24-hour hotlines and also numerous lifestyle and family factors. The strongest effect is that of target setting by the team and the perceived targets by the individual patient. These factors must be influenced by the content and quality of diabetes education provided to the patients.

Summary and guidance

There is universal agreement that education is of crucial importance in developing and maintaining standards of care. Clinical experience from centres of excellence around the world and the results of scientifically validated research provide evidence that purely educational interventions have a modest effect on glycaemic control but they have a greater effect on psychosocial functioning.

Educational and psychosocial interventions are usually inextricably interwoven and when used together in certain studies have been shown to have positive effects.

Evidence has been described which indicates that improvements in diabetes care for children and adolescents, particularly in the psychoeducational domains, are more likely if the following features exist or are available:

• HCPs who are enthusiastic, motivating, charismatic educators (**C**) [29, 31, 33, 41, 49, 75], (**B**) [46, 54], (**E**) [55]
• Carefully designed structured education (**E**) [26]
• Cultural environments that are more conducive than others to assist in the process of transmitting positive educational messages (**C**) [74]
• Interdisciplinary teams that are experienced and specialise in managing diabetes with dedicated time and resources for more frequent (**E**) [52, 75], longer duration contacts (**A**) [52], (**E**) [22]
• The educational style is patient centred, empowering patients and family to take charge of their own diabetes self-management (**E**) [2, 3, 20–24]
• Diabetes education that:
  – teaches adjustment of insulin in daily management (**C**) [11, 75, 76]
  – sets clear targets for good glycaemic control (HbA1c) (**C**) [76]
• Psychoeducational interventions should be based on clear theoretical principles (**A**) [34]
• Interventions appear to be most effective when integrated into routine clinical care especially as an adjunct to intensive insulin management (**C**) [29, 31, 32, 41, 49]
• Interventions should maintain the support of and involve parents, carers and family because most successful interventions involve elements of behavioural counselling (**A, B**) [37–40, 44, 45]
• The educational and behavioural approaches that appear to be most frequently used are related to:
  – problem-solving (**A, B**) [36, 37, 44, 45]
  – communication skills (**C**) [36]
  – family counselling including conflict resolution (**A, B**) [37–40, 44, 45]
  – coping skills training including stress management (**B**) [41–43, 47]
  – motivational interviewing (**C**) [48]
  – enhancement of self-efficacy (**A**) [52]
  – empowerment (**E**) [2]
• Consideration should be given to training, education and support in the use of new technologies in providing educational variety and new motivation to young people with diabetes.

References

1 Bliss M. A continuing epilogue. *The Discovery of Insulin.* Paul Harris Publishing, Edinburgh, 1983: 242.
2 Anderson RM, Funnell MM. Patient empowerment: reflections on the challenge of fostering the adoption of a new paradigm. *Patient Educ Couns* 2005; **57**: 153–7.
3 Assal JP. Revisiting the approach to treatment of long-term illness: from the acute to the chronic state. A need for educational and managerial skills for long-term follow-up. *Patient Educ Couns* 1999; **37**: 99–111.
4 Lestradet H, Besse J, Grenet P. Problems medico-sociaux chez le jeune diabetique. *Le Diabete de l'enfant et de l'adolescent.* Publ Librairie Maloine, Paris, 1968: 289–335.

5 ADA Consensus Statement. Type 2 diabetes in children and adolescents. American Diabetes Association. *Diabetes Care* 2000; **23**: 381–9.

6 Doherty Y, James P, Roberts S. Stage of change counselling. In: Snoek FJ, Skinner TC, eds. *Psychology in Diabetes Care*. John Wiley, Chichester, England, 2002: 99–139.

7 Morris AD, Boyle DI, McMahon AD *et al*. Adherence to insulin treatment, glycaemic control, and ketoacidosis in insulin-dependent diabetes mellitus. The DARTS/MEMO Collaboration. Diabetes Audit and Research in Tayside Scotland. Medicines Monitoring Unit. *Lancet* 1997; **350**: 1505–10.

8 Clement S. Diabetes self-management education. *Diabetes Care* 1995; **18**: 1204–14.

9 Nicolucci A, Cavaliere D, Scorpiglione N *et al*. A comprehensive assessment of the avoidability of long-term complications of diabetes. A case-control study. SID-AMD Italian Study Group for the Implementation of the St. Vincent Declaration. *Diabetes Care* 1996; **19**: 927–33.

10 DCCT Research Group. The effect of intensive treatment of diabetes on the development and progression of long-term complications in insulin-dependent diabetes mellitus. The Diabetes Control and Complications Trial Research Group. *N Engl J Med* 1993; **329**: 977–86.

11 DCCT Research Group. Effect of intensive diabetes treatment on the development and progression of long-term complications in adolescents with insulin-dependent diabetes mellitus: Diabetes Control and Complications Trial. Diabetes Control and Complications Trial Research Group. *J Pediatr* 1994; **125**: 177–88.

12 Holl RW, Swift PG, Mortensen HB *et al*. Insulin injection regimens and metabolic control in an international survey of adolescents with type 1 diabetes over 3 years: results from the Hvidøre Study Group. *Eur J Pediatr* 2003; **162**: 22–9.

13 Diabetes Trials Unit. *UK Prospective Diabetes Study*. Available at: http://www.dtu.ox.ac.uk/index.php?maindoc=/ukpds/

14 DCCT Trials Unit. Retinopathy and nephropathy in patients with type 1 diabetes four years after a trial of intensive therapy. The Diabetes Control and Complications Trial/Epidemiology of Diabetes Interventions and Complications Research Group. *N Engl J Med* 2000; **342**: 381–9.

15 Nathan DM, Lachin J, Cleary P *et al*. Intensive diabetes therapy and carotid intima-media thickness in type 1 diabetes mellitus. *N Engl J Med* 2003; **348**: 2294–303.

16 Mogensen CE. Combined high blood pressure and glucose in type 2 diabetes: double jeopardy. British trial shows clear effects of treatment, especially blood pressure reduction. *BMJ* 1998; **317**: 693–4.

17 Lorenz RA, Bubb J, Davis D *et al*. Changing behavior: practical lessons from the diabetes control and complications trial. *Diabetes Care* 1996; **19**: 648–52.

18 Diabetes UK. *UKPDS – Implications for the Care of People with Type 2 Diabetes*. Available at: http://www.diabetes.org.uk/About_us/Our_Views/Position_statements/UKPDS__Implications_for_the_care_of_people_with_Type_2_diabetes_/

19 Canadian Diabetes Association. *Clinical Practice Guidelines e-Guidelines*. Available at: http://www.diabetes.ca/cpg2003/chapters.aspx

20 NHMRC. *The Australian Clinical Practice Guidelines on the Management of Type 1 Diabetes in Children and Adolescents 2005*. Available at: http://www.chw.edu.au/prof/services/endocrinology/apeg/

21 NICE. *Type 1 Diabetes in Children and Young People: Full Guideline 2004*. Available at: http://www.nice.org.uk/page.aspx?o=CG015childfullguideline

22 Silverstein J, Klingensmith G, Copeland K *et al*. Care of children and adolescents with type 1 diabetes: a statement of the American Diabetes Association. *Diabetes Care* 2005; **28**: 186–212.

23 ISPAD. *Consensus Guidelines for the Management of Type 1 Diabetes Mellitus in Children and Adolescents*. Medical Forum International, Zeist, Netherlands, 2000.

24 Diabetes Education Study Group (DESG). *Basic Curriculum for Health Professionals on Diabetes Therapeutic Education*. Available at: http://www.desg.org/article/articlestatic/50/1/10/

25 Mensing C, Boucher J, Cypress M *et al*. National Standards for Diabetes Self-Management Education. *Diabetes Care* 2005; **28**(suppl 1): S72–9.

26 Diabetes UK DoH. *Structured Patient Education: Report from the Patient Education Working Group*. Available at: http://www.diabetes.org.uk/Document/Reports/StructuredPatientEd.pdf

27 National Institute for Clinical Excellence (NICE). *Guidance on the Use of Patient-Education Models for Diabetes*. Available at: http://www.nice.org.uk/page.aspx?o=TA060guidance

28 Terent A, Hagfall O, Cederholm U. The effect of education and self-monitoring of blood glucose on glycosylated hemoglobin in type I diabetes: a controlled 18-month trial in a representative population. *Acta Med Scand* 1985; **217**: 47–53.

29 Boland EA, Grey M, Oesterle A *et al.* Continuous subcutaneous insulin infusion: a new way to lower risk of severe hypoglycemia, improve metabolic control, and enhance coping in adolescents with type 1 diabetes. *Diabetes Care* 1999; **22**: 1779–84.

30 Daneman D, Siminerio L, Transue D *et al.* The role of self-monitoring of blood glucose in the routine management of children with insulin-dependent diabetes mellitus. *Diabetes Care* 1985; **8**: 1–4.

31 Muhlhauser I, Bruckner I, Berger M *et al.* Evaluation of an intensified insulin treatment and teaching programme as routine management of type 1 (insulin-dependent) diabetes. The Bucharest-Dusseldorf Study. *Diabetologia* 1987; **30**: 681–90.

32 Reichard P, Britz A, Cars I *et al.* The Stockholm Diabetes Intervention Study (SDIS): 18 months' results. *Acta Med Scand* 1988; **224**: 115–22.

33 DAFNE Study Group. Training in flexible, intensive insulin management to enable dietary freedom in people with type 1 diabetes: dose adjustment for normal eating (DAFNE) randomised controlled trial. *BMJ* 2002; **325**: 746.

34 Hampson SE, Skinner TC, Hart J *et al.* Effects of educational and psychosocial interventions for adolescents with diabetes mellitus: a systematic review. *Health Technol Assess* 2001; **5**: 1–79.

35 Northam EA, Todd S, Cameron FJ. Interventions to promote optimal health outcomes in children with type 1 diabetes – are they effective? *Diabet Med* 2006; **23**: 113–21.

36 Satin W, La Greca AM, Zigo MA *et al.* Diabetes in adolescence: effects of multifamily group intervention and parent simulation of diabetes. *J Pediatr Psychol* 1989; **14**: 259–75.

37 Delamater AM, Bubb J, Davis SG *et al.* Randomized prospective study of self-management training with newly diagnosed diabetic children. *Diabetes Care* 1990; **13**: 492–8.

38 Anderson BJ, Brackett J, Ho J *et al.* An office-based intervention to maintain parent-adolescent teamwork in diabetes management: impact on parent involvement, family conflict, and subsequent glycemic control. *Diabetes Care* 1999; **22**: 713–21.

39 Laffel LM, Vangsness L, Connell A *et al.* Impact of ambulatory, family-focused teamwork intervention on glycemic control in youth with type 1 diabetes. *J Pediatr* 2003; **142**: 409–16.

40 Svoren BM, Butler D, Levine BS *et al.* Reducing acute adverse outcomes in youths with type 1 diabetes: a randomized, controlled trial. *Pediatrics* 2003; **112**: 914–22.

41 Grey M, Boland EA, Davidson M *et al.* Coping skills training for youth with diabetes mellitus has long-lasting effects on metabolic control and quality of life. *J Pediatr* 2000; **137**: 107–13.

42 Mendez FJ, Belendez M. Effects of a behavioral intervention on treatment adherence and stress management in adolescents with IDDM. *Diabetes Care* 1997; **20**: 1370–5.

43 Boardway RH, Delamater AM, Tomakowsky J *et al.* Stress management training for adolescents with diabetes. *J Pediatr Psychol* 1993; **18**: 29–45.

44 Wysocki T, Harris MA, Greco P *et al.* Randomized, controlled trial of behavior therapy for families of adolescents with insulin-dependent diabetes mellitus. *J Pediatr Psychol* 2000; **25**: 23–33.

45 Wysocki T, Greco P, Harris MA *et al.* Behavior therapy for families of adolescents with diabetes: maintenance of treatment effects. *Diabetes Care* 2001; **24**: 441–6.

46 Murphy HR, Rayman G, Skinner TC. Psycho-educational interventions for children and young people with type 1 diabetes. *Diabet Med* 2006; **23**: 935–43.

47 Hains AA, Davies WH, Parton E *et al.* A stress management intervention for adolescents with type 1 diabetes. *Diabetes Educ* 2000; **26**: 417–24.

48 Channon S, Smith VJ, Gregory JW. A pilot study of motivational interviewing in adolescents with diabetes. *Arch Dis Child* 2003; **88**: 680–3.

49 Nordfeldt S, Johansson C, Carlsson E *et al.* Prevention of severe hypoglycaemia in type I diabetes: a randomised controlled population study. *Arch Dis Child* 2003; **88**: 240–5.

50 Franklin V, Waller A, Pagliari C *et al.* 'Sweet Talk': text messaging support for intensive insulin therapy for young people with diabetes. *Diabetes Technol Ther* 2003; **5**: 991–6.

51 Liesenfeld B, Renner R, Neese M *et al.* Telemedical care reduces hypoglycemias and improves glycemic control in children and adolescents with type 1 diabetes. *Diabetes Technol Ther* 2000; **2**: 561–7.

52 Howells L, Wilson AC, Skinner TC *et al.* A randomized control trial of the effect of negotiated telephone support on glycaemic control in young people with type 1 diabetes. *Diabet Med* 2002; **19**: 643–8.

53 Winkley K, Ismail K, Landau S *et al.* Psychological interventions to improve glycaemic control in patients with type 1 diabetes: systematic review and meta-analysis of randomised controlled trials. *BMJ* 2006; **333**: 65–8.

54 Deakin TA, Cade JE, Williams R *et al.* Structured patient education: the diabetes X-PERT Programme makes a difference. *Diabet Med* 2006; **23**: 944–54.

55 Skinner TC. What does make the difference? *Diabet Med* 2006; **23**: 933–4.

56 The NHS Health Technology Assessment Programme. *Development and Evaluation of a Psychosocial Intervention for Children and Teenagers Experiencing Diabetes (DEPICTED).* Available at: http://www.ncchta.org/projectdata/1_project_record_not_published.asp?PjtId=1450&SearchText=depicted

57 Anderson RM, Funnell M, Carlson A *et al.* Facilitating self-care through empowerment. In: Snoek FJ, Skinner TC, eds. *Psychology in Diabetes Care.* John Wiley, Chichester, England, 2000: 69–97.

58 Coles C. Diabetes education: letting the patient into the picture. *Pract Diabetes* 1990; **7**: 110–12.

59 Knowles J, Waller H, Eiser C *et al.* The development of an innovative education curriculum for 11–16 yr old children with type 1 diabetes mellitus (T1DM). *Pediatr Diabetes* 2006; **7**: 322–8.

60 Skinner TC, Channon S, Howells L *et al.* Diabetes during adolescence. In: Snoek FJ, Skinner TC, eds. *Psychology in Diabetes Care.* John Wiley & Sons, Chichester, England, 2000: 27.

61 Jacobson AM, Hauser ST, Willett J *et al.* Consequences of irregular versus continuous medical follow-up in children and adolescents with insulin-dependent diabetes mellitus. *J Pediatr* 1997; **131**: 727–33.

62 Kaufman FR, Halvorson M, Carpenter S. Association between diabetes control and visits to a multidisciplinary pediatric diabetes clinic. *Pediatrics* 1999; **103**: 948–51.

63 Edge JA, Swift PG, Anderson W *et al.* Diabetes services in the UK: fourth national survey; are we meeting NSF standards and NICE guidelines? *Arch Dis Child* 2005; **90**: 1005–9.

64 Hoey H, Aanstoot HJ, Chiarelli F *et al.* Good metabolic control is associated with better quality of life in 2,101 adolescents with type 1 diabetes. *Diabetes Care* 2001; **24**: 1923–8.

65 Hanas R. Getting to grips with diabetes. *Type 1Diabetes in Children, Adolescents and Young Adults*, 3rd edn. Class Publishing, London, 2007: 5.

66 Hanson CL, De Guire MJ, Schinkel AM *et al.* Empirical validation for a family-centered model of care. *Diabetes Care* 1995; **18**: 1347–56.

67 White K, Kolman ML, Wexler P *et al.* Unstable diabetes and unstable families: a psychosocial evaluation of diabetic children with recurrent ketoacidosis. *Pediatrics* 1984; **73**: 749–55.

68 Miller GE. The assessment of clinical skills/competence/performance. *Acad Med* 1990; **65**: S63–7.

69 Mortensen HB, Hougaard P. Comparison of metabolic control in a cross-sectional study of 2,873 children and adolescents with IDDM from 18 countries. The Hvidøre Study Group on Childhood Diabetes. *Diabetes Care* 1997; **20**: 714–20.

70 Danne T, Mortensen HB, Hougaard P *et al.* Persistent differences among centers over 3 years in glycemic control and hypoglycemia in a study of 3,805 children and adolescents with type 1 diabetes from the Hvidøre Study Group. *Diabetes Care* 2001; **24**: 1342–7.

71 Battelino T. Risk and benefits of continuous subcutaneous insulin infusion (CSII) treatment in school children and adolescents. *Pediatr Diabetes* 2006; **7**(suppl 4): 20–4.

72 Danne T, von Schutz W, Lange K *et al.* Current practice of insulin pump therapy in children and adolescents – the Hannover recipe. *Pediatr Diabetes* 2006; **7**(suppl 4): 25–31.

73 Adair JG. The Hawthorne effect: a reconsideration of the methodological artefact. *J Appl Psychol* 1984; **69**: 334–45.

74 Greene AC, Tripaldi M, Chiarelli F *et al.* Cross-cultural differences in the management of children and adolescents with diabetes. *Horm Res* 2002; **57**(suppl 1): 75–7.

75 Dorchy H. Insulin regimens and insulin adjustments in diabetic children, adolescents and young adults: personal experience. *Diabetes Metab* 2000; **26**: 500–7.

76 Swift PGF, de Beaufort CE, Skinner TC on behalf of the Hvidøre Study Group. Services provided by the diabetes team: do they affect glycemic outcome? *Pediatr Diabetes* 2006; **7**(suppl 5): OP6 19.

CHAPTER 10

Psychological interventions in childhood diabetes

John W. Gregory & Sue Channon

We should not pretend to understand the world only by the intellect; we apprehend it just as much by feeling. Therefore, the judgment of the intellect is, at best, only the half of truth, as must, if it be honest, also come an understanding of its inadequacy.
—Carl Jung, Swiss psychiatrist and founder of
analytical psychology (1875–1961)

Introduction

The management of diabetes imposes considerable practical and psychological burdens on young people with diabetes. Variations in blood glucose concentrations may impact directly on behaviour and mood (**B**) [1]. Furthermore, the demands of complying with a complex regimen may lead to either overdependence of children on their adult carers (**B**) [2] or adverse effects on behaviour including an increase in suicidal thoughts (**B**) [3]. Coping with diabetes also places particular pressures on the child's family, ranging from grief at diagnosis (**B**) [4] to changes in patterns of communication and increased family conflict with parents experiencing frustration and guilt at failure to achieve optimal outcomes (**E**) [5]. It is therefore unsurprising that childhood diabetes is associated with increased risks of psychological morbidity (**A, B**) [6, 7]. This chapter will therefore review the evidence that psychoeducational interventions impact on metabolic control and measures of mental health in young people with diabetes, in particular highlighting some of the key randomised controlled trials (RCTs) in the field.

By contrast with other aspects of the management of type 1 diabetes mellitus (T1DM) in childhood, psychoeducational interventions have been poorly evaluated until relatively recently. A systematic review in 2001 identified 62, mostly North American, studies of psychosocial and educational interventions of which only 42% were RCTs and none was from the UK (**A**) [8]. The mean (median) effect size was 0.36 (0.37) for psychosocial outcomes and 0.33 (0.18) for glycated haemoglobin. An effect size for HbA1c of 0.18 is equivalent to a reduction in HbA1c of 0.31%, suggesting modest beneficial effects from such interventions. However, the practical implications of these studies were limited by their piecemeal development and lack of theoretical basis, their short-term nature with follow-up rarely beyond a year, lack of targeting and scant economic evaluation. A more recent review of studies published from 1999 to 2005 (**A**) [9] identified a further 24 interventions of which 13 were RCTs. Although characterised by improved quality, effect sizes for psychoeducational and HbA1c outcomes were similar.

Diagnosis

Severity of presentation

In Italy, a non-randomised prevention programme largely focused around posters providing information about the symptoms of diabetes displayed in schools has suggested that it is possible to reduce the risk of presentation in diabetic ketoacidosis (DKA) at diagnosis (**B**) [10].

Treatment at home or in hospital

Once diagnosed with diabetes, there are a few studies that have evaluated the relative benefits of care from diagnosis in those sufficiently well to be treated at home as opposed to hospital. Those that have were of a retrospective nature or uncontrolled and difficult to interpret (**B**) [11, 12] and so there is insufficient evidence to recommend either model of care from the psychoeducational perspective. However, an RCT by Simell *et al.* (**A**) [13] suggests no benefit on metabolic control of long-term (1 mo) over short-term (1 wk) hospitalisation at diagnosis.

Psychoeducational interventions

With respect to the effectiveness of specific psychoeducational interventions at diagnosis, an RCT has shown that whether the family live together within the hospital during that period seems to have no effect on outcome (**A**) [14]. By contrast, another such trial suggested that the deterioration in glycaemic control frequently seen 6–24 months after diagnosis at the end of the 'honeymoon period' may be ameliorated by effective self-management training shortly after diagnosis (**B**) [15]. RCTs at diagnosis have shown a benefit of a family psychosocial intervention delivered out of hospital on family functioning but not glycaemic control (**A**) [16] and that a parent–mentor programme may reduce the impact of diabetes on family life (**A**) [17].

Problems with ongoing management

It is clear that in most clinics, suboptimal outcomes are achieved with the majority of young people with diabetes demonstrating less than ideal blood glucose control, resulting in HbA1c concentrations above the ideal target of 7.5%. A few individuals experience more significant problems with compliance, including poor adherence to recommendations about diet and exercise, failure of blood glucose monitoring, omission of insulin injections, poor clinic attendance and recurrent hospital admissions with either severe hypoglycaemia or DKA.

Comparison of studies that have evaluated psychoeducational interventions to improve outcomes is difficult due to the range of psychological outcome measures evaluated, though most have evaluated effects on glycaemic control. A recent systematic review (**A**) [9] has concluded that with respect to optimising glycaemic control, no particular theoretical basis, or individual intervention, appears to be superior to others, with the possible exception of coping skills training in those who already have good glycaemic control and supportive family backgrounds (**C**) [18]. The range of interventions evaluated by an RCT and the

Table 10.1 Effect sizes for glycated haemoglobin and psychosocial outcomes for each intervention. Effect sizes were averaged across different outcomes within each category within each study

Study	Glycated haemoglobin	Psychosocial
Anderson (A) [19]	0.47	N/A
Anderson (B) [20]	−0.48	0.72
Boardway (A) [21]	N/A	0.11
Brown (B) [22]	−0.11	0.36
Cook (B) [23]	0.19	0.23
Daley (B) [24]	N/A	0.28
Delamater – intervention 1 (B) [15]	0.18	N/A
Delamater – intervention 2 (B) [15]	0.18	N/A
Forsander (A) [16]	−0.11	N/A
Gilbertson (A) [25]	0.23	N/A
Grey (A, B) [26, 27]	0.34	0.48
Hains (C) [28]	−0.31	0.41
Hansson [29]	N/A	0.62
Howells (A) [30]	−0.20	0.42
Laffel (A) [31]	0.50	−0.35
Ludvigsson (A) [32]	0.45	N/A
Marrero (A) [33]	−0.17	N/A
McNabb (C) [34]	0.15	N/A
Olmsted (B) [35]	0.14	0.34
Satin – intervention 1 (A) [36]	1.18	N/A
Satin – intervention 2 (A) [36]	2.03	N/A
Simell (A) [13]	0.23	N/A
Sullivan-Bolyai (A) [17]	N/A	1.08
Sundelin (A) [14]	N/A	0.00
Wysocki (A) [37]	−0.03	0.37
All studies		
Mean	0.21	0.36
Median	0.18	0.36

N/A, not available.

Derived from Hampson *et al.* [8] and Murphy *et al.* [9].

effect sizes of these interventions on HbA1c and psychosocial outcomes identified by two systematic reviews (**A**) [8, 9] are shown in Table 10.1.

Improving HbA1c

Significant heterogeneity in effect sizes of psychoeducational interventions on HbA1c has been reported (**A**) [8]. Typically, RCTs of the effectiveness of psychoeducational interventions on HbA1c have produced modest effect sizes ranging from −0.48 to 0.50 for HbA1c. However, one study that has shown much more dramatic results was that reported by Satin *et al.* (**A**) [36], in which parental simulation of diabetes was compared with usual care following group therapeutic sessions of three to five families at a time during which the families' feelings about diabetes and influence on treatment adherence had been explored. For 1 week in the intervention group, parents were trained by their adolescent offspring to self-administer injections of saline, monitor urine samples and follow appropriate dietary and educational advice. This resulted in effect sizes of 1.18 and 2.03 in two studies, equivalent to an improvement in HbA1c of 2.5–3.0%. These dramatic benefits by comparison with other studies suggest that unique influences of this intervention produced consequences through mechanisms that have not been clarified.

Targeting poor glycaemic control

A few studies have now been published that focus interventions on subgroups of patients, usually adolescents with poor blood glucose control. The only RCT published evaluates a continuous glucose-monitoring system in a small group of individuals with a mean HbA1c of 8.0% using intensive insulin or pump therapy and demonstrates a significant reduction in HbA1c (**A**) [32].

A pilot study has evaluated the effectiveness of an intervention based upon motivational and solution-focused techniques in addition to elements of proven psychotherapeutic treatments including systemic and narrative approaches and cognitive behavioural therapy in a subgroup of adolescents with a mean HbA1c of 10.2% and demonstrated a significant reduction to 8.7% after 4–6 months, the effect being partially maintained for up to a year (**B**) [38]. The wider potential of motivational interviewing is discussed below. Two other recent studies have targeted individuals with poor glycaemic control but with disappointing outcomes. A non-randomised trial of individual home visits and weekly phone calls from a diabetes educator transiently improved diabetes knowledge and HbA1c but had no sustained benefit once this extra support was withdrawn (**A**) [39]. A stress-management intervention in adolescents (**C**) [28] showed small behavioural improvements but no effect on HbA1c by comparison with a waiting-list control group.

In summary, little effort has been invested thus far in targeting interventions in children with poor glycaemic control and those that have demonstrated generally disappointing results. This area requires further research especially in the vulnerable adolescent age group.

Behavioural and other psychosocial interventions

Approximately half the published studies of psychoeducational interventions have an explicit theoretical basis to the intervention. These may be subdivided into those based on family therapy, behavioural principles, social learning theory or other principles such as anchored instruction or social support.

Family interventions

A recent systematic review identified 13 RCT studies that have investigated the potential benefits of family interventions to promote better outcomes in children with T1DM, of mean age approximately 10 years (**A**) [40]. Twelve studies measured effects on metabolic control, of which seven showed an improvement in HbA1c. The overall effect on HbA1c in those studies from which data could be pooled showed a reduction of 0.6% (95% confidence interval −1.2 to −0.1; Figure 10.1) (**A, B, C**) [14, 20, 36, 41–46] whereas the overall effect size on parental-diabetes-knowledge-related outcomes was large (0.94), suggesting a net beneficial effect of such interventions (see section *Family conflict* below). The work of Anderson *et al.* (**B, A**) [20, 31] is of note in that the basis of the intervention

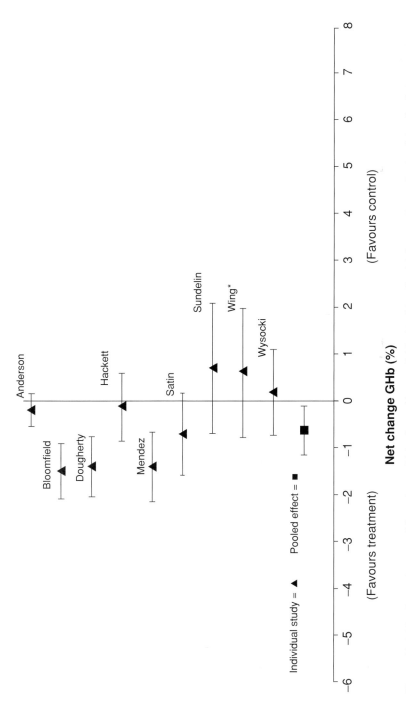

Figure 10.1 Net change (95% confidence intervals) in glycated haemoglobin (GHb) at distal follow-up for studies involving family interventions. The study of Wing *et al.* reports GHb for adults and is not included in the pooled effect. (From Armour *et al.* [40], with permission.)

has developed over more than one trial. These interventions that focus on parent–teenager responsibility for sharing diabetes tasks and ways to avoid conflicts produced a large effect size on psychosocial outcomes (0.72) but initially, a disappointing outcome for HbA1c (effect size −0.48) (**B**) [20]. However, a further study that developed this family-focused teamwork intervention has now shown an improvement in HbA1c (**A**) [31]. These findings suggest that family involvement in diabetes management may prevent the deterioration in glycaemic control seen in adolescence but without increased conflict or deteriorating quality of life.

Unfortunately, the heterogeneity of most study designs evaluating family interventions has made it difficult to determine which key characteristics of such interventions may be responsible for beneficial outcomes. Interventions that target families' abilities to cope with stress or diabetes-related conflict and those which increase diabetes-related knowledge seem to have potential with respect to their psychosocial aspects even if influences on glycaemic control seem less consistent. Longer term outcome studies are required in this area.

Behavioural interventions

Behavioural interventions based on the principles of cognitive behavioural therapy (CBT), either alone (**C, A**) [26, 28, 30, 47, 48] or in combination with behavioural therapy (**B**) [23] or solution-focused theory (**B**) [38], have been evaluated by a number of groups. Whilst these studies have shown mostly moderate benefits on psychosocial outcomes, effects on HbA1c have been more variable. An RCT by Grey *et al.* (**B, A**) [26, 27, 49, 50] has evaluated coping skills training in the context of intensive management based around social problem-solving, social skills, cognitive behavioural modification and conflict resolution. This resulted in moderate improvements in HbA1c and psychosocial outcomes (effect sizes of 0.43 and 0.48, respectively) that were maintained 1 year later. By contrast, two recent studies, one based on negotiated telephone support from a paediatric dietitian (**A**) [30] for an unselected population of young people with diabetes and the other involving stress management for a subgroup with HbA1c values greater than 9.0% whilst showing small psychological benefits, showed no beneficial effects on HbA1c (**C**) [28].

Motivational interviewing has recently been evaluated given that the principles of this technique, which was developed in the addiction field, seem particularly appropriate to the management of teenagers. A pilot study (**C**) [51] has confirmed the value of this behavioural technique with respect to influencing HbA1c concentrations in a group of individuals demonstrating 'readiness-to-change' behaviour with a mean HbA1c of 10.8%. Motivational interviewing has now been more stringently evaluated by the same group using an RCT design (**C**) [47] that compared motivational interviewing with non-specific counselling to allow for contact time with a therapist in a relatively unselected group of teenagers. This study has demonstrated a significant reduction in HbA1c over the 1 year of the intervention, with the benefit being maintained for a further year thereafter.

A number of studies have been published that have evaluated a range of other generic interventions. Svoren *et al.* (**A**) [52] have extended the observations made by the group at the Joslin Diabetes Center (**B, A**) [20, 31] to evaluate the effectiveness of a case-manager and psychoeducational modules to monitor and encourage routine diabetes care. This RCT demonstrated significant reduction in rates of hypoglycaemia and admission to hospital, albeit at the expense of more routine visits to the diabetes centre. An improvement in

HbA1c was seen only in those with higher HbA1c concentrations at the time of entry into the study. Another RCT has shown that videos and brochures designed for self-study to review skills aimed at preventing severe hypoglycaemia may also reduce the risk of severe hypoglycaemic episodes (A) [53]. A small RCT has evaluated the effectiveness of stress management and coping skills (A) [21]. Although diabetes-specific stress was reduced, adherence, coping style, self-efficacy and glycaemic control were unaffected.

Problems of everyday life

Very little work has been done on interventions targeting the mental health needs of young people with diabetes. Most research has reviewed mental health needs and prevalence rather than the effectiveness of interventions to improve mental health outcomes. The rest of this chapter therefore looks at the evidence and, where possible, extrapolates from two other areas: the research on mental health interventions in the general population and interventions that have targeted diabetes-related outcomes but that have had an impact on indices of mental health.

Emergence of independence

The move from dependence on the parent for diabetes care to full independence in self-care is a gradual process that needs to be negotiated over time and matched to the child's cognitive and emotional development. If it is too early and the young person is not ready, the research evidence consistently shows that glycaemic control will deteriorate (B) [54]. This negotiation between the family members can be facilitated by the diabetes service with a positive impact on levels of conflict in the family and HbA1c (see section *Family conflict*) (B) [20]. This approach has been taken forward in the UK by the FACTS (Families Adolescents and Children's Teamwork Study) group (E) [55]. The intervention provides four sessions per year, integrated into routine clinical care. Families are seen in small groups with separate sessions for children and young people in a structured programme that incorporates sessions on dietetics, blood sugar monitoring, communication and independence. Preliminary findings suggest that there is increased agreement between parents and adolescents, more involvement of parents and adolescents in diabetes care and short-term improvements in glycaemic control. An RCT is currently under way (E) [56, 57].

Family conflict

Family factors are significantly associated with metabolic control in children: low levels of conflict, good communication and the appropriate involvement of parent and child in diabetes management are associated with higher regimen adherence (C) [58] and better metabolic control (B) [20].

Whilst recognising that independence in diabetes care too early can have a negative impact on the child's glycaemic control, inclusion of the parents in the care may elicit conflict for some families, either because diabetes is an area of particular difficulty or because of general patterns of interaction existing within the family. A relatively low-intensity intervention (20–30 min following routine clinic appointments every 3–4 months) to improve parent–adolescent teamwork in diabetes management has been shown to reduce family conflict (B) [20]. In an RCT of behavioural family systems therapy (A) [46],

10 sessions over 3 months yielded improvements in parent–adolescent relationships and reduced diabetes-specific conflicts, improvements that were sustained at 12-month follow-up. A recent systematic review of family interventions in people with diabetes concluded that interventions targeting diabetes-related conflict or stress can reduce the number of conflicts in families (**A**) [40].

Peer relationships

Diabetes management occurs across contexts so, whilst familial support is necessary, peer relationships may also play an important part in helping or hindering children with their diabetes care. This could be particularly true in the teenage years, as peer influence steadily increases through childhood and peaks during early adolescence (**B**) [59]. Work on peer relationships and diabetes has shown evidence of both positive and negative effects: when presented with hypothetical social situations, in adolescence there is an increase in choice consistent with peer desires (compared to children) and decrease in regimen adherence (**C**) [60]. More positively, friends have been found to provide more emotional support than families in relation to diabetes (**C**) [61]. In one study, the inclusion of peers in treatment has been associated with reduced diabetes-related conflict in the families and parents reporting better adherence by the teenager (**C**) [48]. However, perceived peer support does not correlate with metabolic control or self-report of adherence (**C**) [62].

Psychological difficulties and psychiatric disorders

It is recognised that living with a chronic condition in childhood increases the likelihood of psychological difficulties. Diabetes is no exception to this and studies have shown a greater prevalence of psychiatric disorder in young people with diabetes compared to the general population (**E**) [63]. There is also a relationship between psychiatric disorder and diabetes outcomes including higher HbA1c, hospitalisations, DKA and severe hypoglycaemia (**B**) [64, 65]. There are several potential mechanisms for this association (described in more detail in Garrison *et al.* (**B**) [64]), including non-adherence leading to psychological difficulties, mental health issues leading to intentional self-harm (e.g. excessive or underuse of insulin), apathy or disordered beliefs leading to poor self-care or an external factor such as family environment underlying both the psychological and the diabetes-management difficulties. The relationship between the two is likely to be bi-directional with difficulties in each area exacerbating the other.

Depression and anxiety

Young people with diabetes have greater rates of depression (**B**) [65], with reports of prevalence two- to threefold higher than in those without diabetes [66] and those with depression have poorer glycaemic control [67]. In a retrospective cohort study using data from 37 children's hospitals in the USA (**B**) [64], it was found that internalising disorders such as anxiety and depression are associated with increases in repeat hospitalisations for diabetes, suggesting that screening for comorbid internalising disorders would help target resources at those most vulnerable to readmission. Despite these clear areas of concern, there is an absence of clinical trials of any therapeutic approach in children and adolescents who have both depression and diabetes. As described in a recent review of the area (E) [68], few adolescents meet the criteria for the diagnosis of depression at any one time. However, there is some evidence that subthreshold manifestations in young people may be just as disabling as syndromatic depression (C) [69], with difficulties including irritability, sadness, sleep disturbance and pessimism. The symptoms may not be at a level to reach criteria for diagnosis but early intervention with high-risk subgroups could be particularly helpful to prevent deterioration, which will then have a significant impact on their diabetes. One intervention that was designed to reduce risk for mental health problems in children with a range of chronic illnesses was the family-to-family network (A) [70]. In a randomised, controlled clinical trial, this study demonstrated modest positive effect in promoting adjustment in 7–11-year-old children through a combination of professional intervention and support contact from mothers whose children had the same condition.

In the general population, both individual and group CBT have been shown in RCTs to be effective in working with depression (A) [71, 72]. In a series of RCTs (A) [73] comparing CBT, family therapy and non-directive support for adolescents, those in the CBT arm showed the greatest improvement, particularly those with comorbid anxiety. However this positive finding for CBT was reduced by adverse family factors, in particular where the mother was also clinically depressed and where there were high levels of family conflict. In the non-directive support arm of the study, there was a higher proportion of both rapid responders and non-responders to treatment. For a diabetes service where access to psychiatric services may be limited, this would suggest that, if possible, providing supportive therapy might be worthwhile whilst waiting for them to be seen or as part of the assessment to decide if a referral is appropriate.

Anxiety disorders are the most common psychiatric disorder in childhood, with prevalence studies showing 8–12% of 4–20-year olds experiencing one or more diagnosable anxiety disorders (A) [74]. Fears and worries are a part of the normal process of development and anxiety disorders (including phobias and obsessive-compulsive disorder) are diagnosed only when the difficulties are disabling and persistent (A) [75]. Individual and group CBT have been demonstrated to be the most effective approach for phobias and generalised anxiety (B) [76]. For obsessive-compulsive disorder this needs to be combined with medication for the best outcomes (E) [77].

In studies where improvements in low mood or levels of anxiety have been reported, these outcomes have not been the specific target of the intervention but rather a positive subsidiary outcome of an intervention that targeted a diabetes-related outcome. For example, Grey *et al.* (B) [50] used a positive coping skills training programme in relation to an intensive insulin regimen. As well as demonstrating positive changes in relation to disease control there were also improvements in psychosocial outcomes. Programmes such as these, which have the potential to impact on a range of outcomes, could be modified to focus on improving coping abilities to reduce stress and depression in the context of diabetes.

Eating disturbance and eating disorders

Disturbed eating behaviour and eating disorders are more common in pre-teen and teenager girls with T1DM (A) [78, 79]. In a multicentre study, eating disorders were found to be more than twice as common among girls with diabetes as in their peers without diabetes (A) [80]. Even mild eating disturbances significantly increase the risk of long-term diabetes-related medical complications (B) [81] and are very common. Binge eating is reported by 60–80% of young women with T1DM (**C**) [82] and up to 38% report insulin omission to assist weight loss (**E**) [83]. Longitudinal studies indicate that early, relatively mild eating disturbances are likely to persist and worsen (**B**) [84]. There is little evidence available of effective interventions with this group of young people. In a psychoeducational intervention over six sessions for adolescent girls with disturbed eating patterns, adapted from a standardised intervention for eating disorders (**B**) [35], there were improvements in dieting and body dissatisfaction compared to the usual treatment control group but there were no improvements in insulin omission or HbA1c levels.

In the general population there is little clinical consensus on the most effective approach to treating eating disorders. Early identification and intervention is important, and any therapeutic input needs to be multifaceted, including family and individual work.

Transition from paediatric to adult services

Transition from adolescence to adulthood is a developmental phase in which lifelong patterns of self-care can become established (**E**) [85]. It is critical for long-term health outcomes that the transition from paediatric to adult services is a 'purposeful and planned movement' as defined by the position statement for the Society for Adolescent Health (**E**) [86]. The importance of this process is also underlined in the National Service Framework for Diabetes Standard 6, which states, '*All young people with diabetes will experience a smooth transition of care from paediatric diabetes services to adult services . . .*' (**E**) [87]. However it is unclear what components are necessary for this to be achieved and there are concerns that a significant proportion of young people become dislocated from the health-care system as a result (**B**) [88].

A multimethod review of transition for young people with chronic illness or disability (**E**) [89] concluded that there is a paucity of high-quality research in this area, with most of the work failing to take account of the multidimensional nature of transition. A review and analysis of 43 transition studies in young people with special health-care needs (**E**) [90] similarly concludes that the research is at a very early stage with most studies being exploratory, using a descriptive or qualitative design.

From the work that has been done, there are some central themes beginning to emerge as the basis for good practice and further research. These fall into two broad, interrelated areas: psychosocial aspects of transition and the organisation of transition.

Psychosocial aspects of transition

The work of Anderson and Wolpert (**E**) [85] takes a developmental perspective and outlines some development-based principles for clinical practice in the young adult period:

1 *The practitioner–patient relationship.* Retrospective studies have shown that irregular clinic attendance and loss to follow-up are important predictors for the ultimate development of complications of diabetes (**C**) [91]. In a comparison between four districts in the Oxford region that employed different transfer methods, prior contact with the adult physician seemed to be an important determinant of future clinic attendance (**B**) [85]. Patients respond more positively to providers who facilitate a problem-solving approach and who use a collaborative model of care provision rather than a traditional authoritarian model that can lead to patient disengagement (**E**) [92]. The focus of the consultation needs to be personally salient for the patient, reflecting their goals rather than the more abstract focus of improving control that may be perceived as too difficult to achieve (**E**) [93].

2 *Recognition of the developmental phase of the patient.* Many services already recognise the impact of pubertal and educational changes on the patient's capacity to engage with self-care. However the developmental picture is more complex than this, encompassing changes in all domains including cognitive, social, emotional, financial and familial across a broad time frame, with individuals often only taking on a fully adult role in their late twenties **(E)** [94]. These competing priorities will detract from a commitment to self-care and so it may be unrealistic to initiate significant changes in early adulthood when receptiveness to change is limited and it is experienced as a time to assert independence that often means a rejection of external control **(E)** [94].

3 *Understanding experience and expectations.* The patient's individual experience within paediatric services will influence the appropriate timing of transfer for them. When the relationship with paediatric care providers is a positive, constructive relationship, it can help individuals weather the impact on their diabetes of changes in other areas of the lives **(E)** [95]. However, if it is a more complex relationship, particularly where there have been difficulties in achieving collaborative working, it may be better for the young person to make a fresh start with the adult provider, particularly when that service has experience with adolescents and young adults **(B)** [96]. At the point of transition it may be valuable to assess the patients' expectations of the change: do they regard it as a pragmatic change with no implications for their behaviour or is it seen as an opportunity for a new start with possibilities of change?

The organisation of transition

In a review of practice, Viner **(E)** [97] outlines six key principles of a good transition programme:

1 *Policy on timing of transfer.* Whilst a flexible approach is important to respond to the developmental readiness of the individual and the particular circumstances of the adult services, a target transfer age is useful, preferably after many of the developmental milestones are passed, e.g. growth is complete, they have left school, etc.

2 *Preparation period and education programme.* The young people should only be transferred once they are able to manage their diabetes largely independently. Young people should be able to contribute to the planning of the process and receive appropriate education to equip them for independence.

3 *Coordinated transfer process.* In the year leading up to transfer, the young person should have a timetable of the process and should attend at least one clinic in the adult service.

4 *Interested and capable adult service.* The transition programme can only be successful if the staff from the adult service are fully engaged with it.

5 *Administrative support.* Resources are required to ensure that the organisational aspects of transition are efficiently managed, e.g. appointments sent, medical records available, etc.

6 *Primary care involvement.* Transition planning needs to include the primary care team that can provide continuity during the transition.

Conclusions

In summary, despite some recent methodological improvements, the literature regarding psychoeducational interventions in childhood T1DM remains difficult to interpret due to low participation rates, small, unrepresentative samples, unstandardised measures of poorly defined constructs, selection bias, varied methods and instruments and multiple components to the intervention, making it difficult in those studies that have produced beneficial outcomes to identify the key elements responsible for these changes (**B**) [98]. Despite the well-recognised interrelationship between psychological health and diabetes outcomes, there is a dearth of intervention research targeting specific mental health difficulties, such as anxiety and depression. There is also very little work with the pre-teenage group in any domain. There needs to be more work on adapting research in other areas, targeting these difficulties, taking note of the Hampson review's conclusion that theoretically driven intervention-generated larger effect sizes than atheoretical ones (**A**) [8]. It is also clear that routine mental health screening as instituted in Royal Children's Hospital, Melbourne (**B**) [99], could help facilitate early identification of high-risk subgroups within the clinic.

References

1 Matyka KA, Wigg L, Pramming S *et al*. Cognitive function and mood after profound nocturnal hypoglycaemia in prepubertal children with conventional insulin treatment for diabetes. *Arch Dis Child* 1999; **81**: 138–42.

2 Evans CL, Hughes IA. The relationship between diabetic control and individual and family characteristics. *J Psychosom Res* 1987; **31**: 367–74.

3 Goldston DB, Kelley AE, Reboussin DM *et al*. Suicidal ideation and behavior and noncompliance with the medical regimen among diabetic adolescents. *J Am Acad Child Adolesc Psychiatry* 1997; **36**: 1528–36.

4 Lowes L, Lyne P, Gregory JW. Childhood diabetes: parents' experience of home management and the first year following diagnosis. *Diabet Med* 2004; **21**: 531–8.

5 Jacobson AM. The psychological care of patients with insulin-dependent diabetes mellitus. *N Engl J Med* 1996; **334**: 1249–53.

6 Blanz BJ, Rensch-Riemann BS, Fritz-Sigmund DI *et al*. IDDM is a risk factor for adolescent psychiatric disorders. *Diabetes Care* 1993; **16**: 1579–87.

7 Kovacs M, Goldston D, Obrosky DS *et al*. Psychiatric disorders in youths with IDDM: rates and risk factors. *Diabetes Care* 1997; **20**: 36–44.

8 Hampson SE, Skinner TC, Hart J *et al*. Effects of educational and psychosocial interventions for adolescents with diabetes mellitus: a systematic review. *Health Technol Assess* 2001; **5**: 1–79.

9 Murphy HR, Rayman G, Skinner TC. Psycho-educational interventions for children and young people with type 1 diabetes. *Diabet Med* 2006; **23**: 935–43.

10 Vanelli M, Chiari G, Ghizzoni L *et al*. Effectiveness of a prevention program for diabetic ketoacidosis in children: an 8-year study in schools and private practices. *Diabetes Care* 1999; **22**: 7–9.

11 Siminerio LM, Charron-Prochownik D, Banion C *et al*. Comparing outpatient and inpatient diabetes education for newly diagnosed pediatric patients. *Diabetes Educ* 1999; **25**: 895–906.

12 Swift PG, Hearnshaw JR, Botha JL *et al*. A decade of diabetes: keeping children out of hospital. *BMJ* 1993; **307**: 96–8.

13 Simell T, Kaprio EA, Maenpaa J *et al*. Randomised prospective study of short-term and long-term initial stay in hospital by children with diabetes mellitus. *Lancet* 1991; **337**: 656–60.

14 Sundelin J, Forsander G, Mattson SE. Family-oriented support at the onset of diabetes mellitus: a comparison of two group conditions during 2 years following diagnosis. *Acta Paediatr* 1996; **85**: 49–55.

15 Delamater AM, Bubb J, Davis SG *et al*. Randomized prospective study of self-management training with newly diagnosed diabetic children. *Diabetes Care* 1990; **13**: 492–8.

16 Forsander GA, Sundelin J, Persson B. Influence of the initial management regimen and family social situation on glycemic control and medical care in children with type I diabetes mellitus. *Acta Paediatr* 2000; **89**: 1462–8.

17 Sullivan-Bolyai S, Grey M, Deatrick J *et al*. Helping other mothers effectively work at raising young children with type 1 diabetes. *Diabetes Educ* 2004; **30**: 476–84.

18 Anderson BJ, Auslander WF, Jung KC *et al*. Assessing family sharing of diabetes responsibilities. *J Pediatr Psychol* 1990; **15**: 477–92.

19 Anderson BJ, Wolf FM, Burkhart MT *et al.* Effects of peer-group intervention on metabolic control of adolescents with IDDM: randomized outpatient study. *Diabetes Care* 1989; **12**: 179–83.

20 Anderson BJ, Brackett J, Ho J *et al.* An office-based intervention to maintain parent-adolescent teamwork in diabetes management: impact on parent involvement, family conflict, and subsequent glycemic control. *Diabetes Care* 1999; **22**: 713–21.

21 Boardway RH, Delamater AM, Tomakowsky J *et al.* Stress management training for adolescents with diabetes. *J Pediatr Psychol* 1993; **18**: 29–45.

22 Brown SJ, Lieberman DA, Germeny BA *et al.* Educational video game for juvenile diabetes: results of a controlled trial. *Med Inform (Lond)* 1997; **22**: 77–89.

23 Cook S, Herold K, Edidin DV *et al.* Increasing problem solving in adolescents with type 1 diabetes: the choices diabetes program. *Diabetes Educ* 2002; **28**: 115–24.

24 Daley BJ. Sponsorship for adolescents with diabetes. *Health Soc Work* 1992; **17**: 173–82.

25 Gilbertson HR, Brand-Miller JC, Thorburn AW *et al.* The effect of flexible low glycemic index dietary advice versus measured carbohydrate exchange diets on glycemic control in children with type 1 diabetes. *Diabetes Care* 2001; **24**: 1137–43.

26 Grey M, Boland EA, Davidson M *et al.* Coping skills training for youth with diabetes mellitus has long-lasting effects on metabolic control and quality of life. *J Pediatr* 2000; **137**: 107–13.

27 Grey M, Boland EA, Davidson M *et al.* Short-term effects of coping skills training as adjunct to intensive therapy in adolescents. *Diabetes Care* 1998; **21**: 902–8.

28 Hains AA, Davies WH, Parton E *et al.* A stress management intervention for adolescents with type 1 diabetes. *Diabetes Educ* 2000; **26**: 417–24.

29 Hansson K, Ryden O, Johnsson P. Parent-rated family climate: a concomitant to metabolic control in juvenile IDDM. *Fam Syst Med* 2006; **12**: 405–13.

30 Howells L, Wilson AC, Skinner TC *et al.* A randomized control trial of the effect of negotiated telephone support on glycaemic control in young people with type 1 diabetes. *Diabet Med* 2002; **19**: 643–8.

31 Laffel LM, Vangsness L, Connell A *et al.* Impact of ambulatory, family-focused teamwork intervention on glycemic control in youth with type 1 diabetes. *J Pediatr* 2003; **142**: 409–16.

32 Ludvigsson J, Hanas R. Continuous subcutaneous glucose monitoring improved metabolic control in pediatric patients with type 1 diabetes: a controlled crossover study. *Pediatrics* 2003; **111**: 933–8.

33 Marrero DG, Vandagriff JL, Kronz K *et al.* Using telecommunication technology to manage children with diabetes: the Computer-Linked Outpatient Clinic (CLOC) Study. *Diabetes Educ* 1995; **21**: 313–19.

34 McNabb WL, Quinn MT, Murphy DM *et al.* Increasing children's responsibility for diabetes self-care: the in control study. *Diabetes Educ* 1994; **20**: 121–4.

35 Olmsted MP, Daneman D, Rydall AC *et al.* The effects of psychoeducation on disturbed eating attitudes and behavior in young women with type 1 diabetes mellitus. *Int J Eat Disord* 2002; **32**: 230–9.

36 Satin W, La Greca AM, Zigo MA *et al.* Diabetes in adolescence: effects of multifamily group intervention and parent simulation of diabetes. *J Pediatr Psychol* 1989; **14**: 259–75.

37 Wysocki T, Harris MA, Greco P *et al.* Randomized, controlled trial of behavior therapy for families of adolescents with insulin-dependent diabetes mellitus. *J Pediatr Psychol* 2000; **25**: 23–33.

38 Viner RM, Christie D, Taylor V *et al.* Motivational/solution-focused intervention improves HbA1c in adolescents with type 1 diabetes: a pilot study. *Diabet Med* 2003; **20**: 739–42.

39 Couper JJ, Taylor J, Fotheringham MJ *et al.* Failure to maintain the benefits of home-based intervention in adolescents with poorly controlled type 1 diabetes. *Diabetes Care* 1999; **22**: 1933–7.

40 Armour TA, Norris SL, Jack L, Jr, *et al.* The effectiveness of family interventions in people with diabetes mellitus: a systematic review. *Diabet Med* 2005; **22**: 1295–1305.

41 Bloomfield S, Calder JE, Chisholm V *et al.* A project in diabetes education for children. *Diabet Med* 1990; **7**: 137–42.

42 Dougherty G, Schiffrin A, White D *et al.* Home-based management can achieve intensification cost-effectively in type I diabetes. *Pediatrics* 1999; **103**: 122–8.

43 Hackett AF, Court S, Matthews JN *et al.* Do education groups help diabetics and their parents? *Arch Dis Child* 1989; **64**: 997–1003.

44 Mendez FX, Olivares J, Ros MC *et al.* Applicability of the Parent's stress reduction strategies on the children with insulin-dependent diabetes mellitus. *Analisis y Modificacion Conducta* 1997; **23**: 669.

45 Wing RR, Marcus MD, Epstein LH *et al.* A 'family-based' approach to the treatment of obese type II diabetic patients. *J Consult Clin Psychol* 1991; **59**: 156–62.

46 Wysocki T, Greco P, Harris MA *et al*. Behavior therapy for families of adolescents with diabetes: maintenance of treatment effects. *Diabetes Care* 2001; **24**: 441–6.

47 Channon S, Huws-Thomas MV, Rollnick S *et al*. Beneficial long-term effects of motivational interviewing (MI) in adolescents with insulin dependent diabetes mellitus: a multicentre randomised controlled trial. *Pediatr Diabetes* 2005; **6**(suppl 3): 29.

48 Greco P, Pendley JS, McDonell K *et al*. A peer group intervention for adolescents with type 1 diabetes and their best friends. *J Pediatr Psychol* 2001; **26**: 485–90.

49 Grey M, Boland EA, Davidson M *et al*. Coping skills training for youths with diabetes on intensive therapy. *Appl Nurs Res* 1999; **12**: 3–12.

50 Grey M, Davidson M, Boland EA *et al*. Clinical and psychosocial factors associated with achievement of treatment goals in adolescents with diabetes mellitus. *J Adolesc Health* 2001; **28**: 377–85.

51 Channon S, Smith VJ, Gregory JW. A pilot study of motivational interviewing in adolescents with diabetes. *Arch Dis Child* 2003; **88**: 680–3.

52 Svoren BM, Butler D, Levine BS *et al*. Reducing acute adverse outcomes in youths with type 1 diabetes: a randomized, controlled trial. *Pediatrics* 2003; **112**: 914–22.

53 Nordfeldt S, Johansson C, Carlsson E *et al*. Prevention of severe hypoglycaemia in type I diabetes: a randomised controlled population study. *Arch Dis Child* 2003; **88**: 240–5.

54 Resnick MD, Bearman PS, Blum RW *et al*. Protecting adolescents from harm. Findings from the National Longitudinal Study on Adolescent Health. *JAMA* 1997; **278**: 823–32.

55 Skinner TC, Murphy H, Hews-Thomas MV. Diabetes in adolescents. In: Snoek FJ, Skinner TC, eds. *Psychology in Diabetes Care*, 2nd edn. J Wiley and Sons, London, 2005: 25–59.

56 Byard AJ, Murphy HR, Skinner TC *et al*. The development evaluation and evolution of a paediatric carbohydrate counting programme from the Family and Teamwork Study (FACTS). *Diabet Med* 2004; **21**(suppl 2): A86.

57 Murphy HR, Skinner TC, Wadham C *et al*. The Families and Children Teamwork Study (FACTS). *Diabet Med* 2004; **21**(suppl 2): A84.

58 Schafer LC, Glasgow RE, McCaul KD *et al*. Adherence to IDDM regimens: relationship to psychosocial variables and metabolic control. *Diabetes Care* 1983; **6**: 493–8.

59 Fuligni AJ, Eccles JS, Barber BL *et al*. Early adolescent peer orientation and adjustment during high school. *Dev Psychol* 2001; **37**: 28–36.

60 Thomas AM, Peterson L, Goldstein D. Problem solving and diabetes regimen adherence by children and adolescents with IDDM in social pressure situations: a reflection of normal development. *J Pediatr Psychol* 1997; **22**: 541–61.

61 La Greca AM, Auslander WF, Greco P *et al*. I get by with a little help from my family and friends: adolescents' support for diabetes care. *J Pediatr Psychol* 1995; **20**: 449–76.

62 Schroff-Pendley J, Kasmen LJ, Miller DL *et al*. Peer and family support in children and adolescents with type 1 diabetes. *J Pediatr Psychol* 2002; **27**: 429–38.

63 Dantzer C, Swendsen J, Maurice-Tison S *et al*. Anxiety and depression in juvenile diabetes: a critical review. *Clin Psychol Rev* 2003; **23**: 787–800.

64 Garrison MM, Katon WJ, Richardson LP. The impact of psychiatric comorbidities on readmissions for diabetes in youth. *Diabetes Care* 2005; **28**: 2150–4.

65 Mayou R, Peveler R, Davies B *et al*. Psychiatric morbidity in young adults with insulin-dependent diabetes mellitus. *Psychol Med* 1991; **21**: 639–45.

66 Kokkonen J, Kokkonen ER. Mental health and social adaptation in young adults with juvenile-onset diabetes. *Nord J Psychiatry* 1995; **49**: 175–81.

67 La Greca AM, Swales T, Klemp S *et al*. Adolescents with diabetes: gender differences in psychosocial functioning and glycaemic control. *Child Health Care* 1995; **24**: 61–78.

68 Stewart SM, Rao U, White P. Depression and diabetes in children and adolescents. *Curr Opin Pediatr* 2005; **17**: 626–31.

69 Lewinsohn PM, Solomon A, Seeley JR *et al*. Clinical implications of 'subthreshold' depressive symptoms. *J Abnorm Psychol* 2000; **109**: 345–51.

70 Chernoff RG, Ireys HT, DeVet KA *et al*. A randomized, controlled trial of a community-based support program for families of children with chronic illness: pediatric outcomes. *Arch Pediatr Adolesc Med* 2002; **156**: 533–9.

71 Harrington R, Whittaker J, Shoebridge P. Psychological treatment of depression in children and adolescents: a review of treatment research. *Br J Psychiatry* 1998; **173**: 291–8.

72 Reinecke MA, Ryan NE, DuBois DL. Cognitive-behavioral therapy of depression and depressive symptoms during adolescence: a review and meta-analysis. *J Am Acad Child Adolesc Psychiatry* 1998; **37**: 26–34.

73 Brent DA, Holder D, Kolko D *et al.* A clinical psychotherapy trial for adolescent depression comparing cognitive, family, and supportive therapy. *Arch Gen Psychiatry* 1997; **54**: 877–85.

74 Bernstein GA, Borchardt CM, Perwien AR. Anxiety disorders in children and adolescents: a review of the past 10 years. *J Am Acad Child Adolesc Psychiatry* 1996; **35**: 1110–19.

75 Dadds MR, Spence SH, Holland DE *et al.* Prevention and early intervention for anxiety disorders: a controlled trial. *J Consult Clin Psychol* 1997; **65**: 627–35.

76 Flannery-Schroeder EC, Kendall PC. group and individual cognitive-behavioral treatments for youth with anxiety disorders: a randomized clinical trial. *Cognit Ther Res* 2000; **24**: 251–78.

77 March JS, Franklin M, Nelson A *et al.* Cognitive-behavioral psychotherapy for pediatric obsessive-compulsive disorder. *J Clin Child Psychol* 2001; **30**: 8–18.

78 Colton P, Olmsted M, Daneman D *et al.* Disturbed eating behavior and eating disorders in preteen and early teenage girls with type 1 diabetes: a case-controlled study. *Diabetes Care* 2004; **27**: 1654–9.

79 Nielsen S. Eating disorders in females with type 1 diabetes: an update of a meta-analysis. *Eur Eat Disord Rev* 2002; **10**: 241–54.

80 Jones JM, Lawson ML, Daneman D *et al.* Eating disorders in adolescent females with and without type 1 diabetes: cross sectional study. *BMJ* 2000; **320**: 1563–1566.

81 Rydall AC, Rodin GM, Olmsted MP *et al.* Disordered eating behavior and microvascular complications in young women with insulin-dependent diabetes mellitus. *N Engl J Med* 1997; **336**: 1849–54.

82 Stancin T, Link DL, Reuter JM. Binge eating and purging in young women with IDDM. *Diabetes Care* 1989; **12**: 601–603.

83 Crow SJ, Keel PK, Kendall D. Eating disorders and insulin-dependent diabetes mellitus. *Psychosomatics* 1998; **39**: 233–43.

84 Bryden KS, Neil A, Mayou RA *et al.* Eating habits, body weight, and insulin misuse: a longitudinal study of teenagers and young adults with type 1 diabetes. *Diabetes Care* 1999; **22**: 1956–60.

85 Anderson BJ, Wolpert HA. A developmental perspective on the challenges of diabetes education and care during the young adult period. *Patient Educ Couns* 2004; **53**: 347–52.

86 Blum RW, Garell D, Hodgman CH *et al.* Transition from child-centered to adult health-care systems for adolescents with chronic conditions. A position paper of the Society for Adolescent Medicine. *J Adolesc Health* 1993; **14**: 570–6.

87 Diabetes NSF Implementation Group. *National Service Framework for Diabetes: Delivery Strategy*, 2002. Available at: http://www.dh.gov.uk/prod_consum_dh/groups/dh_digitalassets/@dh/@en/documents/digitalasset/dh_4032823.pdf

88 Kipps S, Bahu T, Ong K *et al.* Current methods of transfer of young people with type 1 diabetes to adult services. *Diabet Med* 2002; **19**: 649–54.

89 Forbes A, While A, Ullman R, Lewis S, Mathes L, Griffiths P. A multi-method review to identify components of practice which may promote continuity in the transition from child to adult care for young people with chronic illness or disability. *Report for the National Co-ordinating Centre for NHS Delivery and Organisation R&D (NDDSCO)*, 2001.

90 Betz CL. Transition of adolescents with special health care needs: review and analysis of the literature. *Issues Compr Pediatr Nurs* 2004; **27**: 179–241.

91 Jacobson AM, Adler AG, Derby L *et al.* Clinic attendance and glycemic control: study of contrasting groups of patients with IDDM. *Diabetes Care* 1991; **14**: 599–601.

92 Wolpert HA. Working with young adults who have type 1 diabetes. In: Anderson B, Rubin R, eds. *Practical Psychology for Diabetes Clinicians*, 2nd edn. American Diabetes Association, Alexandria, VA, 2002: 161–70.

93 Rollnick S, Mason P, Butler C. *Health Behavior Change: A guide for Practitioners.* Churchill Livingstone, Edinburgh, 1999.

94 Arnett JJ. Emerging adulthood: a theory of development from the late teens through the twenties. *Am Psychol* 2000; **55**: 469–80.

95 Betts PR, Jefferson IG, Swift PG. Diabetes care in childhood and adolescence. *Diabet Med* 2002; **19**(suppl 4): 61–5.

96 Orr DP, Fineberg NS, Gray DL. Glycemic control and transfer of health care among adolescents with insulin dependent diabetes mellitus. *J Adolesc Health* 1996; **18**: 44–7.

97 Viner R. Effective transition from paediatric to adult services. *Hosp Med* 2000; **61**: 341–3.

98 Northam EA, Todd S, Cameron FJ. Interventions to promote optimal health outcomes in children with type 1 diabetes – are they effective? *Diabet Med* 2006; **23**: 113–21.

99 Cameron FJ, Smidts D, Hesketh K *et al*. Early detection of emotional and behavioural problems in children with diabetes: the validity of the Child Health Questionnaire as a screening instrument. *Diabet Med* 2003; **20**: 646–50.

CHAPTER 11

Screening for associated conditions and prevention of complications

Catherine Peters & Jeremy Allgrove

Be not astonished at new ideas; for it is well known to you that a thing does not therefore cease to be true because it is not accepted by many.
—Baruch Spinoza, Dutch philosopher (1632–1677)

Introduction

Since the discovery of insulin and its first use in 1922, it has become apparent that treating diabetes with insulin, whilst life saving, is not the only requirement for a healthy life. Since type 1 diabetes mellitus (T1DM) is principally an autoimmune condition, it is not surprising that other autoimmune diseases may be associated with it. This is now recognised to be the case. However, a balance has to be struck between screening for these and identifying additional problems when they arise. This balance is dependent on how often the condition readily manifests itself (i.e. whether or not it may remain 'silent'), how frequently it occurs and what therapy, if any, is available to treat it (i.e. how cost-effective screening is).

Furthermore, it is now well recognised that complications directly related to the presence of the diabetes itself are common and that good control can prevent or delay the onset of these.

Nevertheless, some patients, however well controlled, still develop complications or have associated problems, such as hypertension, which increase the likelihood of complications developing and it is now well established that these should be screened for in adult patients. The situation is not so clear in children and adolescents. This chapter reviews the data available concerning screening for associated conditions and complications specifically in children and adolescents.

Screening for associated conditions

Thyroid disease

It has long been recognised that there is an increased incidence of autoimmune thyroid disease, particularly hypothyroidism, in T1DM (**B**) [1–5]. Studies have shown that antithyroid antibodies, either thyroid peroxidase (TPO) (**B**) [6–10], most commonly, or thyroglobulin (TgA) (**B**) [11], are present in 8–50% of patients. Only a proportion of patients with positive thyroid antibodies develop biochemical or clinical abnormalities (**B**) [12] and most studies have found that about 4–10% of children and adolescents with

T1DM have associated thyroid disease, as defined by raised thyroid-stimulating hormone (TSH) with or without low free thyroxine (fT_4) (**B**) [13].

TPO antibodies have proved to be the most predictive of thyroid autoimmunity (**B**) [13]. Titres rise with age, particularly after the age of 10 years, and are more common in girls than boys (**A, B**) [11, 14–18]. In some studies (**B**) [19, 20], though not others (**A, B**) [16, 21], the presence of antiglutamic acid dehydrogenase (GAD-65) antibodies increases the likelihood of TgA and particularly TPO antibodies. All racial groups are affected (**A, B**) [16, 22–27], although susceptibility varies between them. Screening for thyroid disease in T1DM was first recommended in 1981 (**B**) [28] and has since been endorsed by many authors. It is now recommended that screening for thyroid disease in T1DM should be undertaken annually (**E**) [29–31].

Screening for thyroid disease

The method of screening is somewhat controversial. Some authors (**B**) [12, 32] recommend that this is done by testing for thyroid antibodies with follow-up of those who are antibody positive. Others have suggested that TPO antibodies and TSH are the most cost-effective methods (**B**) [13]. The measurement of TPO antibodies has been questioned as not having a very high specificity, and some authors suggest that TSH is the most effective method of screening. Some clinics prefer to screen for raised TSH using capillary blood spot sampling, as this does not require venepuncture and is particularly useful in very young patients. If TSH is raised (or undetectable), thyroid antibodies can be done to confirm the diagnosis of autoimmune thyroid disease, even if the fT_4 is normal.

There is no evidence, at least in children with the Hashimoto thyroiditis, to support the treatment of antibody-positive patients who have a normal TSH (**B**) [33], so the identification of positive antithyroid antibodies has no clinical relevance. It therefore follows that the most logical approach is to screen patients annually with TSH ($\pm fT_4$) and to confirm the diagnosis with TPO antibodies if necessary. This was the conclusion of the West Midlands Health Technology Assessment Collaboration (**A**) [34] and is the policy pursued in our clinic. It enables patients whose thyroid function is becoming compromised to be treated during the development of the autoimmune process, often before they become symptomatic. Both the National Institute for Clinical Excellence (NICE) (**E**) [31] and the International Society for Pediatric and Adolescent Diabetes (ISPAD) (**E**) [29] guidelines recommend using thyroid function tests as the best method of annual screening and to repeat these at annual intervals.

The ISPAD guidelines suggest that thyroid antibodies should be done at the time of diagnosis and other authors state that thyroid screening should be undertaken at this time. Ketoacidosis is associated with preferential deiodination of thyroxine to reverse T_3 (**A, B**) [35–37] and if present, it may be associated with a 'sick euthyroid' syndrome that may confuse the picture (**A, B**) [38–40]. Screening for thyroid disease should therefore be delayed until after initial stabilisation and treatment of diabetic ketoacidosis.

Hyperthyroidism

Thyrotoxicosis develops much less frequently than does hypothyroidism in association with T1DM (**B, C**) [18, 41–44]. Occasionally, its occurrence will be detected on TSH screening but it is usually diagnosed on overt clinical grounds.

Coeliac disease

Background and definition

Coeliac disease is caused by an inflammatory reaction to dietary gluten, leading to small intestinal villous atrophy and varying degrees of malabsorption. The European Society of Paediatric Gastroenterology, Hepatology and Nutrition (ESPGHAN) criteria recommend that the diagnosis is made on the basis of small intestinal biopsy related to a gluten challenge (E) [45]. The intestinal changes should resolve after elimination of dietary gluten. Silent coeliac disease is characterised by the typical gut changes seen in coeliac disease, i.e. villous atrophy and crypt hyperplasia, but without symptoms (E) [46].

Prevalence

Coeliac disease was first reported in association with diabetes in 1969 (C) [47] and it is now recognised to be the second most common autoimmune condition associated with diabetes after hypothyroidism. There appear to be wide geographical differences in prevalence with an average prevalence of 4.5% calculated from worldwide screening studies of diabetic children (C) [48 and references 8–33 therein]. The prevalence of coeliac disease appears to be particularly high in regions of Saharan Africa (B) [49], with an estimated prevalence of 16.4% in diabetic children screened in Algeria (B) [50]. Most prevalence data are based on autoantibody screening tests.

The differences in prevalence may be partly explained by genetic susceptibility and the presence of common HLA markers DR3 and DQ2. In European countries, the risk of coeliac disease in diabetic children is increased by the presence of HLA-DQB1*02-DQA1*05 and by TNF-308A (B) [51]. However, at this time, genetic testing and subsequent clinical predictions for the timing of coeliac disease screening in diabetic children are not possible.

Presentation and diagnosis

In patients with diabetes and coeliac disease, up to 88% are diagnosed with diabetes first (C) [52]. Coeliac disease can present at any age in childhood or adulthood, and there may be a period of subclinical or latent coeliac disease with minimal symptoms (E) [46]. However, after the diagnosis of coeliac disease is made, there may have retrospectively been subtle complaints in those thought to be asymptomatic. The risk of the subclinical state is unclear, but children are at risk of developing gluten intolerance at a later date (E) [46].

The classical presentation of a young child with coeliac disease includes failure to thrive, diarrhoea with pale stools, abdominal bloating, buttock wasting and miserable affect, with the onset occurring shortly after the introduction of dietary gluten. The presentation of older children may be more variable with short stature, poor weight gain, diarrhoea and/or constipation, anaemia and delayed puberty (E) [53].

Complications of coeliac disease

Malabsorption can lead to vitamin D deficiency and rickets. Impaired bone mineralisation may also lead to later osteoporosis or osteopaenia (A) [54], and there are reports of an increase in bone fractures in adults with untreated coeliac disease (B) [55].

Untreated coeliac disease may also lead to other complications in adulthood, such as reproductive disorders including infertility (B) [56, 57], and there is an increased risk of non-Hodgkin's lymphoma of the small bowel and other gastrointestinal cancers (**B, A**) [49, 58, 59].

Treatment of coeliac disease

After a diagnosis of coeliac disease is confirmed by small bowel biopsy, patients are advised to commence a gluten-free diet (GFD). This dietary restriction may be particularly difficult for the child with diabetes, but in Europe many food stores have targeted this section of the market with better labelling of products and more availability of specific gluten-free products. In the UK, it is possible to prescribe certain gluten-free products.

Treatment with a GFD in symptomatic patients has been shown to improve the symptoms, signs and complications of coeliac disease. However, the effects of a GFD on diabetic control are less well established. Initial reports of improved hypoglycaemic control were based on children who were diagnosed with coeliac disease associated with malabsorption (**A**) [60], but there have subsequently been reports of improvement in diabetic patients with subclinical coeliac disease (**C**) [61]. There are other studies reporting no effect, improved control and improvement of number of hypoglycaemic episodes (**C**) [48].

Screening

The case for (and against) screening diabetic children for coeliac disease is controversial, and there is no clear consensus. Asymptomatic patients with subclinical disease may be difficult to detect, but some clinicians claim that accurate and astute questioning of the patient should reveal symptoms and signs indicating the possibility of coeliac disease (**E**) [62]. However, some symptoms, such as growth failure or delayed puberty, may be attributed to poor glycaemic control rather than coeliac disease itself (**C**) [61].

The ISPAD guidelines recommend that immunological screening for diabetes should be considered close to the time of diagnosis of diabetes and repeated if clinical circumstances suggest the possibility of coeliac disease (**E**) [29]. They recommend the use of endomyseal antibodies (EMA) as the most specific test but caution that this should be combined with total IgA to exclude false-negative results.

An extensive systematic review studying the role of autoantibody testing for coeliac disease in newly diagnosed children with diabetes was carried out in 2004 on behalf of the National Health Service Health Technology Assessment programme in the UK (**A**) [34]. The panel concluded that IgA EMA appeared to be the most accurate test with the highest pooled positive likelihood ratios and lowest negative likelihood ratio. However, if an enzyme-linked immunosorbent assay was required, tissue transglutaminase (TTG) is the most likely to be accurate. Relatively few (20.9%) of the previous studies have used TTG as a screening test (**A**) [34]. However, it is becoming more commonplace, as it can be automated. Our own studies suggest that some patients may have positive TTG but negative EMA antibodies. These were found to be biopsy negative in all cases, in contrast to those with positive antibodies to both (**C**) [63]. This is supported by other studies which suggest that the presence of antibodies to both antigens is associated with an abnormal biopsy in most cases (**A, B**) [64, 65].

The health economic model used for the health technology assessment report found that screening is cost-effective but was unable to conclude when or how frequently screening should be undertaken. Given that patients with diabetes have a lifelong risk of developing coeliac disease, the optimum interval between screens is yet to be determined. In a 6-year prospective study of 273 diabetic children from diagnosis by Barera *et al.* (**B**) [66], coeliac disease was found in 3.3% of children at diagnosis and a further 2.9% over the next 4 years. No child was found to have coeliac disease after 4 years from diagnosis. This suggests that the greatest detection rate is likely to be in the first few years after diagnosis but later occurrence cannot be excluded.

Screening for other autoimmune conditions

Many of the studies that have looked at the prevalence of thyroid and/or coeliac disease have also considered the presence of antibodies to other organs, particularly gastric parietal cells and adrenal glands. Some of these have demonstrated these antibodies in a high proportion of patients, though less frequently than thyroid or coeliac antibodies (**B, E**) [3, 7, 15, 43, 67, 68].

In practice, the association of the Addison disease with T1DM is rare and, even if adrenal antibodies are present, adrenal function usually remains normal (**B**) [69]. Current guidelines make no recommendations for screening for the Addison disease.

Screening for complications of diabetes

It has long been recognised that diabetes is associated with a variety of complications. They occur in both T1DM and T2DM. The most clinically significant of these are microalbuminuria, which may lead to frank proteinuria and ultimately to chronic renal failure (CRF), retinopathy, which may result in blindness, and macrovascular disease, associated with coronary heart, cerebrovascular and peripheral vascular disease. Although there has been some improvement in the prevalence of these complications in the past few years, diabetes remains the leading cause of dialysis-dependent CRF, blindness and coronary heart disease in Western societies. In addition, peripheral neuropathy may lead to loss of all modalities of sensation that, together with micro- and macrovascular abnormalities, increases the likelihood of ulceration of the leg and contributes to arthropathy and altered microvascular responses to normal stimuli. *Necrobiosis lipoidica* (see below) may also develop and may even be present at diagnosis. Autonomic neuropathy may be associated with absence of the normal nocturnal reduction in blood pressure, loss of normal heart rate variation and abnormal pupillary responses. It may lead to impotence in males. Changes in the skin and limitation of movement of the small joints of the hand have also been described and may be the first indication that microvascular changes are occurring even before these become clinically relevant. Alterations of growth and abnormalities of tooth eruption and propensity to tooth decay may also be associated with diabetes.

The Diabetes Control and Complications Trial (DCCT) (**A**) [70] showed that, in adolescents and young adults, the time taken for clinically significant complications to occur could be increased, and early complications could be reversed, by maintaining good diabetic control or improving poor control. However, the prevalence of complications during the prepubertal years is low. Furthermore, there has been debate as to how much influence the presence of diabetes during the prepubertal years affects the likelihood of developing complications later.

As with any screening programme, the costs and inconvenience must be weighed against the potential benefits, particularly where identifying and treating early complications may prevent the more serious late ones. In adults, the cost benefits of screening for nephropathy, neuropathy, hypertension, retinopathy and hyperlipidaemia are well established and current guidelines recommend a programme of screening for all of these (**E**) [31]. The benefits of screening in children and adolescents, particularly the former, are less clear-cut and, in some cases, there is a lack of agreement. Nevertheless, it is incumbent upon paediatric and adolescent physicians to be aware of the possibility of complications and, where relevant, to screen for them.

Complications for which screening procedures are usually performed

Growth

There are conflicting data about growth parameters at diagnosis. Some authors claim that height is above average (**B**) [71, 72], whilst others claim that this is not the case (**A**) [73]. It may depend on the time over which the diabetes has developed. Several studies to date suggest a trend towards an increase in body mass index (BMI) in children with diabetes at diagnosis (**B, A**) [74–77]. It is suggested that this increase in BMI is one reason for the increasing incidence of diabetes and supports the 'accelerator hypothesis' (**B**) [78]. This effect of increased BMI is particularly noted in children of a younger age (**A**) [77], although there is evidence that in children under the age of 5, there is a decrease in growth parameters after 5 years of diabetes duration (**C**) [79].

Growth and puberty usually progress normally during adolescence even when diabetic control is only 'adequate' (**B**) [80, 81]. However, in older children, particularly pubertal females, there is a trend of weight gain, which may represent poor metabolic control and increased insulin resistance (**B**) [79, 82–84]. This pubertal weight gain seems to stabilise after adolescence with improving metabolic control (**B**) [83].

There are few data on final height in children with diabetes and these studies are conflicting. Some reports suggest that diabetic children can be expected to reach their target final height (**B**) [72], with others suggesting a possible reduction in final height (**A, B**) [84–86]. There is some evidence that blunting of the pubertal growth spurt may occur in diabetic adolescents and this may contribute to a reduced final height (**B, A**) [84, 85]. The reported reduction in final height may also relate to poorer glycaemic control in adolescence (**B**) [86].

Insulin sensitivity varies during adolescence but is negatively related to BMI. Insulin clearance rates are highest during midpuberty when insulin resistance is at its greatest (**B**) [87]. IGF-1 levels do not rise during puberty as much as in normal non-diabetic controls despite higher than normal growth hormone levels and this is related to poor diabetic control (**B, A**) [88, 89] and growth hormone binding protein concentrations are lower than in normal controls. This may reflect a degree of growth hormone resistance during puberty.

Poor diabetes control is associated with slowing of growth after diagnosis and some pubertal delay. In its most extreme form, the Mauriac syndrome, a combination of short stature, delayed puberty and hepatomegaly may rarely develop (**A**) [90].

All of the published guidelines recommend that children should be weighed and measured at each clinic visit, BMI calculated and the results plotted, as part of the surveillance of diabetic care. One of the goals of good care is to ensure that growth and development are as normal as possible, and abnormalities in height of weight may indicate that optimum control is not being achieved or, in some cases, that other associated conditions have supervened (e.g. hypothyroidism or coeliac disease).

Nephropathy

Diabetes may affect both renal glomerular and tubular function (**B**) [91]. The most commonly used method for detecting abnormal function is to measure some modality of microalbuminuria. This can be done either on a random or early morning sample measuring albumin-to-creatinine ratio (ACR) or on a timed sample, taken overnight (**B, E**) [92, 93] or over 24 hours, to measure albumin excretion rate (AER) or total albumin excretion (**B**) [94]. Significant microalbuminuria is usually defined as either a rate >15 μg/min or >30 mg/d or ACR of >2.5 mg/mmol in females or >3.5 mg/mmol in males.

Using one or other of these methods, microalbuminuria has been found to be present in up to 35% of patients and increases with duration of diabetes at least up to 10 years after diagnosis (**B**) [95]. It is rarely identified in children who have had their diabetes for fewer than 5 years (**B**) [96] or those who are prepubertal (**B**) [97]. In many instances the microalbuminuria is intermittent (**B**) [98] and may depend on the time of day at which the sample is taken (**A**) [99]. The presence of persistent microalbuminuria, defined as raised AER on two out of three consecutive occasions within a 3–6-month period, and the risk of progressing to renal failure is increased by the coexistence of hypertension (**A**) [100, 101] and poor diabetic control. Nephropathy may be associated with markers of polyneuropathy (**A**) [102, 103].

Most paediatric guidelines recommend starting to screen annually for microalbuminuria from the age of 11 or 12 years.

Hypertension

A review of the literature by a US working group has led to the development of definitions for hypertension in childhood (**E**) [104]. Blood pressure centiles for sex, age and height have been calculated and hypertension has been defined as an average systolic blood pressure and/or diastolic blood pressure that is ≥95th percentile for age, gender and height on three or more occasions.

It has been recommended that children with pre-hypertension (blood pressure between 90th and 95th centile for age, gender and height) should be encouraged to adopt lifestyle changes, such as diet, weight control and increased exercise, to prevent development of hypertension (**E**) [104]. If a child is proven to be hypertensive, pharmacological treatment is recommended, and the treatment threshold for a child with T1DM should be lower than that for children without diabetes (**E**) [104].

If these recommendations for hypertensive children were implemented in all diabetic patients, then 5–10% of all children with diabetes would fulfil the criteria for pharmacological treatment (**E**) [105]. In a German study of atherogenic risk factors (**B**) [106], only a quarter (2.1%) of the 8.1% patients with hypertension were given antihypertensives.

In order to identify patients with hypertension, recommendations have been made that screening should be undertaken. Current consensus guidelines recommend starting either at diagnosis (**E**) [30] or at the age of 12 years (**E**) [31], although there is little evidence base to support this. It is suggested that the screening should be done annually or more frequently if abnormalities are detected. One study advocates measuring blood pressure every 3–6 months but did not specify a starting time (**E**) [107].

The US working party on childhood hypertension (**E**) [104] recommends that the first-line antihypertensive treatment should be an angiotensin converting enzyme inhibitor. There is evidence that ACE inhibitors may improve microalbuminuria and delay the progression to nephropathy in adults (**E**) [108], and they may therefore be particularly beneficial in the diabetic child because of the greater time of exposure to diabetes.

Ophthalmic complications

Cataracts

Diabetic cataracts occur rarely in childhood but may be present in up to 1% of children (**B, C**) [109, 110]. They may be present at diagnosis (**C**) [111] or appear soon afterwards and are more likely to be associated with:

- a prolonged duration of symptoms before diagnosis
- a very high HbA1c at diagnosis (a reflection of the above)
- female gender
- adolescence
- poor diabetic control (**C**) [112].

The aetiology is not clear but it has been suggested that excessive induction of aldose reductase within the lens of the eye may be responsible (**C**) [112].

Although none of the current clinical guidelines specifically recommends screening for cataracts, the NICE guidelines suggest that they should 'be considered' at clinic visits. They should be easy to detect by routine ophthalmoscopy and should at least be looked for at diagnosis (**C**) [112].

Retinopathy

Diabetic retinopathy is a leading cause of acquired blindness in adults and may initially be asymptomatic. The onset of retinopathy is related to metabolic control (**A**) [113], duration of diabetes and age of onset (**B**) [114, 115]. Hypertension and hyperlipidaemia are also modifiable risk factors (**A, B**) [70, 115, 116]. Children under the age of 10 years are at minimal risk of retinopathy (**B**) [115], but the prevalence rate increases after 5 years from diagnosis in postpubertal patients (**B**) [115]. However, the DCCT showed that improving glycaemic control in those with early retinopathy may cause an initial worsening of the retinopathy but with significant benefits in the long run (**A**) [70, 113].

Current consensus guidelines from the American Academy of Pediatrics (AAP) (**E**) [117] and ISPAD (**E**) [29] recommend annual ophthalmological screening, although the age of onset of screening varies. The AAP suggests an initial ophthalmology examination 3–5 years after diagnosis if older than 9 years and annually thereafter (**E**) [117]. The ISPAD guidelines (**E**) [29] suggest that clinical examination of the eyes and ophthalmoscopy should be performed soon after diagnosis to exclude cataract formation or other disorders, and initial education should be provided. The age of onset of screening is dependent on whether the child is pubertal. The recommendation for prepubertal children is to start screening 5 years after onset or at age 11 years, or at puberty (whichever is earlier). Pubertal children should commence screening 2 years after diagnosis.

A recent study advocated biannual screening in developed countries, arguing that the prevalence of retinopathy has decreased in populations of children with more intensive insulin therapy and that severe retinopathy would not be missed (**B**) [118]. However, some studies suggest that young diabetic patients are still missing out on ophthalmological assessments [119, 120] and, as pointed out by the AAP, the most important point in the development of screening programme is to ensure that the guidelines (whether annually or biannually) are implemented. The most effective method of undertaking screening is to use seven-field fundal photography (**E**) [30], although this may not be available in many clinics for whom indirect ophthalmoscopy or monochromatic single-field photography may have to suffice.

Lipids

Dyslipidaemia is a further risk factor for atherosclerosis and has been demonstrated to be present in up to 28.6% of children and young adults with T1DM (**B**) [106]. Glycaemic control appears to be the main risk factor for abnormal lipid profiles (**B**) [121, 122], and this may be related to the increased glycation of low-density lipoprotein (LDL) particles, which reduces their receptor affinity and limits the clearance of LDL cholesterol from the circulation (**B**) [106].

There is controversy over lipid screening in children. Some guidelines suggest that children should be screened for dyslipidaemia within 6–12 months of diagnosis of diabetes and should be performed every 2–5 years or more frequently if abnormal (**E**) [29]. Others suggest that there is no evidence for such screening (**E**) [31] based on studies of global childhood screening for hypercholesterolaemia (**E**) [123]. However, these studies do not take into consideration the increased risk of dyslipidaemia and macrovascular disease in a diabetic population and there is an increasing consensus that screening for lipid abnormalities is appropriate in children with diabetes. Checking for a family history of vascular disease may also be an important aspect of the screening process in the diabetic clinic.

The ISPAD guidelines recommend treating with lipid-lowering drugs if there is an abnormal lipid profile and another risk factor is present. HMG-CoA reductase inhibitors (statins) are the treatment of choice in adults with hypercholesterolemia and appear safe in children (**E**) [124]. Other studies in children with familial hypercholesterolaemia have shown that this group of drugs is safe and effective (**A**) [125, 126] but there are no studies using these agents in diabetic subjects. However, there is no reason to suppose that they are any less safe. Other lipid-lowering agents have more side-effects and are not recommended in children (**E**) [124].

Foot care

The NICE guidelines (**E**) [31] recommend that all children and young people should be offered an annual 'foot care review'. In practice this is not specifically to identify peripheral neuropathy or peripheral vascular disease (see below) but offers an opportunity to educate patients about good foot care, cutting toenails, properly fitting shoes, etc., and to identify the presence of any skin or foot abnormalities.

Complications for which screening procedures are not regularly performed

Macrovascular disease

Macrovascular complications are leading causes of morbidity in individuals who develop diabetes in childhood, and cardiovascular disease is now the major cause of premature mortality in young adults with diabetes. Compared with the general population, T1DM patients have a 2.7–5.7 increased risk of dying from cardiovascular events, depending on age and sex (**A**) [127, 128].

There is evidence that atherosclerosis develops earlier and is more prevalent in children with diabetes compared with healthy, aged-matched control groups (**A**) [105]. Risk factors for atherosclerosis include obesity, hypertension, dyslipidaemia, poor glycaemic control and smoking. A recent large cross-sectional study of these atherogenic risk factors in diabetic children and young adults found that over 50% of patients in all age groups had at least one of these risk factors (**B**) [106]. In addition there was an increase in the prevalence of all these risk factors with age, suggesting that early intervention is desirable for the long-term health of the diabetic child and adolescent. Cardiovascular risk factor screening in adults with diabetes is commonplace [129] but, as yet, there is no evidence to show that such screening in the paediatric age range is of benefit.

Smoking

It is recommended in guidelines that education is important for the child with diabetes that smoking tobacco will increase the risk of cardiovascular complications (**E**) [29, 31]. Studies in the US indicate that the prevalence of smoking in diabetic and non-diabetic adults is similar and unchanged over the 11 years between 1990 and 2001 (**A**) [130]. In adolescents the rate of smoking in those over 15 years of age is at least 20% in most countries (**A**) [131]. Of more concern is the fact that the prevalence of smoking in adolescents with chronic disease, including T1DM, is as high as that in their non-diabetic peers (**E**) [132]. Although this emphasises the need for intensive education about the risks of smoking to teenagers with diabetes and support to those that wish to stop, the success of such programmes is low (**A**) [131].

Skin changes and limited joint mobility

Thirty years ago, limited joint mobility of the hands was described as being one of the earliest and commonest complications of diabetes (**B**) [133]. It was described in 28% of 7–18-year-old children at a diabetic camp and was unusual below the age of 10 years (**B**) [134]. This complication has diminished in frequency, attributed to better metabolic control (**B**) [135]. Limited joint mobility is not usually particularly troublesome but its importance is as a marker of microvascular disease (**B**) [136], neuropathy (**B**) [137], retinopathy and nephropathy (**B**) [138].

Although there are no specific recommendations to look for limited joint mobility in children, if it does occur, it should raise suspicions of other complications being present.

Neuropathy

Diabetic neuropathy is a major complication of T1DM and can be classified as autonomic, focal or polyneuropathic. The prevalence of diabetic neuropathy in children is unclear, with few large epidemiological studies and no clear diagnostic criteria. Studies using electrophysiological nerve conduction studies estimate a prevalence of subclinical neuropathy in 57% of children (**B**) [139, 140].

Clinical examination for signs of neuropathy may not be as sensitive or specific as nerve conduction studies (**B**) [140], but remain practical for screening. In the DCCT, clinical examination identified subclinical polyneuropathy in 39% of asymptomatic adolescents and young adults (**A**) [70, 113]. The DCCT also suggested that intensive insulin treatment and good metabolic control decreased the prevalence of neuropathy by 38–59%. It is unclear if optimising glucose control reverses early neuropathy. Other factors contributing to neuropathy appear to be older age, puberty and longer duration of diabetes (**B, A**) [141,

142]. Autoimmunity, vascular insufficiency and growth factor deficiencies may also have a role (**E**) [143].

Autonomic neuropathy has been documented in diabetic children and includes abnormal pupillary responses (**A**) [103] and cardiac dysfunction (**A, E**) [144, 145]. However, in most paediatric centres, current screening for neuropathy is limited to clinical assessment for evidence of peripheral neuropathy. The ISPAD recommendations suggest that screening for neuropathy should include careful history for evidence of paraesthesia or pain and examination of skin sensation, vibration and ankle reflexes (**E**) [29].

Necrobiosis lipoidica

The prevalence of necrobiosis lipoidica in diabetic children is low (<1%) [146]. There is a suggestion that children with this condition are at an increased risk for nephropathy and retinopathy (**B**) [147], and it should raise suspicions of these complications being present.

Dental abnormalities

There is evidence that salivary glucose levels are raised in children with diabetes with poor metabolic control, particularly during the first year after diagnosis (**B**) [148]. Older age and poor metabolic control increase the risk of periodontal disease (**A**) [149] and caries (**A**) [150]. Some studies also suggest an increase in dental pathogens in the saliva of diabetic children (**A**) [151]. An association between periodontal disease with duration of diabetes and the presence of diabetic complications has been reported (**B**) [152], probably reflecting poor metabolic control in these patients.

Although there are no studies to determine how frequently diabetic children should have their teeth examined, it is advisable that children with diabetes are encouraged to maintain good oral hygiene, inform their dentist of their diabetes and attend regular dental follow-ups (**E**) [29] and 6-monthly follow-up is recommended (E) [153].

Summary

Diabetes is associated with both a number of other conditions and with complications. Associated conditions are usually those that are also autoimmune mediated. Of these, hypothyroidism is sufficiently serious to demand regular screening and coeliac disease is sufficiently common to consider screening, despite some disagreement as to the efficacy of treatment in the child with diabetes. Longer term studies of coeliac disease in children with diabetes are required. Other autoimmune conditions occur but there is no evidence that screening for them is of value.

Overt vascular complications of diabetes are rare in prepubertal children but become more common during later adolescence. The strength of influence of the duration of prepubertal diabetes on the development of later complications remains the subject of research. Studies have suggested that some complications remain subclinical during adolescence and routine screening for them is not recommended. However, there is increasing consensus on the need for screening for serious complications such as retinopathy and nephropathy because there is strong evidence that good diabetic control can delay the onset of these problems and that, if signs are detected, improving glycaemic control may reverse them.

Finally, although no scientific evidence exists, it would seem good practice to introduce the process of screening for complications in childhood, so that it might help in educating

Table 11.1 Recommended programme of screening for complications and associated conditions in children with diabetes

---

1 Three-monthly or at each clinic visit
    Measure height and weight
    Calculate BMI and plot on chart
    HbA1c (result should be DCCT aligned and available in clinic)
    Assess state of injection sites
2 Annually
    Physical examination:
        Blood pressure (from age 12 yr)
        Retinal examination (from age 12 yr)
        Foot examination (principally for education about foot care)
    Take blood to screen for:
        Thyroid disease (at or shortly after diagnosis and annually thereafter)
        Coeliac disease (at diagnosis and at least every 2–3 yr thereafter)
        Lipids (from age 12 yr)
    Take urine sample for assessment of microalbuminuria either as:
        Albumin-to-creatinine ratio or
        Albumin excretion rate (overnight or 24 h) or
        Total albumin excretion (overnight or 24 h)
3 Other complications to be considered:
    Juvenile cataracts
    Necrobiosis lipoidica
    Addison disease
    Limited joint mobility
    Peripheral or autonomic neuropathy
    Smoking status

---

patients and their carers that careful surveillance will become more essential as the duration of diabetes progresses (Table 11. 1).

References

1 Court S, Parkin JM. Hypothyroidism and growth failure in diabetes mellitus. *Arch Dis Child* 1982; **57**: 622–4.

2 Custro N, Scafidi V, Costanzo G *et al.* Thyroid hormone anomalies in patients with insulin-dependent diabetes mellitus and circulating antithyroid microsomal antibodies. *Minerva Med* 1989; **80**: 427–30.

3 Goldstein DE, Drash A, Gibbs J *et al.* Diabetes mellitus: the incidence of circulating antibodies against thyroid, gastric, and adrenal tissue. *J Pediatr* 1970; **77**: 304–6.

4 Hecht A, Gershberg H. Diabetes mellitus and primary hypothyroidism. *Metabolism* 1968; **17**: 108–13.

5 Papalia D, Vigneri R, Casale P *et al.* Thyroid function in diabetes mellitus. *Folia Endocrinol* 1967; **20**: 81–93.

6 Abrams P, De Leeuw IH, Vertommen J. In new-onset insulin-dependent diabetic patients the presence of anti-thyroid peroxidase antibodies is associated with islet cell autoimmunity and the high risk haplotype HLA DQA1*0301-DQB1*0302 Belgian Diabetes Registry. *Diabet Med* 1996; **13**: 415–19.

7 Barker J, Yu J, Yu L *et al.* Autoantibody subspecificity in type 1 diabetes: risk for organ-specific autoimmunity clusters in distinct groups. *Diabetes Care* 2005; **28**: 850–5.

8 Korpal S, Dorant B, Birkholz D *et al.* Thyroid autoantibodies in children with recently diagnosed insulin-dependent diabetes mellitus. *Endokrynol Diabetol Chor Przemiany MateriiWieku Rozw* 2002; **8**: 73–6.

9 Lindberg B, Ericsson UB, Ljung R *et al.* High prevalence of thyroid autoantibodies at diagnosis of insulin-dependent diabetes mellitus in Swedish children. *J Lab Clin Med* 1997; **130**: 585–9.

10 López Medina JA, López-Jurado Romero de la Cruz R, Delgado García A *et al.* Beta-cell, thyroid and celiac autoimmunity in children with type 1 diabetes. *An Pediatr (Barc)* 2004; **61**: 320–5.

11 Smorawinska A, Walczak M, Korman E *et al.* Anti-thyroid autoantibodies in children with insulin-dependent diabetes mellitus. *Endokrynol Pol* 1989; **40**: 163–70.

12 Kordonouri O, Deiss D, Danne T *et al.* Predictivity of thyroid autoantibodies for the development of thyroid disorders in children and adolescents with type 1 diabetes. *Diabet Med* 2002; **19**: 518–21.

13 Bilimoria K, Pescovitz O, DiMeglio L. Autoimmune thyroid dysfunction in children with type 1 diabetes mellitus: screening guidelines based on a retrospective analysis. *J Pediatr Endocrinol Metab* 2003; **16**: 1111–17.

14 Holl RW, Bohm B, Loos U *et al.* Thyroid autoimmunity in children and adolescents with type 1 diabetes mellitus: effect of age, gender and HLA type. *Horm Res* 1999; **52**: 113–18.

15 De Block CE, De Leeuw IH, Vertommen JJ *et al.* Beta-cell, thyroid, gastric, adrenal and coeliac autoimmunity and HLA-DQ types in type 1 diabetes. *Clin Exp Immunol* 2001; **126**: 236–41.

16 Chang CC, Huang CN, Chuang LM. Autoantibodies to thyroid peroxidase in patients with type 1 diabetes in Taiwan. *Eur J Endocrinol* 1998; **139**: 44–8.

17 Kordonouri O, Klinghammer A, Lang E *et al.* Thyroid autoimmunity in children and adolescents with type 1 diabetes: a multicenter survey. *Diabetes Care* 2002; **25**: 1346–50.

18 Lorini R, d'Annunzio G, Vitali L *et al.* IDDM and autoimmune thyroid disease in the pediatric age group. *J Pediatr Endocrinol Metab* 1996; **9**: 89–94.

19 Bárová H, Perusicová J, Hill M *et al.* Anti-GAD-positive patients with type 1 diabetes mellitus have higher prevalence of autoimmune thyroiditis than anti-GAD-negative patients with type 1 and type 2 diabetes mellitus. *Physiol Res* 2004; **53**: 279–86.

20 De Block CE. Diabetes mellitus type 1 and associated organ-specific autoimmunity. *Verh K Acad Geneeskd Belg* 2000; **62**: 285–328.

21 Chen BH, Chung SB, Chiang W *et al.* GAD65 antibody prevalence and association with thyroid antibodies, HLA-DR in Chinese children with type 1 diabetes mellitus. *Diabetes Res Clin Pract* 2001; **54**: 27–32.

22 Abdullah MA, Salman H, Bahakim H *et al.* Antithyroid and other organ-specific antibodies in Saudi Arab diabetic and normal children. *Diabet Med* 1990; **7**: 50–2.

23 Abe K, Fukui S, Shigemasa C *et al.* The incidences of thyroid autoimmunity in diabetics and in patients with insulin autoimmunity. *Yonago Acta Med* 1976; **20**: 1–6.

24 Burek CL, Rose NR, Guire KE *et al.* Thyroid autoantibodies in black and in white children and adolescents with type 1 diabetes mellitus and their first degree relatives. *Autoimmunity* 1990; **7**: 157–67.

25 Czerniawska E, Szalecki M, Piatkowska E *et al.* Prevalence of thyroid antibodies TPO and ATG at the onset of type 1 diabetes mellitus in children treated in two diabetes centres in Lódz and Kielce. *Med Wieku Rozwoj* 2003; **7**: 223–8.

26 Frasier SD, Penny R, Snyder R *et al.* Antithyroid antibodies in Hispanic patients with type I diabetes mellitus: prevalence and significance. *Am J Dis Child* 1986; **140**: 1278–80.

27 Menon PS, Vaidyanathan B, Kaur M. Autoimmune thyroid disease in Indian children with type 1 diabetes mellitus. *J Pediatr Endocrinol Metab* 2001; **14**: 279–86.

28 Riley WJ, Maclaren NK, Lezotte DC *et al.* Thyroid autoimmunity in insulin-dependent diabetes mellitus: the case for routine screening. *J Pediatr* 1981; **99**: 350–4.

29 ISPAD. *Consensus Guidelines for the Management of Type 1 Diabetes Mellitus in Children and Adolescents.* Medical Forum International, Zeist, Netherlands, 2000.

30 NHMRC. *The Australian Clinical Practice Guidelines on the Management of Type 1 Diabetes in Children and Adolescents,* 2005. Available at: http://www.nhmrc.gov.au/publications/synopses/cp102syn.htm

31 NICE. *Type 1 Diabetes in Children and Young People: Full Guideline 2004.* Available at: http://www.nice.org.uk/page.aspx?o=CG015childfullguideline

32 McKenna MJ, Herskowitz R, Wolfsdorf JI. Screening for thyroid disease in children with IDDM. *Diabetes Care* 1990; **13**: 801–3.

33 Rother KI, Zimmerman D, Schwenk WF. Effect of thyroid hormone treatment on thyromegaly in children and adolescents with Hashimoto disease. *J Pediatr* 1994; **124**: 599–601.

34 Dretzke J, Cummins C, Sandercock J *et al.* Autoantibody testing in children with newly diagnosed type 1 diabetes mellitus. *Health Technol Assess* 2004; **8**: 7–14.

35 Bernasconi S, Vanelli M, Nori G *et al.* Serum TSH, T4, T3, FT4, FT3, rT3, and TBG in youngsters with non-ketotic insulin-dependent diabetes mellitus. *Horm Res* 1984; **20**: 213–17.

36 Lee PD. Thyroid dysfunction in insulin-dependent diabetes mellitus. *Am J Dis Child* 1987; **141**: 604–5.

37 Radetti G, Paganini C, Gentili L *et al.* Altered adrenal and thyroid function in children with insulin-dependent diabetes mellitus. *Acta Diabetol* 1994; **31**: 138–40.

38 Chiarelli F, Tumini S, Verrotti A *et al.* Effects of ketoacidosis and puberty on basal and TRH-stimulated thyroid hormones and TSH in children with diabetes mellitus. *Horm Metab Res* 1989; **21**: 494–7.

39 Gilani BB, MacGillivray MH, Voorhess ML *et al.* Thyroid hormone abnormalities at diagnosis of insulin-dependent diabetes mellitus in children. *J Pediatr* 1984; **105**: 218–22.

40 Tan SH, Lee BW, Low PS *et al.* Assessment of complications in children with insulin-dependent diabetes mellitus. *Ann Acad Med Singapore* 1985; **14**: 266–71.

41 Chambers TL. Coexistent coeliac disease, diabetes mellitus, and hyperthyroidism. *Arch Dis Child* 1975; **50**: 162–4.

42 Kalicka K, Dziatkowiak H, Nazim J *et al.* Thyroid peroxidase antibodies and thyroid diseases in children and adolescents with type 1 diabetes mellitus from Southeast Poland. *Przegl Lek* 2003; **60**: 403–6.

43 Kontiainen S, Schlenzka A, Koskimies S *et al.* Autoantibodies and autoimmune diseases in young diabetics. *Diabetes Res* 1990; **13**: 151–6.

44 Roldán MB, Alonso M, Barrio R. Thyroid autoimmunity in children and adolescents with type 1 diabetes mellitus. *Diabetes Nutr Metab* 1999; **12**: 27–31.

45 Troncone R, Bhatnagar S, Butzner D *et al.* Celiac disease and other immunologically mediated disorders of the gastrointestinal tract. Working Group report of the Second World Congress of Pediatric Gastroenterology, Hepatology and Nutrition. *J Pediatr Gastroenterol Nutr* 2004; **39**(suppl 2): 601–10.

46 Ferguson A, Arranz E, O'Mahony S. Clinical and pathological spectrum of coeliac disease: active, silent, latent, potential. *Gut* 1993; **34**: 150–1.

47 Walker-Smith JA, Grigor W. Coeliac disease in a diabetic child. *Lancet* 1969; **1**: 1021.

48 Holmes GKT. Screening for coeliac disease in type 1 diabetes. *Arch Dis Child* 2002; **87**: 495–8.

49 Catassi C, Rätsch IM, Gandolfi L *et al.* Why is coeliac disease endemic in the people of the Sahara? *Lancet* 1999; **354**: 647–8.

50 Boudraa G, Hachelaf W, Benbouabdellah M *et al.* Prevalence of coeliac disease in diabetic children and their first-degree relatives in west Algeria: screening with serological markers. *Acta Paediatr Suppl* 1996; **412**: 58–60.

51 Sumnik Z, Cinek O, Bratanic N *et al.* Risk of celiac disease in children with type 1 diabetes is modified by positivity for HLA-DQB1*02-DQA1*05 and TNF-308A. *Diabetes Care* 2006; **29**: 858–63.

52 Pocecco M, Ventura A. Coeliac disease and insulin-dependent diabetes mellitus: a causal association? *Acta Paediatr* 1995; **84**: 1432–3.

53 British Society for Gastroenterology. *Guidelines for the Management of Patients with Coeliac Disease.* Available at: http://www.bsg.org.uk/pdf_word_docs/coeliac.doc

54 Mora S, Barera G, Beccio S *et al.* A prospective, longitudinal study of the long-term effect of treatment on bone density in children with celiac disease. *J Pediatr* 2001; **139**: 516–21.

55 Vasquez H, Mazure R, Gonzalez D *et al.* Risk of fractures in celiac disease patients: a cross-sectional, case-control study. *Am J Gastroenterol* 2000; **95**: 183–9.

56 Collin P, Vilska S, Heinonen PK *et al.* Infertility and coeliac disease. *Gut* 1996; **39**: 382–4.

57 Meloni GF, Dessole S, Vargiu N *et al.* The prevalence of coeliac disease in infertility. *Hum Reprod* 1999; **14**: 2759–61.

58 Askling J, Linet M, Gridley G *et al.* Cancer incidence in a population-based cohort of individuals hospitalized with celiac disease or dermatitis herpetiformis. *Gastroenterology* 2002; **123**: 1428–35.

59 Holmes GK, Prior P, Lane MR *et al.* Malignancy in coeliac disease: effect of a gluten free diet. *Gut* 1989; **30**: 333–8.

60 Mohn A, Cerruto M, Lafusco D *et al.* Celiac disease in children and adolescents with type I diabetes: importance of hypoglycemia. *J Pediatr Gastroenterol Nutr* 2001; **32**: 37–40.

61 Thain ME, Hamilton JR, Ehrlich RM. Coexistence of diabetes mellitus and celiac disease. *J Pediatr* 1974; **85**: 527–9.

62 Freemark M, Levitsky L. Screening for celiac disease in children with type 1 diabetes: two views of the controversy. *Diabetes Care* 2003; **26**: 1932–9.

63 Peters C, Allgrove J. Low incidence of biopsy positive coeliac disease following screening in type 1 diabetes. *Pediatr Diabetes* 2006; **7**(suppl 5): 52–3.

64 Hansen D, Bennedbaek FN, Hansen LK *et al.* Thyroid function, morphology and autoimmunity in young patients with insulin-dependent diabetes mellitus. *Eur J Endocrinol* 1999; **140**: 512–18.

65 Hansen D, Bennedbaek FN, Høier M *et al.* A prospective study of thyroid function, morphology and autoimmunity in young patients with type 1 diabetes. *Eur J Endocrinol* 2003; **148**: 245–51.

66 Barera G, Bonfanti R, Viscardi M *et al.* Occurrence of celiac disease after onset of type 1 diabetes: a 6-year prospective longitudinal study. *Pediatrics* 2002; **109**: 833–8.

67 Betterle C, Coco G, Zanchetta R. Adrenal cortex autoantibodies in subjects with normal adrenal function. *Best Pract Res Clin Endocrinol Metab* 2005; **19**: 85–99.

68 Marks S, Girgis R, Couch R. Screening for adrenal antibodies in children with type 1 diabetes and autoimmune thyroid disease. *Diabetes Care* 2003; **26**: 3187–8.

69 Silva RC, Sallorenzo C, Kater CE *et al.* Autoantibodies against glutamic acid decarboxylase and 21-hydroxylase in Brazilian patients with type 1 diabetes or autoimmune thyroid diseases. *Diabetes Nutr Metab* 2003; **16**: 160–8.

70 DCCT Research Group. The effect of intensive treatment of diabetes on the development and progression of long-term complications in insulin-dependent diabetes mellitus. The Diabetes Control and Complications Trial Research Group. *N Engl J Med* 1993; **329**: 977–86.

71 Bognetti E, Riva MC, Bonfanti R *et al.* Growth changes in children and adolescents with short-term diabetes. *Diabetes Care* 1998; **21**: 1226–9.

72 Lebl J, Schober E, Zidek T *et al.* Growth data in large series of 587 children and adolescents with type 1 diabetes mellitus. *Endocr Regul* 2003; **37**: 153–61.

73 Hoskins PJ, Leslie RD, Pyke DA. Height at diagnosis of diabetes in children: a study in identical twins. *BMJ* 1985; **290**: 278–80.

74 Betts P, Mulligan J, Ward P *et al.* Increasing body weight predicts the earlier onset of insulin-dependent diabetes in childhood: testing the 'accelerator hypothesis' (2). *Diabet Med* 2005; **22**: 144–151.

75 Clarke SL, Craig ME, Garnett SP *et al.* Increased adiposity at diagnosis in younger children with type 1 diabetes does not persist. *Diabetes Care* 2006; **29**: 1651–3.

76 Kibirige M, Metcalf B, Renuka R *et al.* Testing the accelerator hypothesis: the relationship between body mass and age at diagnosis of type 1 diabetes. *Diabetes Care* 2003; **26**: 2865–70.

77 Knerr I, Wolf J, Reinehr T *et al.* The 'accelerator hypothesis': relationship between weight, height, body mass index and age at diagnosis in a large cohort of 9,248 German and Austrian children with type 1 diabetes mellitus. *Diabetologia* 2005; **48**: 2501–4.

78 Kordonouri O, Hartmann R. Higher body weight is associated with earlier onset of type 1 diabetes in children: confirming the 'accelerator hypothesis'. *Diabet Med* 2005; **22**: 1783–4.

79 Clarke WL, Vance ML, Rogol AD. Growth and the child with diabetes mellitus. *Diabetes Care* 1993; **16**(suppl 3): 101–6.

80 Clarson C, Daneman D, Ehrlich RM. The relationship of metabolic control to growth and pubertal development in children with insulin-dependent diabetes. *Diabetes Res* 1985; **2**: 237–41.

81 Jackson RL, Holland E, Chatman ID *et al.* Growth and maturation of children with insulin-dependent diabetes mellitus. *Diabetes Care* 1978; **1**: 96–107.

82 Choudhury S, Stutchfield P. Linear growth and weight gain in diabetic children: a cross-sectional and longitudinal evaluation. *J Pediatr Endocrinol Metab* 2000; **13**: 537–44.

83 Domargard A, Sarnblad S, Kroon M *et al.* Increased prevalence of overweight in adolescent girls with type 1 diabetes mellitus. *Acta Paediatr* 1999; **88**: 1223–8.

84 Elamin A, Hussein O, Tuvemo T. Growth, puberty, and final height in children with type 1 diabetes. *J Diabetes Complicat* 2006; **20**: 252–6.

85 Brown M, Ahmed ML, Clayton KL *et al.* Growth during childhood and final height in type 1 diabetes. *Diabet Med* 1994; **11**: 182–7.

86 Penfold J, Chase HP, Marshall G *et al.* Final adult height and its relationship to blood glucose control and microvascular complications in IDDM. *Diabet Med* 1995; **12**: 129–33.

87 Acerini CL, Cheetham TD, Edge JA *et al.* Both insulin sensitivity and insulin clearance in children and young adults with type I (insulin-dependent) diabetes vary with growth hormone concentrations and with age. *Diabetologia* 2000; **43**: 61–8.

88 Danne T, Kordonouri O, Enders I *et al.* Factors influencing height and weight development in children with diabetes. Results of the Berlin Retinopathy Study. *Diabetes Care* 1997; **20**: 281–5.

89 Knip M, Tapanainen P, Pekonen F *et al.* Insulin-like growth factor binding proteins in prepubertal children with insulin-dependent diabetes mellitus. *Eur J Endocrinol* 1995; **133**: 440–4.

90 Mauras N, Merimee T, Rogol AD. Function of the growth hormone-insulin-like growth factor I axis in the profoundly growth-retarded diabetic child: evidence for defective target organ responsiveness in the Mauriac syndrome. *Metabolism* 1991; **40**: 1106–11.

91 Abdel-Shakour S, el-Hefnawy H, el-Yamani MY *et al.* Urinary N-acetyl-beta-D-glucosaminidase in children with diabetes as an early marker of diabetic nephropathy. *East Mediterr Health J* 2002; **8**: 24–30.

92 Al-Hermi BE, Al-Abbasi AM, Rajab M *et al.* Diabetic nephropathy in children with type 1 diabetes mellitus in Bahrain. *Saudi Med J* 2005; **26**: 294–7.

93 Chiari G, Daneman D, Vanelli M. Practical considerations on screening for microalbuminuria in children and adolescents with type 1 diabetes. *Acta Biomed Ateneo Parmense* 2000; **71**: 97–104.

94 Baak MA, Odink RJ, Delemarre van de Waal HA. Microalbuminuria as risk factor for nephropathy in children with insulin-dependent diabetes mellitus. *Ned Tijdschr Geneeskd* 1993; **137**: 1349–52.

95 Schultz CJ, Konopelska B, Dalton RN *et al.* Microalbuminuria prevalence varies with age, sex, and puberty in children with type 1 diabetes followed from diagnosis in a longitudinal study Oxford Regional Prospective Study Group. *Diabetes Care* 1999; **22**: 495–502.

96 Rudberg S, Ullman E, Dahlquist G. Relationship between early metabolic control and the development of microalbuminuria: a longitudinal study in children with type 1 insulin-dependent diabetes mellitus. *Diabetologia* 1993; **36**: 1309–14.

97 Lévy M, Sahler C, Cahané M *et al.* Risk factors for microalbuminuria in children and adolescents with type 1 diabetes. *J Pediatr Endocrinol Metab* 2000; **13**: 613–20.

98 Mullis P, Köchli HP, Zuppinger K *et al.* Intermittent microalbuminuria in children with type 1 diabetes mellitus without clinical evidence of nephropathy. *Eur J Pediatr* 1988; **147**: 385–8.

99 Koch HC, Burmeister W, Liappis N *et al.* Microalbuminuria in children and adolescents with and without type-I diabetes mellitus IDDM. *Klin Padiatr* 1991; **203**: 167–72.

100 Kordonouri O, Danne T, Hopfenmüller W *et al.* Lipid profiles and blood pressure: are they risk factors for the development of early background retinopathy and incipient nephropathy in children with insulin-dependent diabetes mellitus? *Acta Paediatr* 1996; **85**: 43–8.

101 Kowalewski M, Peczynska J, Glowinska B *et al.* The assessment of 24-hour ambulatory blood pressure monitoring ABPM, microalbuminuria and diabetic autonomous neuropathy in children with type 1 diabetes and hypertension. *Endokrynol Diabetol Chor Przemiany MateriiWieku Rozw* 2006; **12**: 103–6.

102 dos Santos LHC, Bruck I, Antoniuk S *et al.* Evaluation of sensorimotor polyneuropathy in children and adolescents with type I diabetes: associations with microalbuminuria and retinopathy. *Pediatr Diabetes* 2002; **3**: 101–8.

103 Karavanaki K, Baum JD. Coexistence of impaired indices of autonomic neuropathy and diabetic nephropathy in a cohort of children with type 1 diabetes mellitus. *J Pediatr Endocrinol Metab* 2003; **16**: 79–90.

104 National High Blood Pressure Education Program Working Group on High Blood Pressure in Children and Adolescents. The fourth report on the diagnosis, evaluation, and treatment of high blood pressure in children and adolescents. *Pediatrics* 2004; **114**: 555–76.

105 Dahl-Jorgensen K, Larsen JR, Hanssen KF. Atherosclerosis in childhood and adolescent type 1 diabetes: early disease, early treatment? *Diabetologia* 2005; **48**: 1445–53.

106 Schwab K, Doerfer J, Hecker W *et al.* Spectrum and prevalence of atherogenic risk factors in 27,358 children, adolescents, and young adults with type 1 diabetes: cross- sectional data from the German diabetes documentation and quality management system DPV. *Diabetes Care* 2006; **29**: 218–25.

107 Sochett E, Daneman D. Early diabetes-related complications in children and adolescents with type 1 diabetes: implications for screening and intervention. *Endocrinol Metab Clin North Am* 1999; **28**: 865–82.

108 Navaneethan S, Querques M, Bonifati C *et al.* Antihypertensive agents in patients with diabetes: trade-off between renal and cardiovascular protection. *Diabetes Educ* 2006; **32**: 596–602.

109 Falck A, Laatikainen L. Diabetic cataract in children. *Acta Ophthalmol Scand* 1998; **76**: 238–40.

110 Montgomery EL, Batch JA. Cataracts in insulin-dependent diabetes mellitus: sixteen years' experience in children and adolescents. *J Paediatr Child Health* 1998; **34**: 179–82.

111 Lang-Muritano M, La Roche GR, Stevens JL *et al.* Acute cataracts in newly diagnosed IDDM in five children and adolescents. *Diabetes Care* 1995; **18**: 1395–6.

112 Datta V, Swift PG, Woodruff GH *et al.* Metabolic cataracts in newly diagnosed diabetes. *Arch Dis Child* 1997; **76**: 118–20.

113 DCCT Research Group. Effect of intensive diabetes treatment on the development and progression of long-term complications in adolescents with insulin-dependent diabetes mellitus: Diabetes Control and Complications Trial. Diabetes Control and Complications Trial Research Group. *J Pediatr* 1994; **125**: 177–88.

114 Holl RW, Lang GE, Grabert M *et al.* Diabetic retinopathy in pediatric patients with type-1 diabetes: effect of diabetes duration, prepubertal and pubertal onset of diabetes, and metabolic control. *J Pediatr* 1998; **132**: 790–4.

115 Klein R, Klein BE, Moss SE *et al.* The Wisconsin Epidemiologic Study of Diabetic Retinopathy. IX: four-year incidence and progression of diabetic retinopathy when age at diagnosis is less than 30 years. *Arch Ophthalmol* 1989; **107**: 237–43.

116 Tight blood pressure control and risk of macrovascular and microvascular complications in type 2 diabetes: UKPDS 38. UK Prospective Diabetes Study Group. *BMJ* 1998; **317**: 703–13.

117 Lueder GT, Silverstein J. Screening for retinopathy in the pediatric patient with type 1 diabetes mellitus. *Pediatrics* 2005; **116**: 270–3.

118 Maguire A, Chan A, Cusumano J *et al.* The case for biennial retinopathy screening in children and adolescents. *Diabetes Care* 2005; **28**: 509–13.

119 McCarty CA, Taylor KI, McKay R *et al.* Diabetic retinopathy: effects of national guidelines on the referral, examination and treatment practices of ophthalmologists and optometrists. *Clin Experiment Ophthalmol* 2001; **29**: 52–8.

120 Witkin SR, Klein R. Ophthalmologic care for persons with diabetes. *JAMA* 1984; **251**: 2534–7.

121 Erciyas F, Taneli F, Arslan B *et al.* Glycemic control, oxidative stress, and lipid profile in children with type 1 diabetes mellitus. *Arch Med Res* 2004; **35**: 134–40.

122 Maahs D, Maniatis A, Nadeau K *et al.* Total cholesterol and high-density lipoprotein levels in pediatric subjects with type 1 diabetes mellitus. *J Pediatr* 2005; **147**: 544–6.

123 Newman TB, Browner WS, Hulley SB. The case against childhood cholesterol screening. *JAMA* 1990; **264**: 3039–43.

124 Rodenburg J, Vissers M, Daniels S *et al.* Lipid-lowering medications. *Pediatr Endocrinol Rev* 2004; **2**: 171–80.

125 de Jongh S, Ose L, Szamosi T *et al.* Efficacy and safety of statin therapy in children with familial hypercholesterolemia: a randomized, double-blind, placebo-controlled trial with simvastatin. *Circulation* 2002; **106**: 2231–7.

126 Stein EA, Illingworth DR, Kwiterovich PO, Jr, *et al.* Efficacy and safety of lovastatin in adolescent males with heterozygous familial hypercholesterolemia: a randomized controlled trial. *JAMA* 1999; **281**: 137–44.

127 Laing SP, Swerdlow AJ, Slater SD *et al.* The British Diabetic Association Cohort Study, II: cause-specific mortality in patients with insulin-treated diabetes mellitus. *Diabet Med* 1999; **16**: 466–71.

128 Laing SP, Swerdlow AJ, Slater SD *et al.* The British Diabetic Association Cohort Study, I: all-cause mortality in patients with insulin-treated diabetes mellitus. *Diabet Med* 1999; **16**: 459–65.

129 NICE. *Type 1 Diabetes in Adults: Quick Reference Guide.* Available at: http://www.nice.org.uk/guidance/CG15/quickreference/pdf/English

130 Ford E, Mokdad A, Gregg E. Trends in cigarette smoking among US adults with diabetes: findings from the Behavioral Risk Factor Surveillance System. *Prev Med* 2004; **39**: 1238–42.

131 Thomas R, Perera R. School-based programmes for preventing smoking. *Cochrane Database Syst Rev* 2006; Issue **3**: Art no CD001293.

132 Tyc VL, Throckmorton-Belzer L. Smoking rates and the state of smoking interventions for children and adolescents with chronic illness. *Pediatrics* 2006; **118**: e471–87.

133 Grgic A, Rosenbloom AL, Weber FT *et al.* Joint contracture: common manifestation of childhood diabetes mellitus. *J Pediatr* 1976; **88**: 584–8.

134 Rosenbloom AL, Silverstein JH, Lezotte DC *et al.* Limited joint mobility in diabetes mellitus of childhood: natural history and relationship to growth impairment. *J Pediatr* 1982; **101**: 874–8.

135 Lindsay JR, Kennedy L, Atkinson AB *et al.* Reduced prevalence of limited joint mobility in type 1 diabetes in a U.K. clinic population over a 20-year period. *Diabetes Care* 2005; **28**: 658–61.

136 Rosenbloom AL, Silverstein JH, Lezotte DC *et al.* Limited joint mobility in childhood diabetes mellitus indicates increased risk for microvascular disease. *N Engl J Med* 1981; **305**: 191–4.

137 Starkman HS, Gleason RE, Rand LI *et al.* Limited joint mobility (LJM) of the hand in patients with diabetes mellitus: relation to chronic complications. *Ann Rheum Dis* 1986; **45**: 130–5.

138 Garg SK, Chase HP, Marshall G *et al.* Limited joint mobility in subjects with insulin dependent diabetes mellitus: relationship with eye and kidney complications. *Arch Dis Child* 1992; **67**: 96–9.

139 Hyllienmark L, Brismar T, Ludvigsson J. Subclinical nerve dysfunction in children and adolescents with IDDM. *Diabetologia* 1995; **38**: 685–92.

140 Nelson D, Mah JK, Adams C *et al.* Comparison of conventional and non-invasive techniques for the early identification of diabetic neuropathy in children and adolescents with type 1 diabetes. *Pediatr Diabetes* 2006; **7**: 305–10.

141 Abad F, Díaz G, Rodríguez I *et al.* Subclinical pain and thermal sensory dysfunction in children and adolescents with type 1 diabetes mellitus. *Diabet Med* 2002; **19**: 827–31.

142 Riihimaa PH, Suominen K, Tolonen U *et al.* Peripheral nerve function is increasingly impaired during puberty in adolescents with type 1 diabetes. *Diabetes Care* 2001; **24**: 1087–92.

143 Trotta D, Verrotti A, Salladini C *et al.* Diabetic neuropathy in children and adolescents. *Pediatr Diabetes* 2004; **5**: 44–57.

144 Suys BE, Huybrechts SJ, De Wolf D *et al.* QTc interval prolongation and QTc dispersion in children and adolescents with type 1 diabetes. *J Pediatr* 2002; **141**: 59–63.

145 Verrotti A, Giuva PT, Morgese G *et al.* New trends in the etiopathogenesis of diabetic peripheral neuropathy. *J Child Neurol* 2001; **16**: 389–94.

146 De Silva BD, Schofield OM, Walker JD. The prevalence of necrobiosis lipoidica diabeticorum in children with type 1 diabetes. *Br J Dermatol* 1999; **141**: 593–4.

147 Verrotti A, Chiarelli F, Amerio P *et al.* Necrobiosis lipoidica diabeticorum in children and adolescents: a clue for underlying renal and retinal disease. *Pediatr Dermatol* 1995; **12**: 220–3.

148 Twetman S, Nederfors T, Stahl B *et al.* Two-year longitudinal observations of salivary status and dental caries in children with insulin-dependent diabetes mellitus. *Pediatr Dent* 1992; **14**: 184–8.

149 de Pommereau V, Dargent-Pare C, Robert JJ *et al.* Periodontal status in insulin-dependent diabetic adolescents. *J Clin Periodontol* 1992; **19**: 628–32.

150 Siudikiene J, Machiulskiene V, Nedzelskiene I. Dietary and oral hygiene habits in children with type I diabetes mellitus related to dental caries. *Stomatologija* 2005; **7**: 58–62.

151 Siudikiene J, Machiulskiene V, Nyvad B *et al.* Dental caries and salivary status in children with type 1 diabetes mellitus, related to the metabolic control of the disease. *Eur J Oral Sci* 2006; **114**: 8–14.

152 Al Shammari KF, Al Ansari JM, Moussa NM *et al.* Association of periodontal disease severity with diabetes duration and diabetic complications in patients with type 1 diabetes mellitus. *J Int Acad Periodontol* 2006; **8**: 109–14.

153 Iughetti L, Marino R, Bertolani MF *et al.* Oral health in children and adolescents with IDDM: a review. *J Pediatr Endocrinol Metab* 1999; **12**: 603–10.

CHAPTER 12

Type 2 diabetes mellitus – genetics, diagnosis and management. Polycystic ovarian syndrome

John Porter & Timothy G. Barrett

In all things it is a good idea to hang a question mark now and then on the things we have taken for granted.
— Bertrand Russell, British philosopher, logician and mathematician (1872–1970)

Genetics of type 2 diabetes mellitus

John Porter

The World Health Organization defines type 2 diabetes mellitus (T2DM) as 'characterised by disorders of insulin action and insulin secretion, either of which may be the predominant feature' [1]. Under the World Health Organization definition, other specific types of diabetes (which used to be considered as subtypes of T2DM) are distinct from T2DM. These rare forms of diabetes will not be further considered in this chapter (see Chapter 13 for a detailed discussion of these).

The importance of genetic and environmental factors in T2DM

Whilst the evidence of the importance of genetics in the development of T1DM is strong [2], the situation with T2DM is rather less clear. There is an increased risk of T2DM in siblings of patients than in the general population ($\sim$10% vs 3%) [3], and initial twin studies seemed to show strong concordance between monozygotic but not dizygotic twins, suggesting a major effect of genetics on developing T2DM. This suggestion was further strengthened by the finding that some ethnic groups, such as the Pima Native Americans, are particularly at risk for T2DM [3a]. However, twin studies have been flawed in many cases by the use of a clinic-based, rather than population (i.e. twin)-based, approach that tends to recruit patients with more severe diabetes and by the use of different definitions of diabetes in the initial twin versus the second twin. The situation is further complicated by the rising prevalence of T2DM in the background population, which increases the risk that concordance in twins may be a chance finding. Finally, there is evidence that the intrauterine environment may have an effect on the development of T2DM, and this may be influenced by twin-to-twin transfusion, which is specific to monozygotic twins. It is perhaps not surprising therefore that recent studies in twins have been less convincing of monozygotic/dizygotic concordance [4, 5].

Table 12.1 Variants with the strongest evidence for association with T2DM

Gene	Variant amino acid	Odds ratio for T2DM	Prevalence of risk allele	Chromosome
PPARγ	P12A	~1.25	~ 85%	3p25
KCNJ11	E23K	~1.2	~40%	11p15.1
CAPN10	Multiple SNPs	~1.2		2q37
HNF4A	Multiple SNPs	1.1–2.1		20q12–q13.1
TCF7L2	DG10S478	1.45 (heterozygote)	38%	10q25.2
		2.41 (homozygote)	7%	
Insulin	VNTR	?		11p15.5

The rapid increase in the burden of T2DM over recent years is not disputed, and many consider that this is in part due to an increased incidence of diabetes. There is certainly evidence that T2DM is being diagnosed in younger age groups, and in particular in the paediatric age group where historically T2DM was not found. This change is too rapid to reflect a genetic shift, and it suggests that other factors, most notably lifestyle changes, are to blame. This theory is supported by the findings that ethnic groups from areas with relatively low diabetes prevalence rates who migrate to areas of high prevalence quickly develop diabetes prevalence similar to the native population [5a]. It appears most likely that a calorie-rich and exercise-deficient lifestyle produces an overrich intrauterine environment and postnatal obesity, which in combination with an individual's genetic susceptibility to insulin resistance and beta-cell deficiency, in both antenatal and postnatal life, produces T2DM.

Investigation of the genetics of T2DM

The genetic nature of T2DM has been investigated via two main approaches: firstly, the use of genome-wide scans to identify candidate genes by position and secondly, the analysis of biologically plausible candidate genes. Both approaches have generated many association studies, but few of these have been consistently positive when tested on large numbers in multiple populations. This may reflect differences in genetic susceptibility between populations or chance findings associated with multiple testing.

Genome-wide scanning

The basic principle of genome-wide scanning is that by genotyping multiple polymorphic markers throughout the genome in a large number of families with the condition of interest, an area common to all families can be defined. The gene responsible for the condition should then be within this area. In a complex polygenic condition such as T2DM, rather than a single area of interest, multiple areas are expected, and the probability of these areas being linked to susceptibility genes rather than being chance findings can be calculated. Unfortunately, to be adequately powered, genome-wide scans in polygenic conditions require large numbers of families.

Many genome-wide scans have been performed in several different populations world-wide. A selection of the more recent studies is shown in Table 12.1. There have been several peaks common to multiple genome-wide scans. Investigation of two of these has led to the findings of two susceptibility genes for T2DM: calpain-10 and *HNF4A*.

Calpain-10

Calpain-10 is a calcium-activated protease involved in a number of cellular functions, particularly intracellular signalling. A genome-wide scan in Mexican-Americans with T2DM identified a locus on chromosome 2q. Linkage-disequilibrium mapping was used to narrow the area of interest down and calpain-10 emerged as the candidate gene able best to explain the linkage to 2q [6]. This was interesting, as calpain-10 did not at the time seem a good biological candidate as a T2DM causative gene. In Mexican-Americans the strongest susceptibility was caused by a haplotype of three intronic polymorphisms, but this association was not confirmed in several other populations studied. A study in the UK found a separate single-nucleotide polymorphism (SNP-44) in calpain-10 in linkage disequilibrium with a non-synonymous coding polymorphism (T504A) that would also account for the diabetes susceptibility, and which was more likely to have functional significance. Meta-analysis of all published SNP-44 association studies suggested an association with T2DM, with an overall odds ratio of 1.2 [7]. These associations between T2DM and calpain-10 have prompted research into the role of calpain-10 in glucose homeostasis. Although the function of calpain-10 is still only partially understood, it appears that it may be important in the mitochondrial response to glycolysis, the transport of insulin to the plasma membrane and insulin secretion [8].

HNF4A *promoter variants*

The *HNF4A* gene encodes a transcription factor, HNF4α, which is expressed in liver and pancreas. Mutations in *HNF4A* were found to be causative for maturity-onset diabetes of the young (MODY-1) in 1996 [9]. As MODY has some similarities to T2DM, the MODY genes were investigated as biological candidates for T2DM susceptibility genes. However this approach did not produce the expected yield and initial investigation of *HNF4A* did not show a clear association with T2DM [10, 11], despite 20q (the location for *HNF4A*) being noted as a peak in several genome scans. The finding of a distant upstream alternative promoter in *HNF4A* [12] provided a further candidate for linkage to T2DM, and indeed when linkage to 20q was explored further with a series of SNPs across the area, polymorphisms near the alternative promoter were found to associate with T2DM risk in two independent studies with different populations [13, 14].

TCF7L2

A foretaste of the possible future of genetics research was the finding of a new gene associated with diabetes by the biopharmaceutical company deCode in 2006 [15]. The company had performed a genome-wide scan in the Icelandic population that reported evidence of linkage to 10q [16], a region already highlighted by a study in Mexican-Americans [17]. By a comprehensive single-marker-association analysis, the company found a single marker *DG10S478* that was associated with T2DM in Icelandic, Danish and American populations. This marker is in an intron of *TCF7L2*, a gene coding for a transcription factor in the Wnt intracellular signalling pathway. *TCF7L2* may be having an effect on T2DM or may be in linkage disequilibrium to another effector gene. *TCF7L2* regulates proglucagon expression in enteroendocrine tissues. An important product of proglucagon is glucagon-like peptide 1 (GLP-1), one of the executors of the incretin effect [18]. The effect of carrying any of the susceptibility alleles at *DG10S478* is a ~1.5-fold increase in the risk of T2DM, and carrying two increases this to ~2.4 times the risk. This suggests a significant health risk, although this association needs to be explored more fully.

Investigation of candidate genes

The second method of investigation of the genetic basis of T2DM that has been used is the investigation of biologically plausible candidate genes. The plethora of genes involved in the processes of intracellular signalling in the beta cell, insulin production and secretion, and end-organ response to insulin, provide numerous candidate genes for T2DM. Many of these candidates have been investigated, but to date few have proven to be associated with T2DM.

HNF1A

The genes for MODY were obvious candidates to investigate as susceptibility genes for T2DM. Mutations in *HNF1A* are the commonest cause of MODY in the UK. Investigation of *HNF1A* in European populations did not, however, yield a major T2DM susceptibility gene. By contrast, in the Oji-Cree people of Canada, who have the third highest prevalence of diabetes in the world, a mutation in *HNF1A* (G319S) was found to associate with early onset of T2DM. Possession of the heterozygous mutation increases the risk of diabetes in the Oji-Cree by 2 and the homozygous mutation by 4. However, even in the Oji-Cree, 60% of those with T2DM do not possess the *S*319 allele, so this mutation has only a minor impact.

NEUROD1

NEUROD1 is a helix-loop-helix transcription factor involved in pancreatic embryogenesis and insulin secretion. *NEUROD1* binds to the insulin gene promoter in conjunction with E47, another helix-loop-helix protein, and increases insulin gene expression. *NEUROD1* knockout mice exhibit pancreatic dysgenesis and diabetes. Investigation of *NEUROD1* in 94 families with T2DM and apparent autosomal dominant inheritance revealed two families in which mutations in *NEUROD1* segregated with diabetes [19]. Further studies have shown that *NEUROD1* mutations are a minor cause of T2DM and MODY, and do not have a major impact on T2DM.

Insulin gene

The insulin gene was clearly a good candidate for conferring T2DM susceptibility. Investigation of the insulin gene has shown association between variation in the gene and T1DM, and there were initial reports of association between the area in the insulin gene with a variable number of tandem repeats (*VNTR*) and insulin resistance and T2DM, which appeared to be confirmed by a meta-analysis of six previous studies [20]. Further investigation of this association using the Warren resource of parent–offspring trios showed a parent of origin effect, with diabetic offspring more likely to have inherited a type III *VNTR* allele from his or her father than predicted (69% vs 50% predicted) [21]. This result suggested that the insulin *VNTR* effect is mediated through imprinting of the insulin gene. Disconcertingly, a study of 1462 Danes with T2DM failed to show any increase in the type III allele of the insulin *VNTR* [22]. However a more recent study from the Framingham Heart Study seems to confirm the importance of the *VNTR* as a susceptibility locus but did not show any parent of origin effect [23].

PPARγ

PPARγ is a transcription factor predominantly expressed in adipose tissue but has also been shown to be expressed in small quantities in liver, muscle and pancreas [24]. It has become increasingly clear that PPARγ has a vital role in the regulation of body fat distribution and insulin sensitivity, acting to promote energy storage as a thrifty response. Interest in PPARγ as a T2DM candidate gene stemmed from the fact that the thiazolidinedione class of drugs act through PPARγ stimulation and improve hypertension, blood glucose control and insulin sensitivity in patients with T2DM [25]. Inactivating mutations in the gene for PPARγ (*PPARG*) in humans have been found in rare forms of diabetes with lipodystrophy [26–28]. Taken together, these findings suggest that increasing activity of PPARγ is inversely proportional to insulin sensitivity. A common polymorphism in *PPARG* (Pro12Ala), which decreases the activity of PPARγ, has however been shown to be associated with high insulin sensitivity and decreased susceptibility to T2DM [29, 30]. This apparent paradox is due to the multiple effects of PPARγ; loss of function of PPARγ causes decreased lipogenesis and increased fatty acid oxidation; both processes result in decreased adipocyte hypertrophy and decreased free fatty acids, and hence increased insulin sensitivity whilst PPARγ stimulation increases production of small insulin-sensitive adipocytes and reduces hepatic glucose production [31]. Early studies of Pro12Ala were inconclusive, but larger studies have provided more evidence that possession of the proline allele increases the risk of developing T2DM by ~1.25 times. This is a low relative risk (RR) but the proline allele is so common in most ethnic groups (~80% of individuals) that it has a significant effect on the population risk [32].

KCNJ11

The beta-cell potassium channel is intimately involved in regulation of insulin secretion. The channel is composed of four inwardly rectifying potassium channels (Kir 6.2 gene *KCNJ11*) and four sulphonylurea receptor subunits *SUR1* gene [33]. Mutations in *KCNJ11* have been shown to cause both infantile hyperinsulinaemia (inactivating mutations) [34] and neonatal diabetes (activating mutations) [35]. Interest in the role of Kir 6.2 in insulin secretion led to consideration of *KCNJ11* as a candidate gene for T2DM. Early studies did not show any association between variation in *KCNJ11* and T2DM, but two studies did show such an association in French and British subjects [36, 37]. Larger studies and meta-analyses have strengthened the evidence that the k allele present in ~60% of white Europeans increases the risk of developing T2DM ~1.2-fold [38–40], although one study found that the allele is in linkage disequilibrium with a variant in *SUR1*, raising the possibility that variation in *SUR1* may be the underlying cause of an increase in T2DM in the populations studied [41].

Summary

The genetics of T2DM are complex. Research strategies to date have focused on genome-wide scanning and evaluation of plausible candidate genes. As the methods and tools for investigating complex genetic disease improve, it seems likely that more of the genome's and proteome's variation can be analysed in the hunt for the susceptibility factors that influence an individual's risk of T2DM.

Treatment of T2DM in childhood

Timothy G. Barrett

Introduction

T2DM in childhood is a relatively new phenomenon, with the first cases described only in 1979 [42]. Since then, children with T2DM diabetes have been reported from many countries around the world; the prevalence is increasing and relates to the rise in childhood obesity seen in many Western and developing countries. In children, it is most often related to obesity, and other cardiovascular risk factors may be present. T2DM results from a combination of insulin resistance, increased hepatic glucose output and progressive decline of glucose-stimulated insulin secretion. In healthy children, insulin secretion involves a basal component, which maintains normal fasting plasma glucose, and a prandial component, which sharply increases insulin secretion in response to a glucose load. This limits hepatic glucose release and inhibits gluconeogenesis. One of the earliest defects in T2DM is reduction in the prandial component of insulin secretion, through loss of the first-phase insulin response. This can be insidious in adults and probably children, with a decrease in the prandial component of insulin release by as much as 50% by the time T2DM is diagnosed [43]. Consequently, postprandial glucose rises above the normal range are an early abnormality in T2DM. Abnormal fasting glucose can be a late sign, indicating that a marked deterioration in beta-cell function has already occurred [44].

Guidelines for the management of T2DM

Although there is a very small literature on optimum treatment of T2DM in children, and almost none on outcomes, there is a wealth of data available on adults with T2DM. Thus the paediatrician has access to a large evidence base, and the experience of his or her adult colleagues guide the management of children. This section will review some of this evidence and relate it to the special case of T2DM in children.

T2DM has no clear definition, but pragmatically it can be considered as tissue insulin resistance, with a significant and progressive insulin secretory defect. It is known that insulin resistance is associated with multiple cardiovascular risk factors; consequently, T2DM in childhood is likely to be associated with earlier micro- and macrovascular complications than seen with childhood-onset T1DM. In addition, the insidious onset of T2DM, and a variable asymptomatic period before presentation, means that vascular complications may already be present at diagnosis. This was originally shown in the Pima Indian children with T2DM and has now been shown in a larger cohort of T2DM children from the Treatment Options for Type 2 Diabetes in Adolescence and Youth (TODAY) study: of 240 children enrolled into this study with T2DM, 26% had hypertension, 60% had dyslipidaemia and 17% had both (**B**) [45]. There is also evidence that even stricter glycaemic control is required for insulin-resistant patients with T2DM than for those with T1DM: the UK Prospective Diabetes Study (UKPDS) showed that a reduction in average HbA1c from 7.9 to 7.0% resulted in a 25% decrease in microvascular complications (**A**) [46], and reducing blood pressure below 144/82 resulted in a 44% reduction in the risk of stroke and 36% reduction in the risk of heart failure (**A**) [47].

Bearing the above evidence in mind, recent policy initiatives have emphasised the importance of good glycaemic control in T2DM (**A**) [48]. There are now well-defined targets to work towards in T2DM, most recently an ADA–EASD (American Diabetes Association–European Association for the Study of Diabetes) consensus algorithm for the management of hyperglycaemia in T2DM (**E**) [49]. This algorithm suggests that an HbA1c target of less than 7.0% should be aimed for, with an HbA1c less than 6.0% (normal) being the 'gold standard'. Aiming for a normal HbA1c is probably not appropriate in children because of the risk of hypoglycaemia; however, our challenge is to make an HbA1c of 7.0% a realistic aim for our patients.

The treatment goals for childhood T2DM are to:

1 achieve glycaemic control to target HbA1c ≤7.0% without severe hypoglycaemic episodes

2 reduce body mass index (BMI) to <95th centile for age and sex

3 encourage exercise to increase cardiovascular fitness towards 60 minutes of moderate-to-vigorous exercise daily (**E**) [50]

4 look for and treat associated comorbidities, e.g. hypertension, hyperlipidaemia and microalbuminuria

The evidence for reducing HbA1c to 7.0% has been cited above. Obesity is an established cardiovascular risk factor; this definition of obesity is widely used in North America and is less likely to underestimate obesity than the International Obesity Task Force cut-off values. However a lower centile cut-off might be appropriate for obese children with T2DM from ethnic minorities. The exercise guideline is a recent recommendation based on an exhaustive literature review and is for healthy children. Obese children will struggle to achieve this ambitious goal, but any increase in exercise is probably of benefit to cardiovascular health.

Lifestyle changes

There is clear evidence from the Finnish Diabetes Prevention Study and the Diabetes Prevention Program that intensive lifestyle interventions can reduce insulin resistance, slow the rate of progression to T2DM and improve glycaemic control (**A**) [51, 52]. The first step in managing young people with T2DM is to encourage lifestyle changes. Paediatricians are used to the concept of multidisciplinary care teams in the management of their patients; they work in partnership with their patients to develop individual care plans with clearly defined treatment objectives and targets. These might include regular self-monitoring of blood glucose, HbA1c measurement at each clinic visit, annual fasting lipid and blood pressure measurement, weight monitoring and advice on stopping smoking. There is a need to develop structured education packages for children with T2DM both at diagnosis and during ongoing management. Of great importance is explaining to children and parents that they are likely to require insulin therapy within 10 years of diagnosis (**A**) [53]. Children and parents need to understand that treatment for T2DM involves a stepwise progression to maintain glycaemic control and that commencement of insulin is not an indication that they have failed.

The Royal College of Paediatrics and Child Health has published guidelines for diet and exercise advice for the prevention of obesity, which are also very useful for obese children with T2DM (Tables 12.2 and 12.3) (**E**) [54]. There is good evidence that children with obesity have reduced exercise tolerance and that goals have to be realistic; any increase in activity, however small, is an advance, and children should be encouraged to increase their activity levels in a graded programme. A recent literature review suggested that school-age youth should participate daily in 60 minutes or more of moderate-to-vigorous physical

Table 12.2 Royal College of Paediatrics and Child
Health (RCPCH) guidelines on dietary advice for obesity

- Reduce energy intake to estimated average requirements
- Reduce fat to 30%
- Have regular mealtimes and avoid grazing/TV snacks
- Have smaller portions
- Avoid using food as reward
- Eat healthy snacks, e.g. fruit instead of crisps/sweets
- Eat less energy dense food, e.g. semi-skimmed milk
- Eat whole foods which take time to eat
- Have at least five   portions fruit and vegetables per day
- Have low-calorie drinks (water)
- Have grill/boil/bake foods, no frying

Table 12.3 RCPCH guidelines for physical exercise
in obesity

- Any ↑activity helps
- 30–60 min a day
- Sustainable, e.g. walking, cycling and climbing stairs
- Active lifestyle for whole family
- Walk or cycle to school
- Encourage active play
- Reduce television viewing and computer games

---

activity that is developmentally appropriate, enjoyable, and involves a variety of activities
(**E**) [50]. The authors suggested that brisk walking, bicycling and active outdoor playing
would achieve this requirement.

Oral therapy with one agent

Adult studies suggest that lifestyle changes are unlikely to reduce HbA1c by more than 1%
initially [46]. However, in the author's experience, greater improvements in HbA1c can
be achieved in children with T2DM. If at diagnosis, HbA1c is above 7.0%, then an oral
hypoglycaemic agent should be introduced in addition to lifestyle changes. Newly diagnosed children who have osmotic symptoms or whose HbA1c is above 8.5% should be
prescribed insulin and oral therapy at diagnosis. Metformin is the first-line drug treatment
for children with T2DM, as it has cardioprotective properties, is an insulin sensitiser and
has a low risk of hypoglycaemia [55]. It is licensed for use in children and has an excellent
safety record, having been in clinical use for over 60 years. It acts on insulin receptors in
the liver, muscle and adipose tissue, and has multiple effects, including decreasing hepatic
gluconeogenesis, increasing insulin-stimulated glucose uptake in muscle and adipose tissue and reducing appetite. One clinical trial of metformin in children with T2DM showed
a reduction in HbA1c of 1.1% after 4 months (**B**) [56]. The disadvantages of metformin include a high risk of side-effects (nausea, abdominal pain, diarrhoea, bloating and a metallic
taste in the mouth). These side-effects are exacerbated if metformin is taken on an empty
stomach. The arrival of a slow-release preparation of metformin, and liquid preparations
(500 mg/5mL) allowing titration starting with lower doses, should reduce the incidence of
these side-effects. A reasonable starting dose in children would be metformin 200 mg orally

twice a day with meals, increasing gradually every 2 weeks until the maximum tolerated dose (**E**). Metformin is not usually tolerated in doses greater than 1 g 8- or 12-hourly. The contraindications to metformin use include renal and hepatic impairment (liver enzymes >twice the upper limit of normal). Lactic acidosis is a rare side-effect seen if metformin accumulates in the body, such as in impaired renal function. Metformin is contraindicated in people with uncontrolled heart failure (e.g. some children with Alstrom syndrome and cardiomyopathy), renal impairment, advanced liver disease and any predisposition to hypoxaemia, such as sepsis. Metformin may also enhance the likelihood of ovulation in teenagers with PCOS, so the risks of pregnancy should be explained and contraceptive advice offered.

Oral therapy with two agents

If after 3 months of oral therapy with metformin the HbA1c remains above the target level of 7.0%, a second agent should be introduced. The current National Institute of Clinical Excellence (NICE) guidelines suggest the use of a glitazone as a replacement for either metformin or an insulin secretagogue (**E**) [48]. However, these guidelines are currently being revised, and there is some logic to adding a glitazone to metformin, as this combination targets insulin resistance and consequently may benefit cardiovascular risk factors. This is supported by the results of the PROactive study (**B**) [57]. Thiazolidinediones act on the nuclear receptor peroxisome proliferator-activated receptor gamma (PPARϒ). This receptor is strongly expressed in adipose tissue, and its downstream pathway increases transcription of various insulin-sensitive genes involved in lipid and glucose metabolism. The net effect is a lowering of insulin resistance. The original drug in this class troglitazone was withdrawn due to hepatotoxicity. The two drugs currently available in the UK are pioglitazone and rosiglitazone. In adult studies, glitazones, either alone or in combination with metformin, have been shown to reduce HbA1c by 1–1.5%, but the glucose-lowering effect may take 3–6 months to reach maximum effect. There may also be benefits in blood pressure and cholesterol reduction. The side-effects include fluid retention, so are contraindicated in heart failure (e.g. diabetes in cardiomyopathy such as Alstrom syndrome) and weight gain due to increased subcutaneous fat. Other contraindications include hepatic or renal impairment.

Alternative second-line agents to glitazones include the sulphonylureas, meglitinide analogues and alpha-glucosidase inhibitors. There is almost no evidence of the effects of their use in children.

Sulphonylureas

Sulphonylureas bind to receptors on the K^+/ATP channels, causing them to close; this depolarises the beta-cell membrane, which opens Ca^{++} channels, allowing influx of calcium and insulin exocytosis. These drugs work by increasing insulin secretion, so require residual pancreatic beta-cell function. Sulphonylurea binding persists on its receptors for long periods, so that the earlier sulphonylureas have prolonged effects, including hypoglycaemia. Hypoglycaemia is still the main side-effect of this class of drugs, and families and children need to be educated about hypoglycaemia if sulphonylureas are being considered as treatment. The first generation of these drugs was tolbutamide, and the second generation include glibenclamide, gliclazide, glimepiride, glipizide and gliquidone. Studies in adults have shown them to reduce HbA1c by 1–2%. NICE guidelines recommend a sulphonylurea as initial therapy in adults with T2DM, who are normal weight or underweight (**B**)

[48]. In children with obesity-related T2DM, sulphonylureas are a second-line treatment in combination with metformin. Gliclazide is popular in the UK, and there is a once-a-day modified release preparation available, which is associated with less hypoglycaemia than the standard generic 80 mg tablets.

Meglitinide analogues

These are short-acting insulin secretagogues that also bind to the K^+/ATP channels, causing them to close and initiate insulin release from the pancreatic beta cells. They act within 10–30 minutes and have a duration of action from 2 to 4 hours. They have been used with meals to enhance insulin secretion. They may be less likely to cause hypoglycaemia due to their shorter duration of action but are less effective in controlling basal hyperglycaemia. Repaglinide has been used in adults with T2DM alone or in combination with metformin. Nateglinide is used only with metformin. There are no published data on their use in children.

Alpha-glucosidase inhibitors

Acarbose is the only drug available in the UK in this class, and it inhibits gastrointestinal alpha-glucosidase, an enzyme that breaks down ingested carbohydrates. It can reduce the postprandial rise in blood glucose but is associated with unacceptable side-effects for most teenagers (flatulence, bloating and diarrhoea).

Insulin therapy

Insulin has been available for use in children for over 80 years; paediatricians have extensive experience of its use in children with T1DM; and its effectiveness in glucose reduction and side-effects of hypoglycaemia are well known. The significant insulin resistance in T2DM means that hypoglycaemia is not as prevalent as in T1DM. Adults with T2DM are thought to have lost around 50% of pancreatic beta-cell function by the time of diagnosis, and most require supplemental insulin within 5 years. In a study of children with T2DM from North America, 50% had an insulin requirement by 5 years after diagnosis [58]. As well as an increase in hypoglycaemia, important side-effects in children with T2DM are increased appetite and weight gain.

Young people should be considered for insulin therapy if 3 months of dual oral therapy do not achieve an HbA1c less than 7.0% (B). Treatment with metformin can be continued, but any secretagogues should be discontinued if rapid-acting insulin is included in the regime. There is a recognition in adult T2DM practice that patients have not been managed aggressively enough and that the average adult with T2DM has been exposed to about 10 years of excess glycaemic burden, defined as an HbA1c above 7.0%, from diagnosis to initiation of insulin therapy as a result of 'clinician inertia' (B) [59]. It is becoming increasingly recognised that elevated postprandial glucose makes an important, independent contribution to overall glucose control and plays a role in the pathogenesis of diabetes complications [43]. There is evidence that the contribution to HbA1c is predominantly by fasting blood glucose concentrations as HbA1c rises above 7.3%, whereas postprandial blood glucose is the principal contributing factor at lower HbA1c levels [60].

The theoretical ideal insulin regime currently available to address these problems is basal-bolus therapy using analogues (E). The basal component choices include insulin glargine and insulin detemir. These have a longer duration of action than the traditional

Table 12.4 Recommended actions for patients who are not achieving target HbA1c with insulin regimes

---

- Review individualised care plan
- Review lifestyle modifications
- Review diet and carbohydrate counting
- Ensure metformin dose is maximised
- Titrate insulin doses up to achieve target fasting and postprandial glucose levels
- Consider continuous blood glucose monitoring
- Consider switching from twice daily premixed insulin to basal bolus if not already done so
- Check compliance with oral and injected medication
- Check insulin injection technique and device working properly
- Check correct storage of insulin, in date, etc.
- Check injection sites for lipohypertrophy

---

neutral pH Hagedorn (NPH) insulin and a flatter insulin profile over 24 hours. The rapid-acting insulin analogues aspart, lispro and glulisine are designed to mimic more closely the endogenous prandial insulin secretion compared with short-acting human insulin. The basal insulin dose should be titrated to achieve a target fasting glucose less than 7.0 mmol/L. Home blood glucose monitoring should include postprandial measurements; the International Diabetes Federation recommends a target postprandial glucose of less than 7.5 mmol/L [61] and the American Diabetes Association a target of less than 10 mmol/L (**B**) [62]. The major 2-hour postprandial blood glucose excursion should be determined (usually after the main meal) and, if above target, the preceding dose of rapid-acting insulin titrated up until target is achieved. Clearly, patients should be taught carbohydrate counting to facilitate appropriate insulin adjustment.

Although the above description is for a theoretical ideal insulin regimen, this may either be unacceptable to patients or not suitable due to domestic, school or work difficulties. Acceptable alternatives would be twice daily administration of premixed insulins and a basal insulin with an oral secretagogue, such as a repaglinide before meals. Studies comparing basal insulin glargine/oral hypoglycaemic agent preparations with premixed insulins have not shown a clear advantage of one regimen over the other. Some patients might find it more acceptable to have a stepwise progression of treatment, adding first a basal long-acting insulin to oral agents and then preprandial short-acting insulin analogues. For young people who are not achieving target HbA1c with either a basal-bolus regime or twice daily premixed insulin, some suggested actions are given in Table 12.4.

Treatment of comorbidities

T2DM is associated in children with a metabolic syndrome phenotype, and so is associated with several cardiovascular disease risk factors. All affected children should have regular eye examinations and urinary microalbumin excretion estimation. This review will discuss only dyslipidaemia and hypertension.

Dyslipidaemia

Dyslipidaemia in T2DM is characterised by raised triglycerides, low high-density lipo-protein (HDL) cholesterol and increased small dense, atherogenic low-density lipoprotein (LDL) cholesterol. Raised LDL cholesterol and lowered HDL cholesterol are established and modifiable risk factors for the development of cardiovascular disease. An adult with diabetes has a risk for cardiovascular disease close to that of a non-diabetic person with a previous myocardial infarction (**A**) [63]. Adults with T2DM have an absolute risk of cardiovascular disease of 20% or more over 10 years. However, the risk is not known for children with T2DM. The closest comparison we have is a 10-year study of 589 patients with childhood-onset T1DM aged over 18 years at baseline and followed for 10 years (**B**) [64]. The RR for cardiovascular disease was 1.8 with LDL cholesterol >2.6 mmol/L (>100 mg/dL) and 2.3 with LDL cholesterol >3.4 mmol/L (>130 mg/dL). For triglycerides the RR was 2.5 with triglyceride >2.3 mmol/L (>90 mg/dL) and 3.3 with triglyceride >3.9 mmol/L (>150 mg/dL). These data suggest that childhood-onset diabetes is associated with an increased risk for cardiovascular disease if dyslipidaemia is present, and therefore treatment to lower lipids is logical.

The first-line treatment is always a reduced fat diet and exercise, weight reduction if growth is completed and glycaemic control. After non-pharmacological treatments, the most effective class of drugs are 3-hydroxy-3-methylglutaryl coenzyme A (HMG-CoA) reductase inhibitors (statins). These work by competitively inhibiting HMG-CoA, an enzyme involved in cholesterol synthesis, especially in the liver. They are particularly effective in lowering LDL cholesterol and increasing the concentrations of HDL cholesterol. However, they are not as effective as fibrates in reducing triglycerides.

NICE (**E**) [65] has recommended the use of statins as lipid-lowering agents for patients who meet the following criteria:

all patients over 18 years with diabetes plus one other risk factor:

- treated hypertension
- retinopathy
- nephropathy
- features of the metabolic syndrome
- high-risk family history.

Clearly, many children under 18 years with T2DM have multiple risk factors and should be considered for statin therapy. The treatment target is to achieve total cholesterol levels <4 mmol/L and LDL cholesterol <2 mmol/L (**E**) [65]. The side-effects include abdominal pain, flatulence, nausea and vomiting, and altered liver function tests. Atorvastatin, pravastatin and simvastatin are now all listed in the British National Formulary for Children for hyperlipidaemia.

Fibrates such as fenofibrate act mainly by decreasing serum triglycerides and raise HDL-cholesterol concentrations with less effect on LDL cholesterol. Some of the actions of fibrates are mediated through PPARα receptors; consequently, they have multiple actions, including increasing insulin sensitivity and decreasing vascular inflammation. Although theoretically they should be ideal for the dyslipidaemia in T2DM, a recent study of 10,000 adults with T2DM showed a reduction in cardiovascular events, but no effect on total mortality (**A**) [66]. They tend to have more side-effects than statins, and data on use in childhood are very limited. Fibrates remain a second-line treatment in adults after statins. Liver function should be monitored 3-monthly and, as with statins, both these classes of drugs should be avoided in pregnancy.

Hypertension

Hypertension is a frequent accompaniment of T2DM in obese children and an independent risk factor for progression to cardiovascular disease. In the UKPDS, control of hypertension was more important than blood glucose control in decreasing the frequency of cardiac events (**A**) [47]. The same Pittsburgh study of childhood-onset T1DM quoted above showed that a systolic blood pressure ≥120–129 mmHg was associated with an RR of 2.5 for cardiovascular disease (**B**) [64].

All children with diabetes should have blood pressure estimated at least annually using an appropriate-size cuff. This may mean using a thigh cuff in the most obese children. As body size is an important determinant of blood pressure in children, charts of normal values often give blood pressure values in relation to height centiles [67]. If the systolic or diastolic blood pressure is elevated above the 90th centile for age, sex and height on two or more occasions, an early morning urine collection should be collected to screen for microalbuminuria. The first-line treatment is diet and exercise advice as for newly diagnosed T2DM. If these measures have no effect after 3 months, then treatment with an angiotensin converting enzyme (ACE) inhibitor should be considered. These drugs block ACE, which reduces the production of angiotensin II, a potent vasoconstrictor. Lisinopril is an example of this class of drug. The most important side-effects are severe hypotension, renal impairment and a dry cough. The risk of hypotension can be minimised by starting with an initial low dose, such as 2.5 mg once daily. The usual maintenance dose is 10–20 mg once daily. Newer drugs include the angiotensin-II-receptor antagonists, such as losartan, and do not seem to cause the dry cough that may occur with ACE inhibitors.

Non-alcoholic fatty liver

Non-alcoholic fatty liver disease (NAFLD) is the term used to define a range of alcohol-like liver injuries that occur without alcohol abuse and include non-alcoholic steatohepatitis and NAFLD-induced cirrhosis. The term NAFLD is usually used for the liver injuries associated with the metabolic syndrome, but a precise definition has not yet been agreed [68]. The prevalence is unknown in childhood, but it is closely linked to obesity, the metabolic syndrome and T2DM in childhood. Insulin resistance is believed to be the underlying cause, as peripheral insulin resistance leads to influx of free fatty acids to the liver. This occurs by both decreased suppression of lipolysis and increased lipogenesis in the liver. The subsequent accumulation of fat within the hepatocytes leads to the development of hepatic insulin resistance. There is a lack of follow-up data on the outcomes of NAFLD in children; however, adult data show slow progression to cirrhosis over several years or decades. The children most at risk for NAFLD are likely to be those obese children with abnormal glucose tolerance, or with multiple cardiovascular risk factors. The initial investigation should be liver function tests (LFTs): children with persistently (>1 yr) abnormal LFTs (pragmatically more than 1.5 times the upper limit of normal) should undergo a systematic assessment to exclude other forms of chronic liver disease [69]. The diagnosis of NAFLD can only be confirmed by liver biopsy. The current best treatment is lifestyle modification, in terms of increased physical activity and the promotion of a healthy, balanced diet. Vitamin E has been recommended as an antioxidant and metformin as an insulin sensitiser.

Management algorithm (Figure 12.1)

T1DM may be confused with T2DM. Any child in whom T2DM is suspected, who presents with osmotic symptoms, ketonuria, dehydration or ketoacidosis, should be treated with insulin immediately. Insulin can always be weaned off after the acute episode if necessary. These children can present with acute metabolic decompensation and withholding insulin may be fatal. Diabetic ketoacidosis in T2DM is treated in the same way as for

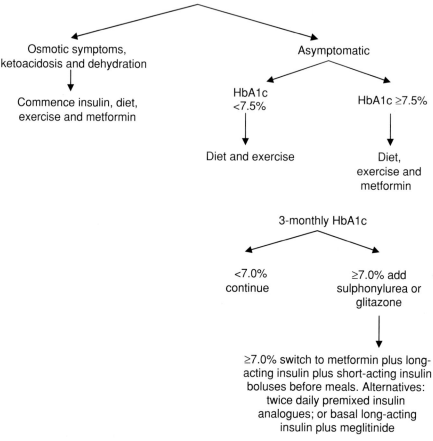

Figure 12.1 Algorithm for the diagnosis of T2DM (evidence of insulin resistance, autoantibody negative).

T1DM. Metformin can be started when the diabetic ketoacidosis has resolved and insulin continued or weaned off depending on glycaemic control. For asymptomatic patients with only moderately raised HbA1c, a trial of diet and exercise is usually the best policy to obtain the maximum benefit from these lifestyle changes before adding in drug therapy. Metformin is the first-line drug treatment. If there is no response, it is worth checking compliance. Finally, insulin should be added for patients with persistently poor glycaemic control. Insulin works best when used in combination with an agent that increases insulin sensitivity.

Polycystic ovarian syndrome

Polycystic ovarian syndrome (PCOS) is a heterogeneous clinical entity affecting 5–10% of women worldwide, making it one of the commonest endocrine disorders of young women and the commonest cause of infertility in this age group. The original description of amenorrhoea with polycystic ovaries was made by Stein and Leventhal more than 60 years ago

[70]. The cardinal features were anovulation, presenting with oligomenorrhoea or amenorrhoea and infertility, and hyperandrogenaemia, presenting with hirsutism, acne and alopecia. In retrospect, the features were probably the same as Achard–Thiers syndrome, the 'diabetes of the bearded lady' [71]. Since then it has become apparent that there are fundamental metabolic disturbances integral to the syndrome that lead to significant cardiovascular risk. These include obesity, insulin resistance, beta-cell dysfunction, impaired glucose tolerance and T2DM, dyslipidaemia, hypertension, obstructive sleep apnoea, a procoagulant state and endothelial dysfunction. In one recent study, 40% of women with PCOS demonstrated glucose intolerance, and 7.5% of these women had overt T2DM [72]. Conversely, 50% of women with T2DM have been reported to have evidence of polycystic ovaries [73]. PCOS is a major risk factor for the development of T2DM in women of all ages. A new area of concern is the recognition of PCOS in teenage girls with T1DM. With increasing weight gain, they become insulin resistant and are made hyperinsulinaemic with exogenous insulin, especially with aggressive insulin regimens [74].

Pathophysiology

There is clearly a genetic component to the development of PCOS, based on observed familial clustering [75]. Female first-degree relatives of women with PCOS have a significantly increased prevalence of PCOS (**A**) [76]. A more extreme version of hyperandrogenism, severe insulin resistance, and *acanthosis nigricans*, designated HAIR-AN, or type A insulin resistance, was described in adolescent girls (**C**) [77], due to mutations in the insulin receptor gene [78]. However, several studies failed to detect mutations in the insulin receptors of women with the much commoner PCOS [79, 80]. Women with PCOS have significantly higher fasting insulin levels compared with age-matched and BMI-matched controls [81]. The exact site of abnormality in the insulin-signalling cascade in PCOS is not known. The insulin resistance has some relation to overweight and obesity, and there is a hyperbolic relation between insulin sensitivity and increasing BMI, with decreasing insulin sensitivity with increasing BMI [82]. However, obesity is not the only cause of insulin resistance in PCOS: insulin resistance is higher and the glucose disposition index is lower in women with PCOS and a family history of T2DM [83]. In addition, insulin resistance also occurs in non-obese women with PCOS and normal glucose tolerance [84]. Even lean women with PCOS are as insulin resistant as obese women without PCOS, and obese PCOS women are as insulin resistant as patients with T2DM.

Insulin resistance and hyperandrogenaemia potentiate each other so that it was not clear which was the underlying abnormality. However, in experiments with gonadotrophin-releasing hormone agonists, it was shown that suppression of hyperandrogenaemia does not improve peripheral or hepatic insulin resistance in PCOS (**B**) [85]. However, if insulin levels are lowered, for instance with metformin, then androgen levels are lowered (**B**) [86]. What is clear is that the hyperinsulinism consistent with insulin resistance precedes and facilitates the androgen excess observed in PCOS. Human ovaries have abundant insulin and IGF-1 receptors, and insulin stimulates ovarian androgen production: theca cells from PCOS patients produce testosterone in response to insulin at higher levels compared with non-PCOS theca cells (**C**) [87]. In PCOS, the ovaries appear to be hypersensitive to insulin action and have augmented androgen production, which is surprising given that there is widespread tissue insulin resistance (**E**) [88]. Sex-hormone-binding globulin (SHBG) is a glycoprotein produced in the liver which acts as a carrier for sex hormones, with a high binding affinity for testosterone and dihydrotestosterone. Insulin is thought to lower

SHBG levels by acting directly to reduce hepatic SHBG synthesis: decreased basal levels of SHBG are seen in PCOS, with a more significant reduction in obese women with PCOS. The hyperinsulinaemia in PCOS lowers the SHBG levels and enhances the expression of hyperandrogenaemia [89].

Insulin resistance is known to rise during puberty, resolving by Tanner stage 5 [90]. However, in girls with premature adrenarche, this pubertal rise in insulin resistance is greatly exaggerated [91], and these girls appear to be at significantly higher risk for developing functional hyperandrogenism and PCOS [92].

Definition

There is not yet a consensus on the diagnostic criteria for PCOS, but minimal criteria are considered to be hyperandrogenism and ovulatory dysfunction in the absence of other hypothalamopituitary, ovarian or adrenal disease. Of interest, polycystic ovaries on ultrasound are not required to make the diagnosis. These have been defined as the presence on ultrasound of eight or more subcapsular follicular cysts ≤10 mm in diameter and increased ovarian stroma. Polycystic ovaries are present in 20–25% or randomly selected women, so their presence in the absence of ovulatory dysfunction or hyperandrogenism is not sufficient to diagnose PCOS [93].

A recent consensus working group [94] has put forward a definition of PCOS based on the presence of two out of three features:
• oligo- or anovulation
• clinical and/or biochemical signs of hyperandrogenism
• polycystic ovaries and exclusion of other aetiologies (congenital adrenal hyperplasia, androgen-secreting tumours and the Cushing syndrome).

Hyperinsulinism may manifest with mild or moderate acanthosis nigricans. Hyperandrogenism may present with excessive hirsutism and/or acne. Raised androgens (testosterone and/or androstenedione) is the most consistent biochemical abnormality in PCOS. Increased adrenal androgen production (e.g. dehydroepiandrosterone sulphate) may often coexist. SHBG is frequently reduced, and a threshold level of <37 nmol/L has been suggested for the diagnosis of PCOS (sensitivity 87.5% and specificity 86.8%) [95].

A common presentation in adult practice is with anovulatory infertility. However in the teenage age group, menstrual disturbance is often the presenting feature. Oligomenorrhoea is an excellent marker for PCOS, and 85% of oligomenorrhoeic women can be assumed to have PCOS. Young women with PCOS have more pronounced irregularity of menstrual cycles than is usual for that age group, and the irregularity may include either amenorrhoea or prolonged heavy periods. Abnormalities of gonadotrophin secretion are also characteristic of PCOS, in particular an elevated luteinizing hormone (LH) or an elevated luteinizing hormone (LH)-to-follicle-stimulating hormone (FSH) ratio [96]. However, serum LH levels may be normal in up to 40% of women with PCOS [97].

At least 60% of adolescent girls with features of the metabolic syndrome have concomitant PCOS, and multiple cardiovascular risk factors are two to three times more common in women with PCOS than in healthy controls. Of all women with PCOS, about 55–60% have normal glucose tolerance, 30% have impaired glucose tolerance and 5–10% have T2DM. Between 30 and 80% of obese PCOS, women will develop T2DM by 30 years of age. The prevalence of glucose intolerance increases with increasing BMI. Women with PCOS have a higher prevalence of cardiovascular disease on long-term follow-up than their healthy peers [98]. The cardiovascular abnormalities include lower HDL cholesterol, increased carotid intima-media artery thickness, reduced vascular-flow-mediated dilatation and an RR for coronary heart disease of 1.5 and for fatal myocardial infarction of 1.9.

Treatment

Therapy for PCOS can be divided into acute and chronic therapy. Acute therapy is aimed at managing the infertility, improving the menstrual cycles and treating the acne and hirsutism. Chronic therapy is aimed at managing the cardiovascular risk factors including glucose intolerance and T2DM.

Acute management

The first principle of management is lifestyle intervention to reduce calorie intake, increase exercise and achieve weight reduction. Several studies have shown the beneficial effects on menstrual abnormalities, fertility rate, hirsutism and acanthosis nigricans (**B, C**) [99–101]. These improvements seem to be maximised in women who lost more than 5% of their body weight. The intervention has to be a combination of diet and exercise programmes. The main beneficial effects of weight loss in PCOS appear to be mediated via reduction of hyperinsulinism, improved insulin sensitivity and consequently reduced androgen levels. However, none of these parameters changed significantly in women who failed to restore a normal ovulation pattern (**B**) [99].

After lifestyle, the choices are between oral contraceptives, antiandrogens and insulin sensitisers. Oral contraceptives (OCP) can regularise the menstrual cycle and promote ovulation. They also reduce serum androgen levels, hirsutism and acne. In these respects, they are more effective than insulin sensitisers. The disadvantages of oral contraceptives are that they may worsen insulin resistance, increase the risk of cardiovascular disease and increase triglyceride levels. Cyproterone acetate has been popular as an antiandrogen in PCOS. In a study of the effectiveness of Dianette (OCP plus cyproterone) versus metformin (**A**) [102], Dianette caused worsening of insulin resistance. There is a concern about putting young people on cyproterone at the age of 14 years and the long-term effects over decades of use in terms of cardiovascular risk. If oral contraceptives are chosen as treatment for PCOS, it is advisable to undertake a baseline oral glucose tolerance test and fasting lipids and repeat after 3–4 months on treatment. Insulin sensitisers have been shown to help ovulation in infertile women with PCOS, and metformin can enhance ovulation in 80% of women. Traditionally, women have been advised to stop metformin once they have conceived. However, there is some evidence of an increased rate of miscarriage in women with PCOS once they have become pregnant and stopped metformin.

Chronic management

The mainstay of chronic management is to reduce the long-term risks for cardiovascular disease. All patients should be screened for cardiovascular risk factors at baseline, including blood pressure and lipids and an oral glucose tolerance test. Insulin sensitisers in PCOS have been shown to reduce insulin resistance and improve glucose tolerance, and there is evidence that they slow progression to T2DM and cardiovascular disease (**B**) [103]. Metformin is the drug of choice: it improves peripheral insulin sensitivity and attenuates hyperandrogenaemia in both lean and obese women with PCOS, restoring normal menses in a large proportion of previously amenorrhoeic women (**B**) [104]. The alternatives include thiazolidinediones; there is some evidence that these drugs can improve carotid intima-media artery thickness.

References

1 World Health Organization Department of Noncommunicable Disease Surveillance. *Definition, Diagnosis and Classification of Diabetes Mellitus and its Complications. Report of a WHO Consultation Part 1: Diagnosis and Classification of Diabetes Mellitus.* Geneva, 1999. Available at: http://www.diabetes.com.au/pdf/who_report.pdf

2 Field LL. Genetic linkage and association studies of type I diabetes: challenges and rewards. *Diabetologia* 2002; **45**: 21–35.

3 Medici F, Hawa M, Ianari A *et al.* Concordance rate for type II diabetes mellitus in monozygotic twins: actuarial analysis. *Diabetologia* 1999; **42**: 146–50.

3a Knowler WC, Bennett PH, Hamman RF *et al.* Diabetes incidence and prevalence in Pima Indians: a 19-fold greater incidence than in Rochester, Minnesota. *Am J Epidemiol* 1978; **108**: 497–505.

4 Hopper JL. Is type II (non-insulin-dependent) diabetes mellitus not so 'genetic' after all? *Diabetologia* 1999; **42**: 125–7.

5 Poulsen P, Kyvik KO, Vaag A *et al.* Heritability of type II (non-insulin-dependent) diabetes mellitus and abnormal glucose tolerance – a population-based twin study. *Diabetologia* 1999; **42**: 139–45.

5a Feltblower RG, Bodansky HJ, McKinney PA *et al.* Trends in the incidence of type 1 diabetes in South Asians in Bradford, UK. *Diabet Med* 2002; **19**: 162–6.

6 Horikawa Y, Oda N, Cox NJ *et al.* Genetic variation in the gene encoding calpain-10 is associated with type 2 diabetes mellitus. *Nat Genet* 2000; **26**: 163–75.

7 Weedon MN, Schwarz PE, Horikawa Y *et al.* Meta-analysis and a large association study confirm a role for calpain-10 variation in type 2 diabetes susceptibility. *Am J Hum Genet* 2003; **73**: 1208–12.

8 Turner MD, Cassell PG, Hitman GA. Calpain-10: from genome search to function. *Diabetes Metab Res Rev* 2005; **21**: 505–14.

9 Yamagata K, Furuta H, Oda N *et al.* Mutations in the hepatocyte nuclear factor-4alpha gene in maturity-onset diabetes of the young (MODY1). *Nature* 1996; **384**: 458–60.

10 Moller AM, Urhammer SA, Dalgaard LT *et al.* Studies of the genetic variability of the coding region of the hepatocyte nuclear factor-4alpha in Caucasians with maturity onset NIDDM. *Diabetologia* 1997; **40**: 980–3.

11 Rissanen J, Wang H, Miettinen R *et al.* Variants in the hepatocyte nuclear factor-1alpha and -4alpha genes in Finnish and Chinese subjects with late-onset type 2 diabetes. *Diabetes Care* 2000; **23**: 1533–8.

12 Thomas H, Jaschkowitz K, Bulman M *et al.* A distant upstream promoter of the HNF-4alpha gene connects the transcription factors involved in maturity-onset diabetes of the young. *Hum Mol Genet* 2001; **10**: 2089–97.

13 Love-Gregory LD, Wasson J, Ma J *et al.* A common polymorphism in the upstream promoter region of the hepatocyte nuclear factor-4 alpha gene on chromosome 20q is associated with type 2 diabetes and appears to contribute to the evidence for linkage in an ashkenazi jewish population. *Diabetes* 2004; **53**: 1134–40.

14 Silander K, Mohlke KL, Scott LJ *et al.* Genetic variation near the hepatocyte nuclear factor-4 alpha gene predicts susceptibility to type 2 diabetes. *Diabetes* 2004; **53**: 1141–9.

15 Grant SF, Thorleifsson G, Reynisdottir I *et al.* Variant of transcription factor 7-like 2 (TCF7L2) gene confers risk of type 2 diabetes. *Nat Genet* 2006; **38**: 320–3.

16 Reynisdottir I, Thorleifsson G, Benediktsson R *et al.* Localization of a susceptibility gene for type 2 diabetes to chromosome 5q34-q35.2. *Am J Hum Genet* 2003; **73**: 323–35.

17 Duggirala R, Blangero J, Almasy L *et al.* Linkage of type 2 diabetes mellitus and of age at onset to a genetic location on chromosome 10q in Mexican Americans. *Am J Hum Genet* 1999; **64**: 1127–40.

18 Kreymann B, Williams G, Ghatei MA *et al.* Glucagon-like peptide-1 7-36: a physiological incretin in man. *Lancet* 1987; **2**: 1300–4.

19 Malecki MT, Jhala US, Antonellis A *et al.* Mutations in NEUROD1 are associated with the development of type 2 diabetes mellitus. *Nat Genet* 1999; **23**: 323–8.

20 Ong KK, Phillips DI, Fall C *et al.* The insulin gene VNTR, type 2 diabetes and birth weight. *Nat Genet* 1999; **21**: 262–3.

21 Huxtable SJ, Saker PJ, Haddad L *et al.* Analysis of parent-offspring trios provides evidence for linkage and association between the insulin gene and type 2 diabetes mediated exclusively through paternally transmitted class III variable number tandem repeat alleles. *Diabetes* 2000; **49**: 126–30.

22 Hansen SK, Gjesing AP, Rasmussen SK *et al.* Large-scale studies of the HphI insulin gene variable-number-of-tandem-repeats polymorphism in relation to Type 2 diabetes mellitus and insulin release. *Diabetologia* 2004; **47**: 1079–87.

23 Meigs JB, Dupuis J, Herbert AG *et al.* The insulin gene variable number tandem repeat and risk of type 2 diabetes in a population-based sample of families and unrelated men and women. *J Clin Endocrinol Metab* 2005; **90**: 1137–43.

24 Kim HI, Ahn YH. Role of peroxisome proliferator-activated receptor-gamma in the glucose-sensing apparatus of liver and beta-cells. *Diabetes* 2004; **53**(suppl 1): S60–5.

25 Suter SL, Nolan JJ, Wallace P *et al.* Metabolic effects of new oral hypoglycemic agent CS-045 in NIDDM subjects. *Diabetes Care* 1992; **15**: 193–203.

26 Barroso I, Gurnell M, Crowley VE *et al.* Dominant negative mutations in human PPARgamma associated with severe insulin resistance, diabetes mellitus and hypertension. *Nature* 1999; **402**: 880–3.

27 Hegele RA, Cao H, Frankowski C *et al.* PPARG F388L, a transactivation-deficient mutant, in familial partial lipodystrophy. *Diabetes* 2002; **51**: 3586–90.

28 Savage DB, Tan GD, Acerini CL *et al.* Human metabolic syndrome resulting from dominant-negative mutations in the nuclear receptor peroxisome proliferator-activated receptor-gamma. *Diabetes* 2003; **52**: 910–17.

29 Deeb SS, Fajas L, Nemoto M *et al.* A Pro12Ala substitution in PPARgamma2 associated with de-creased receptor activity, lower body mass index and improved insulin sensitivity. *Nat Genet* 1998; **20**: 284–7.

30 Yen CJ, Beamer BA, Negri C *et al.* Molecular scanning of the human peroxisome proliferator activated receptor gamma (hPPAR gamma) gene in diabetic Caucasians: identification of a Pro12Ala PPAR gamma 2 missense mutation. *Biochem Biophys Res Commun* 1997; **241**: 270–4.

31 Yamauchi T, Kamon J, Waki H *et al.* The mechanisms by which both heterozygous peroxisome proliferator-activated receptor gamma (PPARgamma) deficiency and PPARgamma agonist improve insulin resistance. *J Biol Chem* 2001; **276**: 41245–54.

32 Altshuler D, Hirschhorn JN, Klannemark M *et al.* The common PPARgamma Pro12Ala polymorphism is associated with decreased risk of type 2 diabetes. *Nat Genet* 2000; **26**: 76–80.

33 Aguilar-Bryan L, Clement JP, Gonzalez G *et al.* Toward understanding the assembly and structure of KATP channels. *Physiol Rev* 1998; **78**: 227–45.

34 Thomas P, Ye Y, Lightner E. Mutation of the pancreatic islet inward rectifier Kir6.2 also leads to familial persistent hyperinsulinemic hypoglycemia of infancy. *Hum Mol Genet* 1996; **5**: 1809–12.

35 Gloyn AL, Pearson ER, Antcliff JF *et al.* Activating mutations in the gene encoding the ATP-sensitive potassium-channel subunit Kir6.2 and permanent neonatal diabetes. *N Engl J Med* 2004; **350**: 1838–49.

36 Gloyn AL, Hashim Y, Ashcroft SJ *et al.* Association studies of variants in promoter and coding regions of beta-cell ATP-sensitive K-channel genes SUR1 and Kir6.2 with Type 2 diabetes mellitus (UKPDS 53). *Diabet Med* 2001; **18**: 206–12.

37 Hani EH, Boutin P, Durand E *et al.* Missense mutations in the pancreatic islet beta cell inwardly rectifying K+ channel gene (KIR6.2/BIR): a meta-analysis suggests a role in the polygenic basis of type II diabetes mellitus in Caucasians. *Diabetologia* 1998; **41**: 1511–15.

38 Gloyn AL. Glucokinase (GCK) mutations in hyper- and hypoglycemia: maturity-onset diabetes of the young, permanent neonatal diabetes, and hyperinsulinemia of infancy. *Hum Mutat* 2003; **22**: 353–62.

39 Hansen SK, Nielsen EM, Ek J *et al.* Analysis of separate and combined effects of common variation in KCNJ11 and PPARG on risk of type 2 diabetes. *J Clin Endocrinol Metab* 2005; **90**: 3629–37.

40 Nielsen EM, Hansen L, Carstensen B *et al.* The E23K variant of Kir6.2 associates with impaired post-OGTT serum insulin response and increased risk of type 2 diabetes. *Diabetes* 2003; **52**: 573–7.

41 Florez JC, Burtt N, de Bakker PI *et al.* Haplotype structure and genotype-phenotype correlations of the sulfonylurea receptor and the islet ATP-sensitive potassium channel gene region. *Diabetes* 2004; **53**: 1360–8.

42 Savage PJ, Bennett PH, Senter RG *et al.* High prevalence of diabetes in young Pima Indians: evidence of phenotypic variation in a genetically isolated population. *Diabetes* 1979; **28**: 937–42.

43 Gerich JE. Clinical significance, pathogenesis, and management of postprandial hyperglycemia. *Arch Intern Med* 2003; **163**: 1306–16.

44 Lebovitz HE. Postprandial hyperglycaemic state: importance and consequences. *Diabetes Res Clin Pract* 1998; **40**(suppl): S27–8.

45 White N, Pyle L, Tamborlane W *et al.* Clinical characteristics and co-morbidities in a large cohort of youth with type 2 diabetes mellitus (T2DM) who volunteered for the Treatment Options for Type 2 Diabetes in Adolescence and Youth (TODAY) study. *Diabetes* 2006; **55**(suppl 1).

46 UKPDS. Intensive blood-glucose control with sulphonylureas or insulin compared with conventional treatment and risk of complications in patients with type 2 diabetes (UKPDS 33). UK Prospective Diabetes Study (UKPDS) Group. *Lancet* 1998; **352**: 837–53.

47 UKPDS. Tight blood pressure control and risk of macrovascular and microvascular complications in type 2 diabetes: UKPDS 38. UK Prospective Diabetes Study Group. *BMJ* 1998; **317**: 703–13.

48 McIntosh A, Hutchinson A, Home PD *et al. Clinical Guidelines and Evidence Review for Type 2 Diabetes: Management of Blood Glucose*, 2001. Available at: http://www.nice.org.uk/pdf/NICE_full_blood_glucose.pdf

49 Nathan DM, Buse JB, Davidson MB *et al.* Management of hyperglycaemia in type 2 diabetes: a consensus algorithm for the initiation and adjustment of therapy. A consensus statement from the American Diabetes Association and the European Association for the Study of Diabetes. *Diabetologia* 2006; **49**: 1711–21.

50 Strong WB, Malina RM, Blimkie CJ *et al.* Evidence based physical activity for school-age youth. *J Pediatr* 2005; **146**: 732–7.

51 Knowler WC, Barrett-Connor E, Fowler SE *et al.* Reduction in the incidence of type 2 diabetes with lifestyle intervention or metformin. *N Engl J Med* 2002; **346**: 393–403.

52 Tuomilehto J, Lindstrom J, Eriksson JG *et al.* Prevention of type 2 diabetes mellitus by changes in lifestyle among subjects with impaired glucose tolerance. *N Engl J Med* 2001; **344**: 1343–50.

53 Wright A, Burden AC, Paisey RB *et al.* Sulfonylurea inadequacy: efficacy of addition of insulin over 6 years in patients with type 2 diabetes in the U.K. Prospective Diabetes Study (UKPDS 57). *Diabetes Care* 2002; **25**: 330–6.

54 Royal College of Paediatrics and Child Health. *RCPCH Guideline Appraisal – Management of Obesity in Children and Young People.* Available at: http://www.rcpch.ac.uk/publications/clinical_docs/Obesity.pdf

55 UKPDS. Effect of intensive blood-glucose control with metformin on complications in overweight patients with type 2 diabetes (UKPDS 34). UK Prospective Diabetes Study (UKPDS) Group. *Lancet* 1998; **352**: 854–65.

56 Jones KL, Arslanian S, Peterokova VA *et al.* Effect of metformin in pediatric patients with type 2 diabetes: a randomized controlled trial. *Diabetes Care* 2002; **25**: 89–94.

57 Dormandy JA, Charbonnel B, Eckland DJ *et al.* Secondary prevention of macrovascular events in patients with type 2 diabetes in the Proactive Study (Prospective pioglitAzone Clinical Trial in macroVascular Events): a randomised controlled trial. *Lancet* 2005; **366**: 1279–89.

58 Grinstein G, Aponte L, Vuguin P *et al.* Presentation and 5-year follow-up of non-insulin dependent diabetes mellitus (NIDDM) in minority youth. *Abstract presented at the 81st Annual Meeting of the Endocrine Society, San Diego, California.* OR 25-5, 1999.

59 Brown JB, Nichols GA, Perry A. The burden of treatment failure in type 2 diabetes. *Diabetes Care* 2004; **27**: 1535–40.

60 Monnier L, Lapinski H, Colette C. Contributions of fasting and postprandial plasma glucose increments to the overall diurnal hyperglycemia of type 2 diabetic patients: variations with increasing levels of HbA(1c). *Diabetes Care* 2003; **26**: 881–5.

61 Alberti G. A desktop guide to type 2 diabetes mellitus. European Diabetes Policy Group 1998–1999. International Diabetes Federation European Region. *Exp Clin Endocrinol Diabetes* 1999; **107**: 390–420.

62 American Diabetes Association. Standards of medical care for patients with diabetes mellitus. *Diabetes Care* 1994; **17**: 616–23.

63 Haffner SM, Lehto S, Ronnemaa T *et al.* Mortality from coronary heart disease in subjects with type 2 diabetes and in nondiabetic subjects with and without prior myocardial infarction. *N Engl J Med* 1998; **339**: 229–34.

64 Orchard TJ, Forrest KY, Kuller LH *et al.* Lipid and blood pressure treatment goals for type 1 diabetes: 10-year incidence data from the Pittsburgh Epidemiology of Diabetes Complications Study. *Diabetes Care* 2001; **24**: 1053–9.

65 NICE. *Statins for the Prevention of Cardiovascular Disease.* Technology Appraisal 94. Available at: www.nice.org.uk/TA094

66 Keech A, Simes RJ, Barter P *et al.* Effects of long-term fenofibrate therapy on cardiovascular events in 9795 people with type 2 diabetes mellitus (the FIELD study): randomised controlled trial. *Lancet* 2005; **366**: 1849–61.

67 Rosner B, Prineas RJ, Loggie JM *et al.* Blood pressure nomograms for children and adolescents, by height, sex, and age, in the United States. *J Pediatr* 1993; **123**: 871–86.

68 McAvoy N, ferguson JW, Campbell IW *et al.* Non-alcoholic fatty liver disease: natural history, pathogenesis and treatment. *Br J Diabetes Vasc Dis* 2006; **6**: 251–60.

69 Baumann U, Brown R. Non-alcoholic fatty liver in childhood. *Br J Diabetes Vasc Dis* 2006; **6**: 264–8.

70 Stein I, Leventhal M. Amenorrhoea associated with bilateral polycystic ovaries. *Am J Obstet Gynecol* 1935; **29**: 181–91.

71 Achard C, Thiers J. Le virilisme pilaire et son association a l'insuffisance glycolitique (diebete des femmes a barb). *Bull Acad Natl Med* 1921; **86**: 51–64.

72 Legro RS, Kunselman AR, Dodson WC *et al.* Prevalence and predictors of risk for type 2 diabetes mellitus and impaired glucose tolerance in polycystic ovary syndrome: a prospective, controlled study in 254 affected women. *J Clin Endocrinol Metab* 1999; **84**: 165–9.

73 Conn JJ, Jacobs HS, Conway GS. The prevalence of polycystic ovaries in women with type 2 diabetes mellitus. *Clin Endocrinol (Oxf)* 2000; **52**: 81–6.

74 Codner E, Soto N, Lopez P *et al.* Diagnostic criteria for polycystic ovary syndrome and ovarian morphology in women with type 1 diabetes mellitus. *J Clin Endocrinol Metab* 2006; **91**: 2250–6.

75 Franks S, Gharani N, McCarthy M. Genetic abnormalities in polycystic ovary syndrome. *Ann Endocrinol (Paris)* 1999; **60**: 131–3.

76 Govind A, Obhrai MS, Clayton RN. Polycystic ovaries are inherited as an autosomal dominant trait: analysis of 29 polycystic ovary syndrome and 10 control families. *J Clin Endocrinol Metab* 1999; **84**: 38–43.

77 Kahn CR, Flier JS, Bar RS *et al.* The syndromes of insulin resistance and acanthosis nigricans: insulin-receptor disorders in man. *N Engl J Med* 1976; **294**: 739–45.

78 O'Rahilly S, Choi WH, Patel P *et al.* Detection of mutations in insulin-receptor gene in NIDDM patients by analysis of single-stranded conformation polymorphisms. *Diabetes* 1991; **40**: 777–82.

79 Conway GS, Avey C, Rumsby G. The tyrosine kinase domain of the insulin receptor gene is normal in women with hyperinsulinaemia and polycystic ovary syndrome. *Hum Reprod* 1994; **9**: 1681–3.

80 Talbot JA, Bicknell EJ, Rajkhowa M *et al.* Molecular scanning of the insulin receptor gene in women with polycystic ovarian syndrome. *J Clin Endocrinol Metab* 1996; **81**: 1979–83.

81 Chang RJ, Nakamura RM, Judd HL *et al.* Insulin resistance in nonobese patients with polycystic ovarian disease. *J Clin Endocrinol Metab* 1983; **57**: 356–9.

82 Kahn SE. The relative contributions of insulin resistance and beta-cell dysfunction to the pathophysiology of type 2 diabetes. *Diabetologia* 2003; **46**: 3–19.

83 Ehrmann DA, Sturis J, Byrne MM *et al.* Insulin secretory defects in polycystic ovary syndrome: relationship to insulin sensitivity and family history of non-insulin-dependent diabetes mellitus. *J Clin Invest* 1995; **96**: 520–7.

84 Dunaif A, Segal KR, Futterweit W *et al.* Profound peripheral insulin resistance, independent of obesity, in polycystic ovary syndrome. *Diabetes* 1989; **38**: 1165–74.

85 Dunaif A, Green G, Futterweit W *et al.* Suppression of hyperandrogenism does not improve peripheral or hepatic insulin resistance in the polycystic ovary syndrome. *J Clin Endocrinol Metab* 1990; **70**: 699–704.

86 Ehrmann DA, Cavaghan MK, Imperial J *et al.* Effects of metformin on insulin secretion, insulin action, and ovarian steroidogenesis in women with polycystic ovary syndrome. *J Clin Endocrinol Metab* 1997; **82**: 524–30.

87 Nestler JE, Jakubowicz DJ, de Vargas AF *et al.* Insulin stimulates testosterone biosynthesis by human thecal cells from women with polycystic ovary syndrome by activating its own receptor and using inositolglycan mediators as the signal transduction system. *J Clin Endocrinol Metab* 1998; **83**: 2001–5.

88 Poretsky L. On the paradox of insulin-induced hyperandrogenism in insulin-resistant states. *Endocr Rev* 1991; **12**: 3–13.

89 Rajkhowa M, Bicknell J, Jones M *et al.* Insulin sensitivity in women with polycystic ovary syndrome: relationship to hyperandrogenemia. *Fertil Steril* 1994; **61**: 605–12.

90 Moran A, Jacobs DR, Jr, Steinberger J *et al.* Insulin resistance during puberty: results from clamp studies in 357 children. *Diabetes* 1999; **48**: 2039–44.

91 Ibanez L, Potau N, Zampolli M *et al.* Hyperinsulinemia in postpubertal girls with a history of premature pubarche and functional ovarian hyperandrogenism. *J Clin Endocrinol Metab* 1996; **81**: 1237–43.

92 Oppenheimer E, Linder B, DiMartino-Nardi J. Decreased insulin sensitivity in prepubertal girls with premature adrenarche and acanthosis nigricans. *J Clin Endocrinol Metab* 1995; **80**: 614–18.

93 Farquhar CM, Birdsall M, Manning P *et al.* The prevalence of polycystic ovaries on ultrasound scanning in a population of randomly selected women. *Aust N Z J Obstet Gynaecol* 1994; **34**: 67–72.

94 Rotterdam ESHRE & ASRM-sponsored PCOS Consensus Workshop Group. Revised 2003 consensus on diagnostic criteria and long-term health risks related to polycystic ovary syndrome. *Fertil Steril* 2004; **81**: 19–25.

95 Escobar-Morreale HF, Asuncion M, Calvo RM *et al.* Receiver operating characteristic analysis of the performance of basal serum hormone profiles for the diagnosis of polycystic ovary syndrome in epidemiological studies. *Eur J Endocrinol* 2001; **145**: 619–24.

96 Morales AJ, Laughlin GA, Butzow T *et al.* Insulin, somatotropic, and luteinizing hormone axes in lean and obese women with polycystic ovary syndrome: common and distinct features. *J Clin Endocrinol Metab* 1996; **81**: 2854–64.

97 Conway GS, Jacobs HS, Holly JM *et al.* Effects of luteinizing hormone, insulin, insulin-like growth factor-I and insulin-like growth factor small binding protein 1 in the polycystic ovary syndrome. *Clin Endocrinol (Oxf)* 1990; **33**: 593–603.

98 Wild S, Pierpoint T, McKeigue P *et al.* Cardiovascular disease in women with polycystic ovary syndrome at long-term follow-up: a retrospective cohort study. *Clin Endocrinol (Oxf)* 2000; **52**: 595–600.

99 Huber-Buchholz MM, Carey DG, Norman RJ. Restoration of reproductive potential by lifestyle modification in obese polycystic ovary syndrome: role of insulin sensitivity and luteinizing hormone. *J Clin Endocrinol Metab* 1999; **84**: 1470–4.

100 Kiddy DS, Hamilton-Fairley D, Bush A *et al.* Improvement in endocrine and ovarian function during dietary treatment of obese women with polycystic ovary syndrome. *Clin Endocrinol (Oxf)* 1992; **36**: 105–11.

101 Pasquali R, Antenucci D, Casimirri F *et al.* Clinical and hormonal characteristics of obese amenorrheic hyperandrogenic women before and after weight loss. *J Clin Endocrinol Metab* 1989; **68**: 173–9.

102 Morin-Papunen LC, Vauhkonen I, Koivunen RM *et al.* Insulin sensitivity, insulin secretion, and metabolic and hormonal parameters in healthy women and women with polycystic ovarian syndrome. *Hum Reprod* 2000; **15**: 1266–74.

103 Sattar N, Hopkinson ZE, Greer IA. Insulin-sensitising agents in polycystic-ovary syndrome. *Lancet* 1998; **351**: 305–7.

104 Diamanti-Kandarakis E, Kouli C, Tsianateli T *et al.* Therapeutic effects of metformin on insulin resistance and hyperandrogenism in polycystic ovary syndrome. *Eur J Endocrinol* 1998; **138**: 269–74.

CHAPTER 13

Rare forms of diabetes

Julian Shield, Maciej T. Malecki, Nicola A. Bridges &
Jeremy Allgrove

> *The ability to ask questions is the greatest resource in learning the truth.*
>
> —Anon

Neonatal diabetes (genetics and management)

Julian Shield

Introduction

Neonatal diabetes is a rare condition affecting 1: 4–500,000 live births a year (**E**) [1]. Whilst rare, the last 10–15 years have witnessed dramatic advances in both the understanding of its genetic basis and the treatment. Although still carrying the nomenclature suggesting a neonatal disease, it has become increasingly obvious that any child under 6 months of age developing diabetes is unlikely to have autoimmune-based type 1 diabetes mellitus (T1DM) and is liable to have one of the monogenic gene disorders linked to neonatal-onset diabetes (**B**) [2]. As might be expected, nearly all the genes associated with this condition are intimately linked to fetal and infant pancreatic development. Neonatal diabetes can, for good prognostic and clinical reasons, be subdivided into a transient (TNDM) and permanent (PNDM) form. The details are summarised in Table 13.1.

Insulin promoter factor 1 deficiency (OMIM 260370)

Frequency: rare
Stoffers *et al.* described a child with permanent neonatal diabetes and pancreatic exocrine insufficiency due to pancreatic agenesis (**C**) [3]. The proband was homozygous for a mutation (Pro63fsdelC) in *insulin promoter factor 1* (*IPF-1*), a gene involved in the master control of exocrine and endocrine pancreatic development, being responsible for the co-ordinated development of the pancreas *in utero* and also for the continued functional integrity of pancreatic beta islet cells. Within the extended family were eight individuals from six generations with early-onset diabetes akin to T2DM. These were identified as heterozygotes for the same mutation. The illness resultant on heterozygosity was reassigned as maturity-onset diabetes of the young (MODY) 4 (**C**) [4]. Only one further case report of pancreatic agenesis has been ascribed to an *IPF-1* mutation and this was a compound heterozygous mutation of the gene (**C**) [5].

Table 13.1 Main types of neonatal diabetes, their genetic basis, comorbidities, treatment, outcome and relative frequencies as potential diagnoses

Gene	Chromosome	Associated features	Outcome and treatment	Frequency of reports and clinical likelihood	OMIM number
IPF-1	13q21.1	Pancreatic agenesis	Insulin and exocrine replacement therapy for life, outcome seemingly good	Rare	#260370
Probable ZAC	6q24	Macroglossia and umbilical herniae	Resolution usually within 3 mo; relapse around adolescence in ≈50%	Commonest form of TNDM	%601410
FOXP3	Xp11.23	Enteropathy with severe failure to thrive; other autoimmune phenomena such as hypothyroidism and autoimmune haemolytic anaemia	Poor prognosis; bone marrow transplantation and immunosuppression have been tried with equivocal success	Fairly common	#304790
Glucokinase	7p15-13	None identified	Lifelong insulin therapy	Relatively rare	*138079
EIF2AK3	2p12	Renal insufficiency, mental retardation, hepatomegaly, spondyloepiphyseal dysplasia	Early death; diabetes requires insulin	Fairly uncommon	#226980
PTF1A	10p12.3	Joint contractures, 'beaked nose' and low-set dysplastic ears: absent pancreas at post-mortem	Early death from respiratory failure	Rare	#609069

Gene	Locus	Features	Treatment/course	Frequency	OMIM
KCN11J	11p15.1	Severe mutations have associated neurological features, such as epilepsy and learning difficulties (DEND)	Majority respond to treatment with sulphonylureas (90%)	Commonest form of PNDM and rarer form of TNDM	*600937
ABCC8	11p15.1	Possibly minor neurological features in some cases	Majority TNDM, permanent cases respond to sulphonylureas as do transient cases in relapse	Moderately frequent	#606176
HNF1β	17cen-q21.3	Renal cysts	Long-term insulin therapy	Rare	#137920
GLIS3	9p24.3-23	Congenital hypothyroidism and glaucoma; liver fibrosis and cystic kidney disease; facial dysmorphism	50% dead by 2 yr of age; oldest surviving case now aged 22 yr	Rare (three families and six cases)	#610199

- An *asterisk* (*) before an entry number indicates a gene of known sequence.
- A *number symbol* (#) before an entry number indicates that it is a descriptive entry, usually of a phenotype, and does not represent a unique locus. The reason for the use of the '#' sign is given in the first paragraph of the OMIM entry. Discussion of any gene(s) related to the phenotype resides in another entry(ies), as described in the first paragraph.
- A *plus sign* (+) before an entry number indicates that the entry contains the description of a gene of known sequence and a phenotype.
- A *per cent sign* (%) before an entry number indicates that the entry describes a confirmed Mendelian phenotype or phenotypic locus for which the underlying molecular basis is not known.

Treatment

Due to the complete absence of pancreatic tissue, exocrine function is compromised, requiring the use of pancreatic enzyme supplementation in addition to lifelong insulin therapy. There are no extra-pancreatic-associated features.

Chromosome 6q anomalies (OMIM 601410)

Frequency: common

Transient diabetes in infancy that resolves within the first 3 months of life is a well-recognised phenomenon. Clinically, these children are born after significant intrauterine growth retardation, developing diabetes at a mean age of 3 days. The diabetes is characterised by severe hyperglycaemia and dehydration but little or no ketosis (**B**) [6]. Associated anomalies include umbilical herniae and relative macroglossia. This condition remains the most frequent single cause of neonatal diabetes (**E**) [7].

In 1995 two patients were identified with paternal uniparental (iso)disomy (UPD) of chromosome 6q24, causing transient neonatal diabetes (**C**) [8]. Effectively, the child inherited two copies of the same chromosome 6 from the father, with no contribution from the mother. The process of UPD can uncover autosomal recessive conditions, as the child can inherit two copies of a single mutation of a recessive gene carried on one of the parent of origin's chromosomes or it can imply that a gene or genes are imprinted, whereby the parent of origin affects a gene's functional phenotype. In simple terms, imprinted genes are switched off by the addition of a methyl group(s) generally in the promoter region, preventing gene transcription that can be either on the maternal or paternal copy of a gene. Anomalies in 6q are due to disorders of imprinting. Two copies of paternal chromosome 6, an unbalanced duplication (extra copy) of paternal 6q24 (**B, C**) [9, 10] that can be inherited, or loss of imprinting (loss of methylation) from maternal 6q24 all cause TNDM (**A**) [11] due to overexpression of gene(s) within the TNDM locus. At the American Diabetes Association meeting in 2006, Polychronakos and Xiaoyu Du presented data on specific and controlled ZAC overexpression on beta-cell function in the insulin 1 gene (INS-1) rat beta-cell line, demonstrating that it was likely to be the gene responsible for TNDM in 6q anomalies (**B**) [12].

All children with 6q anomalies have been associated with a transient form of diabetes in infancy but this has been reported to relapse around the time of adolescence in a majority, although there is probably an element of reporting bias in the quoted levels of around 60% (**B**) [6].

Treatment

All neonates presenting acutely with diabetes should be started on insulin therapy: usually on a continuous infusion so that normoglycaemia and any metabolic decompensation such as acidosis can be addressed swiftly. Once stabilised and an approximately daily requirement of insulin is established, conversion to either subcutaneous, intermittent insulin or continuous pump therapy can be initiated. Although long-acting insulins especially the analogue glargine may prove useful in a basal-bolus regimen (**E**) [13], the best results seem to be obtained using continuous insulin-pump therapy (**E**) [14]. On occasion, when pump therapy has proved logistically difficult, the author has used a three times a day mixed insulin regimen at mealtimes, with some success in those babies undergoing weaning. In the case of 6q anomalies diabetes will be transient, but insulin is required until remission to prevent dehydration and allow normal growth. If a molecular diagnosis of a 6q anomaly is established early in a baby with reasonable glycaemic control, it is tempting to use intermittent subcutaneous injections until remission, as education of the parents in pump therapy can be lengthy and complicated and the diabetes classically resolves over a few weeks or months.

Wolcott–Rallison syndrome (OMIM 226980)

Frequency: relatively uncommon

This is an autosomal recessive disorder characterised by infancy-onset (often within the neonatal period) diabetes associated with a spondyloepiphyseal dysplasia. In addition, there is a constellation of others features, such as hepatomegaly, mental retardation, renal failure and early death (**B**) [15]. In 2000, Delepine *et al.* used two consanguineous families to map the condition to the locus 2p12. Within this locus lay the gene *EIF2AK3* that is highly expressed in islet cells acting as a regulator of protein synthesis. Further analysis within the consanguineous Wolcott–Rallison families confirmed frameshift or amino acid substitution mutations occurring in *EIF2AK3* segregating with the disorder in each family (**C**) [16].

Treatment

Lifelong insulin therapy is required for this condition and the disease is characterised by early death from a number of causes, including renal failure and poorly controlled diabetes.

IPEX (*FOXP3* mutations) (OMIM 304790)

Frequency: fairly common

IPEX is probably the only condition described in children developing diabetes under the age of 6 months in which autoimmunity plays a part. Entitled 'immune dysregulation, polyendocrinopathy, enteropathy, X-Linked syndrome' (IPEX), its major features are early-onset diabetes (often neonatal) and diarrhoea, with small intestinal pathology such as villous atrophy and inflammatory infiltrate. In 2001, the human disease was identified as due to mutations in *FOXP3* (**C**) [17]. T1DM autoantibodies (GAD, IAA and ICA) are frequently described as those directed against the thyroid gland and various other organs (**B**) [18]. Other features frequently described in the human condition other than diabetes, enteropathy and severe failure to thrive include eczema, haemolytic anaemia, thrombocytopaenia and hypothyroidism.

Treatment

Given that immune dysregulation appears to underlie this condition, the obvious routes for treatment have been applied with varying degrees of success. Immunosuppression with cyclosporin or tacrolimus has proved to be of limited value in general, although some patients have responded better than others (**B**) [18]. The immunosuppression has often been at the cost of significant medication toxicity to other organs, such as the kidneys (**E**) [19]. As an alternative, bone marrow transplantation has been attempted in at least four cases with fairly promising effects over the short term on diarrhoea, weight gain and possibly diabetes but three patients subsequently succumbed to infection with evidence of an accompanying lymphoproliferative disorder (**B, C**) [18, 20]. The fourth patient did not have diabetes or a mutation in the coding region of *FOXP3* but did have a deletion in the promoter upstream of the gene and reduced levels of *FOXP3* mRNA. This child remains well 16 months after transplantation with complete clinical and immunological remission (**C**) [21]. Currently, the prognosis has to remain guarded for children with this condition.

Glucokinase mutations

Frequency: rare

MODY-2 is caused by mutations in the glucokinase gene and usually leads to mild hyperglycaemia in affected individuals. Glucokinase is a key regulator of glucose metabolism in islet cells controlling the levels of insulin secretion. However, within two families (Norwegian and Italian) with multiple forms of diabetes in their pedigree, two infants with classical PNDM (presenting on day 1) were identified who were homozygous for missense mutations within the glucokinase gene rendering them completely deficient in glycolytic activity, whilst their apparently consanguineous and mild-to-moderately glucose intolerant parents were heterozygous for the same mutations (**C**) [22, 23]. Further cases of permanent neonatal diabetes secondary to homozygous mutations in glucokinase have now been identified (**C**) [24], all in families with some consanguinity, although the condition is still very rare (**E**) [25]. When there is a history of maternal gestational diabetes, testing for fasting glucose levels in both parents is needed. If both parents have mild glucose intolerance, a screen for glucokinase mutations is then warranted.

Treatment

Lifelong insulin therapy is required.

KCNJ11 permanent neonatal diabetes (OMIM *600937)

Frequency: common

The second most common cause of neonatal diabetes is that induced by heterozygous activating mutations in the *KCNJ11* gene, which encodes the Kir 6.2 subunit of the K_{ATP}channel, a critical regulator of beta-cell insulin secretion (**B**) [26]. Although the majority have been identified to cause permanent neonatal diabetes, a few have been associated with a transient condition akin to that caused by 6q anomalies (**B**) [27].

The babies are born small for gestational age, but not as small as in some other neonatal diabetes conditions (mean birth weight 2.497 (690) g against 1.987 g (510) in 6q anomalies) (**E**) [7]. Thirty per cent have ketoacidosis and all display low insulin levels in the face of quite dramatic hyperglycaemia. The median age of presentation is around 3–4 weeks of age as opposed to 6q anomalies that tend to present in the first week of life, although the spectrum in both conditions is such that birth weight or the age of presentation cannot be used to distinguish between the two conditions. About 20% have associated neurological disease with developmental delay and sometimes epilepsy or muscle weakness reflecting a role for the same potassium channel in the central nervous system. The most severe end of this spectrum has been entitled 'DEND', developmental delay, epilepsy and neonatal diabetes in which children can be severely affected. There is also an intermediate condition (i-DEND) with milder developmental delay and no epilepsy. The mutations causing isolated diabetes produce less change in ATP sensitivity than those associated with diabetes and neurological disease (Q52R and V59G) (**B**) [28].

Treatment

Sulphonylureas, a class of drugs often used in T2DM, close K_{ATP} channels by an ATP-independent mechanism. A recent paper demonstrates that 90% ($n = 44/49$: ages 3 mo–36 yr) of patients with *KCNJ11* gene mutations can be successfully transferred from insulin to oral sulphonylurea therapy, with a highly significant and sustained improvement in glycated haemoglobin (8.1–6.4%). The median dose of glibenclamide (the most commonly used sulphonylurea) is 0.45 mg/kg/d but the range required is quite extensive from 0.05 to 1.5. Although a successful switch to sulphonylureas is not mutation specific, it would appear that those with neurological features are less likely to be successful (**B**) [29]. The effect of sulphonylurea therapy on neurological outcome is currently under investigation.

ABCC8 gene mutations in PNDM (OMIM 606176) and TNDM (OMIM 601410)

Frequency: moderately frequent

Recently, it has been identified that activating mutations in the *ABCC8* gene that encodes the sulphonylurea receptor component of the ATP-sensitive (K_{ATP}) channel together with the inward-rectifying potassium-channel subunit *Kir6.2* in the β cell can be responsible for both permanent and more commonly transient neonatal diabetes (**B**) [30, 31].

Treatment

Those few described with permanent neonatal diabetes ($n = 2$) respond effectively to glibenclamide therapy (0.22 and 0.59 mg/kg/d), whilst this has also proved effective in TNDM cases with later relapse of diabetes (**B**) [30]. Mutations in this gene may also be responsible for some cases of apparent early-onset T2DM in later life.

Permanent neonatal diabetes with cerebellar hypoplasia (OMIM 609069)

Frequency: rare

In 1999, a new recessively inherited disease of neonatal diabetes associated with cerebellar hypoplasia was described (**C**) [32]. The three children of consanguineous Pakistani origin had dysmorphic features (low-set ears, triangular facies, talipes equinovarus and joint stiffness) associated with neonatal diabetes, microcephaly, recurrent apnoeic attacks and absent cerebellar tissue on brain imaging. A further child of North European descent was later identified with an identical phenotype in whom an autopsy demonstrated complete pancreatic agenesis. Further studies on this child and the original family led to the identification of the gene responsible, *PTF1A*. This gene encodes the pancreas transcription factor 1 alpha which is essential for normal pancreatic and cerebellar development (**C**) [33]. So far, all children described with this condition have died in infancy, not from diabetes but associated respiratory failure probably secondary to the brain anomalies.

Other very rare forms of neonatal diabetes

1 In 2004, a probable new autosomal recessive condition of neonatal diabetes with intestinal and biliary anomalies was described. The five children were small for gestational age with neonatal diabetes, atresia of duodenum, jejunum and gall bladder and absence of insulin, glucagon and somatostatin containing cells on pancreatic post-mortem examination.

Four of the five died in the first year of life from seemingly multiorgan failure and/or sepsis (**C**) [34].

2 A similar but possibly different disease has been described with pancreatic agenesis, absent gall bladder and cardiac septal anomalies (**C**) [35, 36].

3 Senee *et al*. described a frameshift mutation or deletions in the transcription factor *GLIS3* in three consanguineous families with neonatal diabetes, congenital hypothyroidism and facial dysmorphology (large, flat, square-shaped face with a thin and bird-shaped curved nose). Additional features seen in some patients included congenital glaucoma, liver fibrosis and cystic kidneys (**C**) [37].

4 In one family, a missense heterozygous mutation of *HNF-1β* was associated with permanent neonatal diabetes and some small cysts in one child but only transient hyperglycaemia with more profound renal dysplasia in the other sibling (**C**) [38].

Maturity-onset diabetes of the young

Maciej Malecki

The progress in molecular genetics over last two decades made all those interested in diabetes research and clinical practice aware of the enormous heterogeneity of this disease. However, the concept of its variety is not entirely new and the clinical differences amongst diabetic patients have been observed over centuries. For example, in the middle of nineteenth century, Bouchardet distinguished two major types of disease (**C**) [39]. The first, with bad prognosis, occurred in young, lean individuals and responded poorly to the only treatment available at that time, which was diet and physical exercise. On the other hand, older, obese persons with diabetes responded much better to this treatment. It took almost another 100 years to realise that even young and lean subjects with diabetes are not all the same. The majority of them required prompt and lifelong insulin treatment to save their lives. There was, however, a much smaller group with a strikingly less severe clinical picture and a better prognosis. Usually, in their families there were a lot of subjects with diabetes of similar clinical picture and the disease was typically passed to the next generations as an autosomal dominant trait. The acronym MODY was given to this form of diabetes (**A**) [40]. The mystery of MODY nature has been recently solved by molecular biology.

Genetics of MODY

Based on the role of genetic factors, diabetes, as many other diseases such as arterial hypertension or hyperlipidaemia, may be divided into two major groups: polygenic and monogenic forms (**E**) [41, 42]. The clinical picture of frequent, complex, multifactorial diabetes, both T1DM and T2DM, is a result of the interaction between the environment and genetic background understood as the contribution of many different genes (see Chapters 3 and 12 respectively for further details). The susceptibility to polygenic forms of diabetes is associated with frequent polymorphisms that influence the expression of genes in the regulatory parts or result in amino acid variants in exons (**E**) [41, 42]. Alleles of those polymorphisms are present in both healthy individuals and diabetic patients, although with different frequencies. Those sequence differences are associated with just a modest increase in the risk of developing the disease. So they can be considered susceptibility variants, but certainly not causative factors that unequivocally determine the disease.

Figure 13.1 Schematic comparison of the influence of genetic and environmental factors on the occurrence of monogenic and polygenic diabetes is shown. In a monogenic form, such as MODY, a mutation with severe biological impact on the function of one protein causes the phenotype. As a result of this mutation, the disease is almost inevitable. Environmental factors are of less importance, they may modify some characteristics of the clinical picture, e.g. the age of diagnosis.

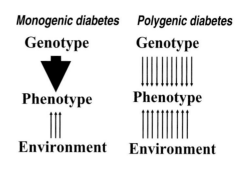

In a polygenic form of disease, such as T2DM, both genetic and environmental factors are necessary for the occurrence of the phenotype. The impact of many genetic polymorphisms and environmental factors, such as sedentary lifestyle and obesity, is being summarised.

In contrast, monogenic forms are a consequence of rare mutations in a single gene (**E**) [41, 42]. Those mutations cause significant changes in the structure and subsequently in the function of a protein or, rarely, a tRNA. Monogenic diseases have enormous impact on the health of specific individuals. However, from the epidemiological perspective, their impact on entire societies is very limited. Genetic background plays a critical role in the pathogenesis of monogenic forms of diabetes, while the environment may only slightly modify the elements of the clinical picture, e.g. age of disease onset (Figure 13.1). They are usually characterised by early age of diagnosis, sometimes in very early childhood, but it may be in adolescence as well, and occasionally by the presence of extra-pancreatic features. Monogenic forms constitute just a small portion of diabetes, but scientific tools available in recent years worked very well in finding those single genes with a big impact on disease development (**E**) [41, 42]. This is a consequence of the fact that monogenic forms have a clearly defined inheritance model and the ascertainment of multigenerational families is relatively straightforward, which makes genetic studies much easier (Figure 13.2). Monogenic diabetes is not frequently met among children and adolescents, unlike cases of autoimmune T1DM (**B**) [43].

However, the right differential diagnosis is of enormous practical importance. The known forms of monogenic diabetes are characterised by either, more frequently, a presence of a defect in insulin secretion or, very rarely, a profound decrease in insulin sensitivity (**E**) [44]. The most frequent monogenic diabetes that is characterised by severe beta-cell defect is MODY. As mentioned above, several decades ago it was noticed that in some families diabetes of moderate clinical picture was inherited as an autosomal dominant trait (**C**) [45]. This means that it occurred in families in several subsequent generations with equal frequency in both genders and was transmitted by both men and women (**E**) [46]. In the years that followed, many such families with diabetes were described and that fact accelerated the genetic studies of this form of disease (**E**) [47]. In addition to an autosomal dominant mode of inheritance, the clinical features linked with MODY included early disease onset, usually in the second or third decade of life, lean body mass as well as impairment in insulin secretion (**E, A**) [47–49].

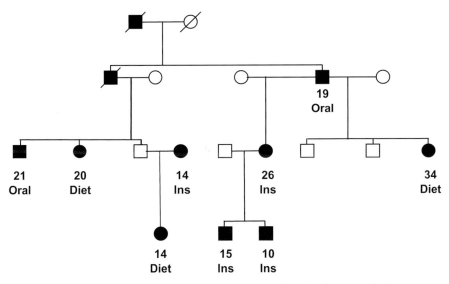

Figure 13.2 An example of a family with MODY is shown. Closed and open symbols represent subjects with diabetes and normal glucose tolerance, respectively. The information about the diabetes age of diagnosis is shown in the first line. Below that is shown the method of treatment. Note that diabetes was diagnosed in four consecutive generations and that it was inherited only from one side of the family. The diagnosis was generally established in the second or third decade of life. In this particular family, the variety of therapeutic options is seen: there are individuals on diet, oral hypoglycaemic agents and insulin.

Even before the pathogenesis of MODY was defined by molecular genetics, it was observed that it did not constitute a uniform entity (**E**) [50]. Among the families with autosomal dominant early-onset diabetes there were some characterised by mild fasting hyperglycaemia, with very moderate post-load glycaemic increment and almost total absence of diabetic complications (**B**) [51]. In contrast, other families had a more severe clinical picture of the disease with substantial impairment in insulin secretion, progressive hyperglycaemia and quite frequent presence of chronic vascular complications (**A,B**) [49, 52, 53]. Indeed, this observation of clinical diversity was later explained by the results of genetic studies that dissected MODY into several forms (**E**) [47]. The term MODY has been very commonly used in hundreds of reports published worldwide every year. However, this name itself was not included in the new classification of diabetes by the American Diabetes Association and World Health Organization (**E**) [54]. Instead of MODY, discrete subtypes of diabetes arising from mutations in specific beta-cell genes and designated as MODY in scientific literature can be found in the section *Other specific types* of this classification (**E**) [54].

Presently, a consensus exists with respect to six genes linked with MODY (**E**) [48, 55]. This list includes hepatocyte nuclear factor *-4α, -1α, -1β* (*HNF-4α, -1α, -1β*), glucokinase, *IPF-1α* and *NEUROD1* (**C, B**) [56–61]. Five proteins coded by those genes are transcription factors present in the beta-cell nucleus; the only exception is glucokinase, the enzyme expressed in the exocrine pancreas and liver (Figure 13.3).

MODY associated with glucokinase gene mutations
Glucokinase is a key regulatory enzyme of the pancreatic beta cells, which catalyses glucose phosphorylation to glucose 6-phosphate. This step is crucial for the energy production

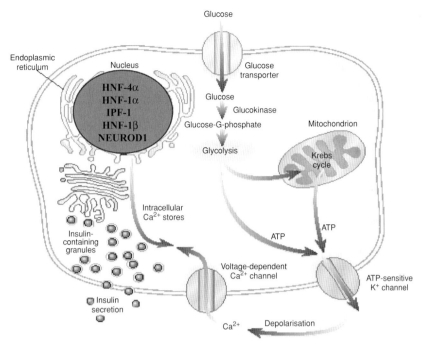

Figure 13.3 The schematic presentation of beta-cell structure and function is shown; the cellular localisation of proteins associated with MODY is marked. Once glucose is transported inside the beta cell by glucose transporter 2 (GLUT-2) protein, a specific transporter, glucokinase enzyme (MODY-2 gene) catalyses its phosphorylation to glucose 6-phosphate. The next steps of glucose metabolism, glycolysis and the Krebs cycle result in the generation of ATP. The rise in its cellular concentration leads to closure of the ATP-sensitive potassium channels, depolarisation of the plasma membrane, opening of the voltage-dependent calcium channels and influx of calcium from extra- and intracellular sources. Subsequently, the fusion of secretory granules containing insulin with the plasma membrane and the release of this hormone into circulation occurs. A heterozygous mutation in the glucokinase gene results in a reduction in activity of this enzyme in the beta cell, causing impaired glucose phosphorylation and subsequently decreased glucose-stimulated insulin release.

The transcription factors associated with MODY – HNF-4α (MODY-1), HNF-1α (MODY-3), IPF-1 (MODY-4), HNF-1β (MODY-5) and NEUROD1 (MODY-6) – function in the nucleus of the beta cell. Each of them regulates the transcription of the insulin gene either directly or indirectly, through effects on the expression of other transcription factors. They also regulate the transcription of many other genes, e.g. encoding transporters and enzymes of glucose metabolism. In addition, those transcription factors are involved in beta-cell development. (Reproduced from Tajans [55] with permission.)

process and subsequently for ATP synthesis and insulin secretion (**B**) [62]. Mutations identified in the glucokinase gene are responsible for impaired glucose sensing by the beta cell that results in an increase of the threshold for insulin secretion and subsequently a modest diabetic phenotype (**E, B**) [63–65]. Abnormalities of glucose metabolism, initially impaired fasting glucose (usually between 6 and 8 mmol/L), are present already in early childhood and they are typically stable during the rest of life. It should be noted that the insulin response to a glucose oral load or a mixed meal is well preserved, and subsequently the incremental rise of glucose level is modest, usually not larger than 3 mmol/L (**B**) [65]. The HbA1c level is slightly elevated, rarely above 7%. The age of diagnosis may vary substantially, even within one family. It depends very much on the moment when glucose is measured for the first time that the subtle abnormalities are noticed. For example, this may occur in childhood in the course of infectious disease such as pneumonia, or during pregnancy with the clinical picture of gestational diabetes (**B**) [66]. Chronic diabetes complications are rare. The expression of the glucokinase is not limited to the beta cell and is also present in the liver. This does not seem to result in clinically noticeable symptoms, although sophisticated investigations can show impairment in glycogen synthesis in glucokinase mutation carriers (**B, A**) [64, 65, 67].

Homozygous mutations in the glucokinase gene cause a complete deficiency of this enzyme and lead to permanent neonatal diabetes mellitus (PNDM). This severe form of PNDM requiring immediate insulin treatment develops in the first few weeks of life and is characterised by low birth weight (**C**) [23].

MODY associated with transcription factors mutations

Transcription factors are a very heterogeneous group of proteins. Their common feature is binding to a specific DNA sequence in the regulatory regions of various genes (**E**) [68]. This way they regulate the expression of many genes and the synthesis of the proteins, including the beta cell's insulin gene, Krebs cycle enzymes and glucose transporters (**B**) [69]. Moreover, it was shown in an animal model that some of these factors also regulate the development of insulin-secreting cells in the fetus (**B**) [70]. Thus, diabetes associated with transcription factors has complicated biological mechanisms that involve the processes of beta-cell development and expression of many genes that impair insulin secretion. This results in a severe phenotype that differs from the glucokinase form with its 'biochemical' pathophysiology (**B**) [71].

Interestingly, there is some degree of heterogeneity among the forms linked with specific transcription factors. Mutations in *HNF*-1α (MODY-3), the most frequent cause of autosomal dominant diabetes, -4α (MODY-1) and -1β genes (MODY-5) cause diabetes that is usually diagnosed in the second and third decades of life and characterised by prominent postprandial hyperglycaemia and the necessity of insulin treatment after some duration of disease (**B**) [71] (see section *Management of MODY* below). These forms of diabetes are frequently accompanied by chronic diabetes complications, which is the consequence of more severe hyperglycaemia than in MODY-2.

Interestingly, some extra-pancreatic manifestations of the mutations in hepatocyte nuclear factors have been described. This phenomenon is called pleiotropy and describes the situation in which a single gene has multiple seemingly unrelated phenotypic effects. This is a result of the fact that HNFs are expressed in several organs, not just in the endocrine pancreas. Some of these manifestations are very remarkable, e.g. developmental abnormalities of uterus and kidney, such as agenesis or multiple cysts, seen frequently in MODY-5 (*HNF*-1β) but rarely in MODY-3 (**C, B**) [72–74]. The other extra-pancreatic features associated with MODY, such as renal tubulopathy and lipid abnormalities, may be rather subtle and thus more difficult to notice in clinical practice (**C, A**) [75, 76]. Diabetes that is a consequence of *IPF*-1α (MODY-4) and *NEUROD1* (MODY-6) genes is very rare, and our knowledge is based on the description of just a few families linked with these subtypes. Table 13.2 summarises the important pathophysiological and clinical features of MODY subtypes.

Table 13.2 Comparison of the clinical features of MODY associated with glucokinase and transcription factors

	Glucokinase mutations	Transcription factors mutations
Age of onset	Variable, usually at the first glucose measurement; it may be as early as in infancy or as late as in the elderly	Typically second or third decade of life
Glucose levels	Fasting hyperglycaemia, stable or with small rise during life	Initially postprandial hyperglycaemia, evident progression in the course of disease
Treatment	Diet is typically sufficient	Diet is frequently not sufficient to control the disease; very good response to sulphonylurea; in some individuals, insulin must be eventually introduced
Complications	Rare	Occur in individuals with long disease duration or poor diabetes control
Extra-pancreatic features	Lack of evident clinical symptoms; some degree of impaired hepatic glycogen synthesis shown in clinical studies	• Low serum concentration of triglycerides, apoAII, apoCIII, and Lp(a) lipoprotein (MODY-1) • Renal tubulopathy, low apoM level, rarely necrobiosis lipoidica, liver adenomatosis or renal agenesis (MODY-3) • Renal cysts, abnormalities of renal and genital development (MODY-5)
Family history	Due to undiagnosed diabetes in some individuals, it involves fewer than three generations or is even negative	Typically involves at least three generations

Management of MODY

A lot is known about the molecular background of MODY and the biological mechanisms that lead to the insulin secretion impairment and the disease development. The clinical picture of specific subforms has been studied in great detail. The important question that should be answered is pertinence to clinical practice. Can a physician working with children and adolescents or with adults use this knowledge for the benefit of the diabetic patients?

Yes, the diagnosis of MODY has important clinical implications. Contrary to typical autoimmune T1DM, we can use alternatives to insulin to treat MODY. In MODY-2, the form associated with the glucokinase gene mutations, diet is sufficient in most of the patients and as long as HbA1c is kept in satisfactory range, some degree of fasting hyperglycaemia can be tolerated (**B**) [64, 71]. It must be noted, however, that, over the course of time, aging and obesity may lead to T2DM being superimposed on an already-existing glucokinase defect. This requires appropriate pharmacological treatment.

The situation is different in subtypes associated with transcription factors since the efficacy of diet is limited and thus pharmacological treatment must be implemented (**B**) [71]. Since sulphonylureas, the oldest group of oral hypoglycaemic agents available worldwide, act on the beta cell, and their specific mechanism of action is associated with enhancing of insulin secretion (**E**) [77], the hypothesis that the latter group are drugs of choice in MODY treatment seemed justified. Several early reports from various populations suggested that the patients with MODY-3 (*HNF-1α*), the most frequent autosomal dominant form of diabetes, be characterised by a specifically prominent therapeutic effect of sulphonylureas (**C**) [78, 79]. However, a clinical, double-blind, randomised study confirming this specific kind of pharmacogenetics in MODY was lacking. The breaking point was the publication of the paper that compared the clinical efficacy of gliclazide (a sulphonylurea) and metformin (a biguanide) in MODY-3 and in complex, late-onset T2DM (**A**) [80]. This study confirmed what had been suspected for years, that the differences in the clinical response to various oral hypoglycaemic agents depend on the cause of diabetes. MODY-3 patients showed better response to gliclazide than the patients with T2DM. The difference was associated with their great insulin secretion increase. An additional factor was high insulin sensitivity in these patients. The effect of metformin on metabolic compensation in MODY-3 patients was similar to that in T2DM and much weaker than for gliclazide.

The researchers attributed their findings to the nature of the beta-cell defect in MODY. *HNF-1α* is responsible for the expression of several genes involved in glucose uptake, glycolysis and mitochondrial metabolism (**B**) [69]. Sulphonylureas act downstream to these defects by binding to the SUR-1 subunit of the beta-cell ATP-dependent potassium channel (**E**) [77]. Thus, they are able to bypass most of these defects and improve the beta-cell functioning. So the genetic cause of MODY-3 is an important determinant of response to oral hypoglycaemic drugs. The pathophysiological similarity suggests that an analogous situation is likely in most of other MODY forms linked to transcription factors (**C, B**) [3, 61, 81].

The legal aspect of sulphonylurea use in children and adolescents should be briefly discussed since these drugs are licensed worldwide only for adults. The European Agency for the Evaluation of Medical Products statement dated 1995 says that, when justified, a physician can use in children drugs licensed for adults (**E**) [82]. It is hard to find a better justification than a molecular diagnosis, such as MODY-3, which provides the basis for very specific pharmacogenetics.

It should be remembered, however, that under these circumstances, sulphonylureas are being used in children and adolescents based on the results of genetic testing. This testing is more and more widely available in various European countries. In some of them testing may by funded by the state health system and in some others it still constitutes part of scientific projects.

The diagnosis of various form of MODY also has prognostic implications for a family. Since MODY is a disease of autosomal dominant inheritance, the probability of passing the gene to a child by a mother or father is 50% (**E**) [46]. The penetration of the mutations, particularly in forms associated with HNFs is very high, which means that eventually almost all the mutation carriers will develop diabetes, although familial factors, including modifying genes, parent of origin and whether or not a mutation carrier was exposed to diabetes *in utero*, may influence the age of diagnosis (**B**) [83, 84]. It should be understood that the efficacy of prevention of MODY, unlike in T2DM, is very limited. It seems, however, that maintaining lean body mass may delay disease onset. In addition, a regular surveillance of blood glucose in non-affected mutation carriers of MODY genes within the family should allow early diagnosis and intervention to maintain good metabolic control from the very onset of the disease in order to prevent chronic diabetic complications.

Other conditions associated with diabetes in childhood

Nicola Bridges

There are several conditions in which diabetes features in one form or another. In the majority of cases this is either mild or does not usually occur until outside the paediatric age range. The ADA classification of diabetes (see Chapter 2) includes most of these. They are listed in Table 13.3 together with the principal features of the diabetes and with reference to their OMIM numbers. Further details on these rare conditions, together with the relevant references relating to the various conditions, can be obtained from the OMIM website (**E/A**) [85]. However, there a few which have a significant relevance to paediatric practice and which bear more detailed discussion. The two most important of these are cystic fibrosis (CF) and Prader–Willi syndrome (P-WS).

Cystic-fibrosis-related diabetes

Introduction

Cystic-fibrosis-related diabetes (CFRD) is a rare cause of diabetes, which has become more common, as improvements in CF care have resulted in increased life expectancy. Recognition of the importance of impaired glucose tolerance and CFRD in prognosis has meant that detection and management of diabetes has assumed a greater relevance in the care of individuals with CF.

Insulin secretion defects in CF

CFRD is found only in individuals with exocrine pancreatic insufficiency. Pathological studies have demonstrated loss of beta cells in CF even without diabetes (**B**) [86]. Loss of insulin secretion has been demonstrated from early childhood, and there is progressive insulin deficiency with age (**A, B**) [87–89]. Insulin secretion is delayed and reduced in response to a glucose load. Baseline insulin secretion is preserved at the onset of diabetes, so fasting glucose levels are usually normal (**A**) [90]. HbA1c can be low in established CFRD, although it still correlates with glucose levels (**B**) [91]. Studies using continuous glucose-monitoring systems have demonstrated significant hyperglycaemia in individuals whose fasting glucose, HbA1c and oral glucose tolerance test (OGTT) are all within normal limits (**C, B**) [92, 93]. HbA1c and fasting glucose are unhelpful in making the diagnosis of CFRD. The primary cause for CFRD is insulin deficiency, but insulin resistance is also a factor in abnormal glucose tolerance (related to chronic inflammation and steroid treatment) (**A**) [87, 94].

European and US register studies from the 1990s reported prevalence of CFRD of 3.1 and 6.1% respectively in all ages (**B**) [95, 96]. Both these studies based prevalence data on whether subjects reported treatment with insulin. If individuals are prospectively screened using OGTT, prevalence is much higher. In one study, 9% of those aged 5–9 years had diabetes, rising to 43% in those over 30 years, with about a third in all age groups with impaired glucose tolerance (**B**) [88]. In 2004 the US patient registry reported a 16.1%

Table 13.3 Principal features of 'other causes' of diabetes

Condition	Chromosome	Gene	Clinical features	OMIM number (see below for symbols)
MODY-1	20q12-q13.1	*HNF-4α*	See above	#125850
MODY-2	7p15-p13	*GCK*	See above	*138079
MODY-3	12q24.2	*HNF-1α*	See above	#600496
MODY-4	13q12.1	*IPF-1*	See above	#606392
MODY-5	17cen-q21.3	*HNF-1β*	See above	#137920
MODY-6	2q32	*NEUROD1*	See above	#606394
Leprechaunism	19p13.2	*Insulin receptor*	Variable but may have severe insulin resistance	#246200
Rabson–Mendenhall syndrome	19p13.2	*Insulin receptor*	Pineal hyperplasia Severe insulin resistance	#262190
Cystic fibrosis	7q31.2	*CFTR*	See above	#219700
Haemochromatosis	6p21.3	*HFE1*	Diabetes usually develops in adulthood	+235200
Stiff-man syndrome	Sporadic		Autoimmune diabetes (60% have anti-GAD antibodies)	%184850
Autoimmune polyendocrine syndrome I (APECED)	21q22.3	*AIRE*	Addison disease Hypoparathyroidism Mucocutaneous candidiasis Autoimmune diabetes	#240300
Autoimmune polyendocrine syndrome II (Schmidt)	Uncertain	*Uncertain*	Polyendocrinopathy Autoimmune diabetes	269200
Down syndrome	47 + 21		Diabetes usually autoimmune	#190685
Turner syndrome	45XO etc.		Diabetes usually autoimmune	
Klinefelter syndrome	47XXY		Diabetes not usually a major feature	

Continued

Table 13.3 *Continued*

Condition	Chromosome	Gene	Clinical features	OMIM number (see below for symbols)
DIDMOAD	MtDNA			#598500
Friedreich ataxia	9q13, 9p23-p11	*FXN*	Diabetes often associated with cardiomyopathy	#229300
Huntington chorea	4p16.3	*Multiple CAG triplet repeats in 'Huntingtin' location*	Diabetes usually type 2	+143100
Laurence–Moon–Biedl syndrome	Heterogeneous		Diabetes usually type 2 secondary to obesity	#209900
Myotonic dystrophy	19q13.2-q13.3	*DMPK, DM and DMK*	Diabetes occurs in 5% of cases	#160900
Prader–Willi syndrome	15q12	*SNRPN and Necdin*	Diabetes usually type 2 (see above)	#176270

- An *asterisk* (*) before an entry number indicates a gene of known sequence.
- A *number symbol* (#) before an entry number indicates that it is a descriptive entry, usually of a phenotype, and does not represent a unique locus. The reason for the use of the '#' sign is given in the first paragraph of the OMIM entry. Discussion of any gene(s) related to the phenotype resides in another entry(ies), as described in the first paragraph.
- A *plus sign* (+) before an entry number indicates that the entry contains the description of a gene of known sequence and a phenotype.
- A *per cent sign* (%) before an entry number indicates that the entry describes a confirmed Mendelian phenotype or phenotypic locus for which the underlying molecular basis is not known.
- *No symbol* before an entry number generally indicates a description of a phenotype for which the Mendelian basis, although suspected, has not been clearly established or that the separateness of this phenotype from that in another entry is unclear.
For further details, see [85]. Available at: http://www.ncbi.nlm.nih.gov/entrez/query.fcgi?db=OMIM

prevalence of CFRD at all ages (**B**) [97], although the increasing age of the CF population has contributed to an increasing prevalence, and increased screening and awareness of diabetes has increased the numbers receiving treatment.

The impact of diabetes and impaired glucose tolerance on clinical state in CF

Life expectancy for individuals with CFRD is reduced compared to unaffected individuals with CF, independent of the effects of bacterial colonisation and underlying mutation (**B**) [98]. The impact is greater for females than males (**B**) [99]. A diagnosis of CFRD is associated with reduced lung function and increased number of infective episodes (**B**) [100]. Nutrition (BMI) and lung function (FEV1 (forced expiratory volume in 1 second) and FVC (forced vital capacity)) start to decline compared with controls up to 5 years before the diagnosis of diabetes and are reduced in CF individuals, with impaired glucose tolerance compared to controls with normal glucose tolerance (**B**) [101–103].

The treatment of diabetes and impaired glucose tolerance in CF

Insulin treatment in CFRD benefits nutrition and lung function and reduces the number of infective episodes (**B, C**) [102–104]. Oral hypoglycaemic agents have been used extensively in CFRD but there is no evidence of benefit to lung function of nutritional status. Sulphonylureas have been demonstrated to maintain adequate glycaemic control in some individuals (**B**) [105]. There have been no studies of insulin-sensitising agents such as metformin or the thiazolidinediones because of concerns about complications in CF.

Studies of insulin treatment have used a variety of different insulin regimens and there is no evidence favouring a particular approach. Improved diabetes management has been suggested as one factor in the trend for longer survival in CF but it is not possible to extract this effect from all the other areas of improved management that have made a difference. Microvascular complications of diabetes have been reported in the CF population (**C**) [106, 107] and, since many patients are likely to survive long enough with diabetes to be at risk of complications, this is a reason to aim for similar glycaemic targets as in other diabetic subjects.

In CF, insulin deficiency is present even in those with normal glucose tolerance on testing (**A**) [90]. There appears to be a gradual progression to impaired glucose tolerance and then diabetes, with a range of clinical factors having an impact on the rate of this process. Insulin deficiency has an adverse effect before the clinical criteria for a diagnosis of diabetes are met, and studies treating subjects with abnormal glucose tolerance but not diabetes have demonstrated a positive effect of insulin on nutrition, lung function and rates of infectious exacerbations (**C**) [92, 108].

Conclusions

CFRD is associated with increased risk of adverse complications and shorter survival. The aim of treatment with insulin is to reverse the adverse impact that loss of the anabolic effect of insulin has on nutrition and lung function. Insulin treatment results in improvements in nutritional and respiratory status, but the longer term effects on survival are not yet known. The diagnostic criteria for diabetes based on glucose levels may not be of help in determining whether treatment is needed in CF, because there is evidence of the adverse effects of insulin deficiency and benefit from treatment in individuals who do not meet these criteria. It is clear that treating the insulin deficiency found in CF with insulin is of clinical benefit but further studies are needed to guide when to start treatment and optimum treatment strategies.

Prader–Willi syndrome

Jeremy Allgrove

Introduction

Prader–Willi syndrome (P-WS) was first described in 1956 (**C**) [109]. The syndrome is characterised by an infant who remains very floppy and initially feeds poorly so much so that most infants require tube feeding. Some time during the first year after birth, a change occurs, as a result of which the patients develop a large appetite, and it is often difficult to prevent these children from seeking food at the least opportunity. If this is allowed to continue unchecked, gross obesity may result.

Diabetes, which usually resembles T2DM, has become increasingly recognised as a complication of P-WS, has a mean age of onset of 20 years and is present in 25% of adults (**B**) [110]. It has been assumed that this is related to the gross obesity that frequently develops. However, it seems that carbohydrate metabolism in P-WS is different from that in exogenous obesity and that it is not related to increased insulin resistance in the same way. Insulin resistance is not present to the same degree (**A**) [111, 112] but insulin release in response to glucose is impaired and hepatic insulin extraction is increased (**A**) [111]. This is perhaps not surprising, as there are no genes that are strongly linked to T2DM present on chromosome 15 (see Chapter 12).

Growth hormone (GH) is now used regularly for the treatment of short stature in P-WS and is thought to have a beneficial effect on body composition. In children who are not diabetic before treatment, there is usually no adverse effect upon glucose metabolism even after 5 years of treatment (**B**) [113, 114] and the impaired insulin release seen before treatment may improve possibly because of the reduction in total body fat and increase in lean mass. However, the onset of diabetes shortly after initiation of GH treatment is described (**C**) [115] and it is not known whether or not diabetes is made worse by GH therapy if it is already present.

Despite the differences between the diabetes of P-WS and T2DM, treatment of diabetes in P-WS is usually undertaken along the same lines as T2DM; i.e. it begins with oral hypoglycaemic agents, such as metformin. There is also some evidence to suggest that the glitazones may also be of value (**C**) [116] and, in the author's experience, a combination of metformin and roziglitazone has proved to be of value. Nevertheless, insulin may be required, although this may have an adverse effect upon body weight.

Conclusion

P-WS is a cause of significant morbidity and mortality. Diabetes develops in an increasing proportion of patients and is being seen in childhood. The aetiology of the diabetes is not the same as in exogenous obesity and is more dependent on insulin deficiency. Nevertheless, treatment usually starts with oral hypoglycaemic agents before adding insulin.

Acknowledgements

Maciej Malecki is grateful to his many colleagues in USA, UK, Poland and other countries with whom he has had the privilege to work and to collaborate with in the field of genetic diabetes research and to the Polish Ministry of Science and Higher Education for supporting the research on monogenic diabetes over recent years.

He also thanks Dr Paul Greenlaw for his editorial help.

References

1 Shield JP, Gardner RJ, Wadsworth EJ et al. Aetiopathology and genetic basis of neonatal diabetes. *Arch Dis Child Fetal Neonatal Ed* 1997; **76**: F39–42.
2 Iafusco D, Stazi MA, Cotichini R et al. Permanent diabetes mellitus in the first year of life. *Diabetologia* 2002; **45**: 798–804.
3 Stoffers DA, Zinkin NT, Stanojevic V et al. Pancreatic agenesis attributable to a single nucleotide deletion in the human IPF1 gene coding sequence. *Nat Genet* 1997; **15**: 106–10.

4 Stoffers DA, Stanojevic V, Habener JF. Insulin promoter factor-1 gene mutation linked to early-onset type 2 diabetes mellitus directs expression of a dominant negative isoprotein. *J Clin Invest* 1998; **102**: 232–41.

5 Schwitzgebel VM, Mamin A, Brun T *et al.* Agenesis of human pancreas due to decreased half-life of insulin promoter factor 1. *J Clin Endocrinol Metab* 2003; **88**: 4398–406.

6 Temple IK, Gardner RJ, Mackay DJ *et al.* Transient neonatal diabetes: widening the understanding of the etiopathogenesis of diabetes. *Diabetes* 2000; **49**: 1359–66.

7 Slingerland AS, Hattersley AT. Mutations in the Kir6.2 subunit of the KATP channel and permanent neonatal diabetes: new insights and new treatment. *Ann Med* 2005; **37**: 186–95.

8 Temple IK, James RS, Crolla JA *et al.* An imprinted gene(s) for diabetes? *Nat Genet* 1995; **9**: 110–12.

9 Cave H, Polak M, Drunat S *et al.* Refinement of the 6q chromosomal region implicated in transient neonatal diabetes. *Diabetes* 2000; **49**: 108–13.

10 Temple IK, Gardner RJ, Robinson DO *et al.* Further evidence for an imprinted gene for neonatal diabetes localised to chromosome 6q22-q23. *Hum Mol Genet* 1996; **5**: 1117–21.

11 Gardner RJ, Mackay DJ, Mungall AJ *et al.* An imprinted locus associated with transient neonatal diabetes mellitus. *Hum Mol Genet* 2000; **9**: 589–96.

12 Graded overexpression of ZAC impairs glucose stimulated insulin secretion in beta-cells. American Diabetes Association, Washington, 2006, 190-OR.

13 Jeha GS, Venkatesh MP, Edelen RC *et al.* Neonatal diabetes mellitus: patient reports and review of current knowledge and clinical practice. *J Pediatr Endocrinol Metab* 2005; **18**: 1095–102.

14 Polak M, Shield J. Neonatal and very-early-onset diabetes mellitus. *Semin Neonatol* 2004; **9**: 59–65.

15 Senee V, Vattem KM, Delepine M *et al.* Wolcott–Rallison syndrome: clinical, genetic, and functional study of EIF2AK3 mutations and suggestion of genetic heterogeneity. *Diabetes* 2004; **53**: 1876–83.

16 Delepine M, Nicolino M, Barrett T *et al.* EIF2AK3, encoding translation initiation factor 2-alpha kinase 3, is mutated in patients with Wolcott–Rallison syndrome. *Nat Genet* 2000; **25**: 406–9.

17 Wildin RS, Ramsdell F, Peake J *et al.* X-linked neonatal diabetes mellitus, enteropathy and endocrinopathy syndrome is the human equivalent of mouse scurfy. *Nat Genet* 2001; **27**: 18–20.

18 Wildin RS, Smyk-Pearson S, Filipovich AH. Clinical and molecular features of the immunodysregulation, polyendocrinopathy, enteropathy, X linked (IPEX) syndrome. *J Med Genet* 2002; **39**: 537–45.

19 Ruemmele FM, Brousse N, Goulet O. Autoimmune enteropathy: molecular concepts. *Curr Opin Gastroenterol* 2004; **20**: 587–91.

20 Baud O, Goulet O, Canioni D *et al.* Treatment of the immune dysregulation, polyendocrinopathy, enteropathy, X-linked syndrome (IPEX) by allogeneic bone marrow transplantation. *N Engl J Med* 2001; **344**: 1758–62.

21 Mazzolari E, Forino C, Fontana M *et al.* A new case of IPEX receiving bone marrow transplantation. *Bone Marrow Transplant* 2005; **35**: 1033–34.

22 Njolstad PR, Sagen JV, Bjorkhaug L *et al.* Permanent neonatal diabetes caused by glucokinase deficiency: inborn error of the glucose-insulin signaling pathway. *Diabetes* 2003; **52**: 2854–60.

23 Njolstad PR, Sovik O, Cuesta-Munoz A *et al.* Neonatal diabetes mellitus due to complete glucokinase deficiency. *N Engl J Med* 2001; **344**: 1588–92.

24 Porter JR, Shaw NJ, Barrett TG *et al.* Permanent neonatal diabetes in an Asian infant. *J Pediatr* 2005; **146**: 131–3.

25 Gloyn AL, Ellard S, Shield JP *et al.* Complete glucokinase deficiency is not a common cause of permanent neonatal diabetes. *Diabetologia* 2002; **45**: 290.

26 Gloyn AL, Pearson ER, Antcliff JF *et al.* Activating mutations in the gene encoding the ATP-sensitive potassium-channel subunit Kir6.2 and permanent neonatal diabetes. *N Engl J Med* 2004; **350**: 1838–49.

27 Gloyn AL, Reimann F, Girard C *et al.* Relapsing diabetes can result from moderately activating mutations in KCNJ11. *Hum Mol Genet* 2005; **14**: 925–34.

28 Proks P, Antcliff JF, Lippiat J *et al.* Molecular basis of Kir6.2 mutations associated with neonatal diabetes or neonatal diabetes plus neurological features. *Proc Natl Acad Sci U S A* 2004; **101**: 17539–44.

29 Pearson ER, Flechtner I, Njolstad PR *et al.* Switching from insulin to oral sulfonylureas in patients with diabetes due to Kir6.2 mutations. *N Engl J Med* 2006; **355**: 467–77.

30 Babenko AP, Polak M, Cave H *et al.* Activating mutations in the ABCC8 gene in neonatal diabetes mellitus. *N Engl J Med* 2006; **355**: 456–66.

31 Proks P, Arnold AL, Bruining J *et al.* A heterozygous activating mutation in the sulphonylurea receptor SUR1 (ABCC8) causes neonatal diabetes. *Hum Mol Genet* 2006; **15**: 1793–1800.

32 Hoveyda N, Shield JP, Garrett C *et al.* Neonatal diabetes mellitus and cerebellar hypoplasia/agenesis: report of a new recessive syndrome. *J Med Genet* 1999; **36**: 700–4.

33 Sellick GS, Barker KT, Stolte-Dijkstra I *et al.* Mutations in PTF1A cause pancreatic and cerebellar agenesis. *Nat Genet* 2004; **36**: 1301–5.

34 Mitchell J, Punthakee Z, Lo B *et al.* Neonatal diabetes, with hypoplastic pancreas, intestinal atresia and gall bladder hypoplasia: search for the aetiology of a new autosomal recessive syndrome. *Diabetologia* 2004; **47**: 2160–7.

35 Ashraf A, Abdullatif H, Hardin W *et al.* Unusual case of neonatal diabetes mellitus due to congenital pancreas agenesis. *Pediatr Diabetes* 2005; **6**: 239–43.

36 Verwest AM, Poelman M, Dinjens WN *et al.* Absence of a PDX-1 mutation and normal gastroduodenal immunohistology in a child with pancreatic agenesis. *Virchows Arch* 2000; **437**: 680–4.

37 Senee V, Chelala C, Duchatelet S *et al.* Mutations in GLIS3 are responsible for a rare syndrome with neonatal diabetes mellitus and congenital hypothyroidism. *Nat Genet* 2006; **38**: 682–7.

38 Yorifuji T, Kurokawa K, Mamada M *et al.* Neonatal diabetes mellitus and neonatal polycystic, dysplastic kidneys: phenotypically discordant recurrence of a mutation in the hepatocyte nuclear factor-1beta gene due to germline mosaicism. *J Clin Endocrinol Metab* 2004; **89**: 2905–8.

39 Bouchardet A. *De la glycosuria ou diabete sucre*. 1875.

40 Tattersall RB, Fajans SS. A difference between the inheritance of classical juvenile-onset and maturity-onset type diabetes of young people. *Diabetes* 1975; **24**: 44–53.

41 McCarthy MI, Hattersley AT. Molecular diagnostics in monogenic and multifactorial forms of type 2 diabetes. *Expert Rev Mol Diagn* 2001; **1**: 403–12.

42 McCarthy MI. Susceptibility gene discovery for common metabolic and endocrine traits. *J Mol Endocrinol* 2002; **28**: 1–17.

43 Ehtisham S, Hattersley AT, Dunger DB *et al.* First UK survey of paediatric type 2 diabetes and MODY. *Arch Dis Child* 2004; **89**: 526–9.

44 Porter JR, Barrett TG. Monogenic syndromes of abnormal glucose homeostasis: clinical review and relevance to the understanding of the pathology of insulin resistance and beta cell failure. *J Med Genet* 2005; **42**: 893–902.

45 Tattersall RB. Mild familial diabetes with dominant inheritance. *Q J Med* 1974; **43**: 339–57.

46 Mange EJ, Mange AP. Human pedigrees. *Basic Human Genetics*, 2nd edn. Sinauer Associates Inc., Sunderland, MA, 1999, pp. 67–92.

47 Tattersall R. Maturity-onset diabetes of the young: a clinical history. *Diabet Med* 1998; **15**: 11–14.

48 Hattersley AT. Maturity-onset diabetes of the young: clinical heterogeneity explained by genetic heterogeneity. *Diabet Med* 1998; **15**: 15–24.

49 Herman WH, Fajans SS, Ortiz FJ *et al.* Abnormal insulin secretion, not insulin resistance, is the genetic or primary defect of MODY in the RW pedigree. *Diabetes* 1994; **43**: 40–6.

50 Tattersall RB, Mansell PI. Maturity onset-type diabetes of the young MODY: one condition or many? *Diabet Med* 1991; **8**: 402–10.

51 Hattersley AT, Turner RC, Permutt MA *et al.* Linkage of type 2 diabetes to the glucokinase gene. *Lancet* 1992; **339**: 1307–10.

52 Bell GI, Xiang KS, Newman MV *et al.* Gene for non-insulin-dependent diabetes mellitus maturity-onset diabetes of the young subtype is linked to DNA polymorphism on human chromosome 20q. *Proc Natl Acad Sci U S A* 1991; **88**: 1484–8.

53 Velho G, Vaxillaire M, Boccio V *et al.* Diabetes complications in NIDDM kindreds linked to the MODY3 locus on chromosome 12q. *Diabetes Care* 1996; **19**: 915–19.

54 Report of a WHO Consultation. *Definition, Diagnosis and Classification of Diabetes Mellitus and Its Complications.* Geneva, 1999.

55 Fajans SS, Bell GI, Polonsky KS. Molecular mechanisms and clinical pathophysiology of maturity-onset diabetes of the young. *N Engl J Med* 2001; **345**: 971–80.

56 Horikawa Y, Iwasaki N, Hara M *et al.* Mutation in hepatocyte nuclear factor-1 beta gene TCF2 associated with MODY. *Nat Genet* 1997; **17**: 384–5.

57 Stoffers DA, Ferrer J, Clarke WL *et al.* Early-onset type-II diabetes mellitus MODY4 linked to IPF1. *Nat Genet* 1997; **17**: 138–9.

58 Vionnet N, Stoffel M, Takeda J *et al.* Nonsense mutation in the glucokinase gene causes early-onset non-insulin-dependent diabetes mellitus. *Nature* 1992; **356**: 721–2.

59 Yamagata K, Furuta H, Oda N *et al*. Mutations in the hepatocyte nuclear factor-4alpha gene in maturity-onset diabetes of the young (MODY1). *Nature* 1996; **384**: 458–60.

60 Yamagata K, Oda N, Kaisaki PJ *et al*. Mutations in the hepatocyte nuclear factor-1alpha gene in maturity-onset diabetes of the young (MODY3). *Nature* 1996; **384**: 455–8.

61 Malecki MT, Jhala US, Antonellis A *et al*. Mutations in NEUROD1 are associated with the development of type 2 diabetes mellitus. *Nat Genet* 1999; **23**: 323–8.

62 Iynedjian PB, Möbius G, Seitz HJ *et al*. Tissue-specific expression of glucokinase: identification of the gene product in liver and pancreatic islets. *Proc Natl Acad Sci U S A* 1986; **83**: 1998–2001.

63 Bell GI, Pilkis SJ, Weber IT *et al*. Glucokinase mutations, insulin secretion, and diabetes mellitus. *Annu Rev Physiol* 1996; **58**: 171–86.

64 Froguel P, Zouali H, Vionnet N *et al*. Familial hyperglycemia due to mutations in glucokinase: definition of a subtype of diabetes mellitus. *N Engl J Med* 1993; **328**: 697–702.

65 Pearson ER, Velho G, Clark P *et al*. Beta-cell genes and diabetes: quantitative and qualitative differences in the pathophysiology of hepatic nuclear factor-1alpha and glucokinase mutations. *Diabetes* 2001; **50**: S101–7.

66 Ellard S, Beards F, Allen LI *et al*. A high prevalence of glucokinase mutations in gestational diabetic subjects selected by clinical criteria. *Diabetologia* 2000; **43**: 250–3.

67 Velho G, Petersen KF, Perseghin G *et al*. Impaired hepatic glycogen synthesis in glucokinase-deficient (MODY-2) subjects. *J Clin Invest* 1996; **98**: 1755–61.

68 Schrem H, Klempnauer J, Borlak J. Liver-enriched transcription factors in liver function and development. Part I: the hepatocyte nuclear factor network and liver- specific gene expression. *Pharmacol Rev* 2002; **54**: 129–58.

69 Shih DQ, Screenan S, Munoz KN *et al*. Loss of HNF-1alpha function in mice leads to abnormal expression of genes involved in pancreatic islet development and metabolism. *Diabetes* 2001; **50**: 2472–80.

70 Naya FJ, Huang HP, Qiu Y *et al*. Diabetes, defective pancreatic morphogenesis, and abnormal enteroendocrine differentiation in BETA2/neuroD-deficient mice. *Genes Dev* 1997; **11**: 2323–34.

71 Frayling TM, Evans JC, Bulman MP *et al*. Beta-cell genes and diabetes: molecular and clinical characterization of mutations in transcription factors. *Diabetes* 2001; **50**: S94–100.

72 Bingham C, Ellard S, Cole T *et al*. Solitary functioning kidney and diverse genital tract malformations associated with hepatocyte nuclear factor-1beta mutations. *Kidney Int* 2002; **61**: 1243–51.

73 Malecki M, Skupien J, Gorczynska K *et al*. Renal malformations may be linked to mutations in the hepatocyte nuclear factor-1alpha MODY3 gene. *Diabetes Care* 2005; **28**: 2774–6.

74 Montoli A, Colussi G, Massa O *et al*. Renal cysts and diabetes syndrome linked to mutations of the hepatocyte nuclear factor-1 beta gene: description of a new family with associated liver involvement. *Am J Kidney Dis* 2002; **40**: 397–402.

75 Menzel R, Kaisaki PJ, Rjasanowski I *et al*. A low renal threshold for glucose in diabetic patients with a mutation in the hepatocyte nuclear factor-1alpha HNF-1alpha gene. *Diabet Med* 1998; **15**: 816–20.

76 Shih DQ, Dansky HM, Fleisher M *et al*. Genotype/phenotype relationships in HNF-4alpha/MODY1: haploinsufficiency is associated with reduced apolipoprotein AII, apolipoprotein CIII, lipoproteina, and triglyceride levels. *Diabetes* 2000; **49**: 832–7.

77 Gribble FM, Reimann F. Sulphonylurea action revisited: the post-cloning era. *Diabetologia* 2003; **46**: 875–91.

78 Pearson ER, Liddell WG, Shepherd M *et al*. Sensitivity to sulphonylureas in patients with hepatocyte nuclear factor-1alpha gene mutations: evidence for pharmacogenetics in diabetes. *Diabet Med* 2000; **17**: 543–5.

79 Søvik O, Njølstad P, Følling I *et al*. Hyperexcitability to sulphonylurea in MODY3. *Diabetologia* 1998; **41**: 607–8.

80 Pearson E, Starkey B, Powell R *et al*. Genetic cause of hyperglycaemia and response to treatment in diabetes. *Lancet* 2003; **362**: 1275–81.

81 Pearson ER, Pruhova S, Tack CJ *et al*. Molecular genetics and phenotypic characteristics of MODY caused by hepatocyte nuclear factor 4alpha mutations in a large European collection. *Diabetologia* 2005; **48**: 878–85.

82 Committee for Proprietary Medicines (CPMP). *Note for Guidance on Clinical Investigation of Medicinal Products in Children*. Human Medicines Evaluation Unit, London, 1997. Available at: http://www.emea.europa.eu/pdfs/human/ich/271199en.pdf

83 Klupa T, Warram J, Antonellis A *et al.* Determinants of the development of diabetes maturity-onset diabetes of the young-3 in carriers of HNF-1alpha mutations: evidence for parent-of-origin effect. *Diabetes Care* 2002; **25**: 2292–301.

84 Stride A, Shepherd M, Frayling T *et al.* Intrauterine hyperglycemia is associated with an earlier diagnosis of diabetes in HNF-1alpha gene mutation carriers. *Diabetes Care* 2002; **25**: 2287–91.

85 NCBI. *OMIM – Online Mendelian Inheritance in Man.* Available at: http://www.ncbi.nlm.nih.gov/entrez/query.fcgi?db=OMIM

86 Iannucci A, Mukai K, Johnson D *et al.* Endocrine pancreas in cystic fibrosis: an immunohistochemical study. *Hum Pathol* 1984; **15**: 278–84.

87 Austin A, Kalhan SC, Orenstein D *et al.* Roles of insulin resistance and beta-cell dysfunction in the pathogenesis of glucose intolerance in cystic fibrosis. *J Clin Endocrinol Metab* 1994; **79**: 80–5.

88 Moran A, Doherty L, Wang X *et al.* Abnormal glucose metabolism in cystic fibrosis. *J Pediatr* 1998; **133**: 10–17.

89 Solomon MP, Wilson DC, Corey M *et al.* Glucose intolerance in children with cystic fibrosis. *J Pediatr* 2003; **142**: 128–32.

90 Yung B, Noormohamed FH, Kemp M *et al.* Cystic fibrosis-related diabetes: the role of peripheral insulin resistance and beta-cell dysfunction. *Diabet Med* 2002; **19**: 221–6.

91 Brennan AL, Gyi KM, Wood DM *et al.* Relationship between glycosylated haemoglobin and mean plasma glucose concentration in cystic fibrosis. *J Cyst Fibros* 2006; **5**: 27–31.

92 Dobson L, Hattersley AT, Tiley S *et al.* Clinical improvement in cystic fibrosis with early insulin treatment. *Arch Dis Child* 2002; **87**: 430–1.

93 Jefferies C, Solomon M, Perlman K *et al.* Continuous glucose monitoring in adolescents with cystic fibrosis. *J Pediatr* 2005; **147**: 396–8.

94 Hardin DS, Leblanc A, Marshall G *et al.* Mechanisms of insulin resistance in cystic fibrosis. *Am J Physiol Endocrinol Metab* 2001; **281**: E1022–8.

95 Konstan MW, Butler SM, Schidlow DV *et al.* Patterns of medical practice in cystic fibrosis: part I. Evaluation and monitoring of health status of patients. Investigators and Coordinators of the Epidemiologic Study of Cystic Fibrosis. *Pediatr Pulmonol* 1999; **28**: 242–7.

96 Navarro J, Rainisio M, Harms HK *et al.* Factors associated with poor pulmonary function: cross-sectional analysis of data from the ERCF. European Epidemiologic Registry of Cystic Fibrosis. *Eur Respir J* 2001; **18**: 298–305.

97 Cystic Fibrosis Foundation. *Patient Registry 2004 Annual Report.* Bethesda, Maryland, 2005. Available at: http://www.cff.org/ID=4573/TYPE=2676/2004%20Patient%20Registry%20Report.pdf

98 Koch C, Rainisio M, Madessani U *et al.* Presence of cystic fibrosis-related diabetes mellitus is tightly linked to poor lung function in patients with cystic fibrosis: data from the European Epidemiologic Registry of Cystic Fibrosis. *Pediatr Pulmonol* 2001; **32**: 343–50.

99 Milla CE, Billings J, Moran A. Diabetes is associated with dramatically decreased survival in female but not male subjects with cystic fibrosis. *Diabetes Care* 2005; **28**: 2141–4.

100 Marshall BC, Butler SM, Stoddard M *et al.* Epidemiology of cystic fibrosis-related diabetes. *J Pediatr* 2005; **146**: 681–7.

101 Milla CE, Warwick WJ, Moran A. Trends in pulmonary function in patients with cystic fibrosis correlate with the degree of glucose intolerance at baseline. *Am J Respir Crit Care Med* 2000; **162**: 891–5.

102 Nousia-Arvanitakis S, Galli-Tsinopoulou A, Karamouzis M. Insulin improves clinical status of patients with cystic-fibrosis-related diabetes mellitus. *Acta Paediatr* 2001; **90**: 515–19.

103 Rolon MA, Benali K, Munck A *et al.* Cystic fibrosis-related diabetes mellitus: clinical impact of prediabetes and effects of insulin therapy. *Acta Paediatr* 2001; **90**: 860–7.

104 Franzese A, Spagnuolo MI, Sepe A *et al.* Can glargine reduce the number of lung infections in patients with cystic fibrosis-related diabetes? *Diabetes Care* 2005; **28**: 2333.

105 Rosenecker J, Eichler I, Barmeier H *et al.* Diabetes mellitus and cystic fibrosis: comparison of clinical parameters in patients treated with insulin versus oral glucose-lowering agents. *Pediatr Pulmonol* 2001; **32**: 351–5.

106 Rosenecker J, Hofler R, Steinkamp G *et al.* Diabetes mellitus in patients with cystic fibrosis: the impact of diabetes mellitus on pulmonary function and clinical outcome. *Eur J Med Res* 2001; **6**: 345–50.

107 Yung B, Landers A, Mathalone B *et al.* Diabetic retinopathy in adult patients with cystic fibrosis-related diabetes. *Respir Med* 1998; **92**: 871–2.

108 Bizzarri C, Lucidi V, Ciampalini P *et al.* Clinical effects of early treatment with insulin glargine in patients with cystic fibrosis and impaired glucose tolerance. *J Endocrinol Invest* 2006; **29**: RC1–4.

109 Prader A, Labhart A, Willi H. Ein Syndrom von Adipositas, Kleinwuchs, Kryptorchismus und Oligonephrie nach Myatonieartigem Zustand in Neugeborenenalter. *Schweiz Med Wochenschr* 1956; **86**: 1260–1.

110 Butler JV, Whittington JE, Holland AJ *et al.* Prevalence of, and risk factors for, physical ill-health in people with Prader–Willi syndrome: a population-based study. *Dev Med Child Neurol* 2002; **44**: 248–55.

111 Schuster DP, Osei K, Zipf WB. Characterization of alterations in glucose and insulin metabolism in Prader–Willi subjects. *Metabolism* 1996; **45**: 1514–20.

112 Zipf WB. Glucose homeostasis in Prader–Willi syndrome and potential implications of growth hormone therapy. *Acta Paediatr Suppl* 1999; **88**: 115–17.

113 L'Allemand D, Eiholzer U, Schlumpf M *et al.* Carbohydrate metabolism is not impaired after 3 years of growth hormone therapy in children with Prader–Willi syndrome. *Horm Res* 2003; **59**: 239–48.

114 Lindgren AC, Ritzen EM. Five years of growth hormone treatment in children with Prader-Willi syndrome. Swedish National Growth Hormone Advisory Group. *Acta Paediatr Suppl* 1999; **88**: 109–11.

115 Yigit S, Estrada E, Bucci K *et al.* Diabetic ketoacidosis secondary to growth hormone treatment in a boy with Prader–Willi syndrome and steatohepatitis. *J Pediatr Endocrinol Metab* 2004; **17**: 361–4.

116 Yamakita T, Ishii T, Mori T *et al.* Troglitazone ameliorates insulin resistance in a diabetic patient with Prader–Willi syndrome. *Diabetes Res Clin Pract* 1998; **42**: 205–8.

CHAPTER 14

Diabetes and information technology

Kenneth J. Robertson

What is laid down, ordered, factual is never enough to embrace the whole truth: life always spills over the rim of every cup.
—Boris Pasternak, Russian poet and writer (1890–1960)

Introduction

Eventually, information technology (IT) will be ubiquitous in health care, regarded as no more remarkable than the electrical sockets in the wall or the taps on the sink. The cultural change required for this to happen is as great, if not greater, than the improvements in the technology to make possible the capture and sharing of clinical information wherever that may be necessary. Note also that for this to happen in one hospital is challenging, but on a global scale it seems an unattainable goal. However, consider the internet – a new technology only a few years ago and now part of daily life for millions across the world.

Obviously, the impact of IT on health and diabetes, in particular, is enormous and reaches all the way from drug manufacture to the meters used to measure blood glucose. This chapter will consider the main areas where IT is making a major contribution to the improvement of care at the patient and professional level. Inevitably, the evidence base is weak, and the implications of this will also be explored.

Registers

While diabetes registers have been in place in many parts of the world for a long time, the majority are still dependent upon manual registration of patient data with central entry onto a database. Modern IT opens up possibilities of having registers developed as a by-product of care. Registers are no longer just epidemiological or research tools. In Scotland, the Scottish Care Information – Diabetes Collaboration (SCI-DC) has grown from a start in two Health Boards to be a national system that comprises a hospital-based application to manage clinics and a network application that collates this with information from general practice. This 'shared' record drives planning, forms the bedrock of annual national audit (Scottish Diabetes Survey) and provides the demographic details to drive the emergent Scottish Diabetes Retinopathy Screening Programme (**E**) [1]. The network element is now in place in every Health Board in Scotland (14 Boards) and the hospital system is in all the adult services. The paediatric 'module' is being developed and is expected to be implemented fully this year.

In England and Wales, the National Diabetes Audit makes extensive use of IT to gather and collate a minimum dataset about the care of individual patients. For the 2005 report on children and young people (**B**) [2], 64 of 237 paediatric diabetes services provided data but this had doubled since the previous year. One of the most important lessons about the process was that additional IT support will be required for centres so that such central reporting can be a by-product of clinical care.

Clinical record

The mantra of health-care informatics is that 'data for secondary uses should be available as a by-product of care'. This rather utopian ideal can only be made a reality when clinical staff are involved in the design and implementation of the system from the start. A series of steps must be gone through to ensure that the project will be managed properly and that the requirements are well understood. Some of the commonest issues and pitfalls are presented here posed as questions. When contemplating the procurement/development/implementation of a clinical system, it would be reckless to proceed without being able to answer them all in some detail (see Table 14.1).

Data standards, data sharing and coding/terming

Traditionally, speciality clinical systems have been procured and implemented from the perspective only of the one speciality. However, given that patients frequently have comorbidities and will, in any case, inevitably have encounters with other clinical professionals, it is increasingly important to be able to share data with others. Such sharing should be regarded as clinically dangerous unless aforethought has been given to establishing data standards with risk of fields being misfiled, interpreted differently by alternative systems, etc. Properly constructed data standards will address:
• the unambiguous clinical definition of a data item
• the range of entries (numeric or text) that may be captured
• validation rules
• the code or term (often ICD-10 code or SNOMED-CT term) to be used
• how the definition fits with the data requirements of other clinical groups – e.g. height may have been defined as '9.99 m' where the 9 represents any number and the measurement is done with the patient in stocking soles.

For a child of 8 months, the numeric definition would have to specify three decimal places and state something about the measuring method. If these differences are not explicit and understood then transfer of the 'height' record from one system to another will be unsatisfactory. While this may not be a major issue, a similar approach to insulin doses could be dangerous where an adult system would almost certainly record a dose of 0.5 U (in a young child) as 0 U since there is unlikely to be provision for decimal parts of units. Such considerations may appear esoteric but planning is vital.

Cross-speciality sharing will also mean that many generic data items will already have been defined. These will need to be viewed in the context of a child with diabetes and may be usable without modification or require qualification or a new data item. The introduction of systems such as the 'Connecting for Health Care Record Service' in England makes such discussion urgent.

Table 14.1 Critical questions for a clinical system

1 *What is (are) the purpose(s) of the proposed system?*
   - It is likely that the principal purpose will be to create a clinical record of the encounters with patients by members of the diabetes team.
   - Consideration must also be given to the need to provide access to information for other professionals within and out with the current organisation, e.g. general practitioner, other hospital staff, etc.
   - Usually, there are defined local governance requirements and, increasingly, statistics are collated at a regional or national level.

2 *Is the record multidisciplinary and how will the different professionals view each other's entries?*
   - Paediatric diabetes teams generally work very closely and will benefit from having full access to their patients' records.

3 *Who will enter data into the system?*
   - Data quality is likely to be higher where clinicians are using the system as their record – mistakes are noted and resolved – and *ad hoc* queries are more likely to produce useful answers.
   - Where clerical staff enter data (often from handwritten records), there is a high likelihood of transcription errors and misinterpretation of the clinician's intended meaning.
   - Clinicians may argue that they do not have time to enter data directly but this has to be challenged. If one of the requirements is to have real-time data capture then the ergonomics of the system has to be able to support this – logical screen layout, ability to move around sections easily (patients do not always present problems and issues in the expected order) and responsiveness. After all, it is a contractual and ethical obligation to record the clinical process, so time would normally be devoted to do this on paper. It may also be appropriate to consider the type of computer hardware being used – peripatetic staff such as diabetes nurse specialists and dietitians may be better served by the use of mobile devices.

4 *What training will be required and who will provide it?*
   - Most clinical staff now have basic computer skills but these may require to be enhanced before system-specific training.

5 *What benefits are expected?*
   - This may seem like a silly question but identification of perceived benefits will focus both the development and implementation of the system and allow objective testing of their achievement at various stages. This may be especially pertinent to securing revenue funding (see below).

6 *What quality assurance processes are in place to ensure that data are being captured accurately?*
   - The system should have validation at a number of levels – input validation should prevent, for example, ridiculous blood pressures such as 1000/800 being entered.
   - Appropriate fields may be mandatory before progressing to the next stage – care must be taken if using this method, that the appropriate information will always be available to the user.
   - Data integrity is another critical concept. Where definitions and options for data fields change, it is essential that historical information can still be presented in its original context; e.g. if a field is recorded as a number from a list, then changes to the list must not result in the recorded data changing meaning.

7 *What will be the outputs?*
   - A common benefit of clinical applications is the production of discharge or clinic letters for primary care clinicians. This is fine but increasingly the latter expect to receive such information in electronic form.
   - Email solutions may be a short-term approach, although they should only be used within an appropriate security model, e.g. encryption.
   - A better ploy would be to ensure that the data are passed in a form that can be incorporated into other systems and this can be achieved only when technical and semantic (meaning) interoperability has been addressed from the outset.

Continued

Table 14.1 *Continued*

- It may be possible to set up 'standard reports' that can be run regularly but most clinicians will also wish to have an *ad hoc* reporting tool. The functionality and ease of use of such tools should be evaluated carefully before selecting a system because many a system has been praised for its ability to absorb information but damned for its reluctance to give it up.

8 *What clinical leadership will be provided?*
  - The introduction of any new technology into the clinical process requires planning and support. Time and again, software programmes have been deemed to fail, not because of inadequacies in the system but because there was no clear leadership providing guidance, encouragement and occasionally coercion to ensure that the difficulties are overcome and success assured. It is a truism in eHealth that many excellent applications are 'failures', while many mediocre ones succeed because of leadership. Note, however, that this has to be true leadership (appropriate seniority and peer respect) with the new process becoming embedded in the clinical workflow or when the leader moves on, the use of the system will cease. Larger projects must also have formal project management and a 'senior responsible owner' who can ensure that progress is maintained.

9 *How will the system be administered?*
  - Any clinical system will have to be fully supported so that continuity of service is assured (commonly described as 24/7 business continuity), and this is expensive and new to the health-care community.
  - User management will be necessary – simple when there are only a few users on one site but much more complex when users, unknown to the system administrator, are to be registered.
  - Consideration must be given to access rights – often based upon role. Login must be strictly by authenticated users so that audit trails are accurate – there is no point in having sophisticated audit functionality in the system if the first person into the diabetes centre in the morning logs on for everyone.

10 *How will the system be funded?*
  - It is common for clinicians to purchase software with 'soft' money. While this may be straightforward, it is almost invariably a bad move unless supported fully by the local/regional IT professionals who will also ensure fit with the strategy.
  - It is very unusual for clinical software to have only a capital cost and the revenue consequences must be considered too – maintenance and upgrades, as well as training costs as appropriate.
  - The licensing model will very often mean that additional users incur additional costs. There is also the cost of the hardware (computers and servers) to factor in.

Germany offers an excellent example of how coordination at the national level can lead to the provision of high-quality data for the purposes of benchmarking and governance. The DPV (**B**) [3] approach comprises three elements – diabetes documentation software (DPV), semi-annual benchmarking (QC-DPV) and a data pool for diabetes research (DPV-SCIENCE). Improvements in the quality of care have been demonstrated with 183 centres enrolled in the project by 2005 covering some 24,000 patients – more than 75% of children with diabetes in Germany (personal communication).

Electronic reminders and algorithms

One of the features of real-time data-entry clinical systems is that they can be set up to provide support for the process of care. Based upon agreed criteria, the system can offer prompts; e.g. when eye screening or urine testing for microalbuminuria is due. In our clinic, introduction of such a system improved adherence to eye-screening targets from 61 to 89% in 1 year. This is not 100%, however, and the finding was similar to a study by Sequist *et al.* in Boston (**A**) [4], who also found that 76% of clinicians felt that such reminders improved quality of care. This serves to emphasise that the introduction of computerised records without consideration of the processes of care and workflow management, coupled with staff training, will fail to deliver the benefits expected.

Confidentiality and consent

Few areas of eHealth are more fraught and contentious just now than the debate about consent in relation to the use of electronic medical records. European Union countries all have their Data Protection Law based upon the European Directive on Data Protection (95/46/EC) (**E**) [5] but the details vary, so readers should be sure that any advice is based upon local legislation. In the UK (**E**) [6], patients should be informed about the uses to which their information will be put but it is acceptable to assume implied consent when sharing clinical information for the specific purpose of direct care (assuming that the patient has not specified any caveats in relation to particularly sensitive information). However, there has been a debate around this principle in relation to the NHS Care Records Service, in England, where the intention is to make summary information available on a Spine record so that it can be accessed wherever the patient is receiving care. The British Medical Association argues that this record should only be created on an opt-in basis (explicit consent), while the NHS argues that it should be created unless the patient has opted out. While such arguments may appear abstruse, they are at the heart of the move to patients having electronic records. Some legislatures have experimented with giving patients their own records on smartcards but this has not been successful at more than a small pilot level. There is absolute clarity, however, around the use of clinical records for research purposes. Unless the data are anonymised, explicit consent must be sought. To be even more specific – when data are used outside of direct care and the patients are identifiable, it is illegal to do this without the explicit (and preferably written) consent of the patients.

Comorbidity

Patients often have other medical problems besides diabetes and this becomes almost universal during adult years. It is not, therefore, in the best interests of the patients or their health professionals if information about each of their problems is held within independent silos. This is a key problem and central to the emergence of pan-health IT solutions being developed throughout the world. It is fair to say that there is no general solution yet but compliance with the appropriate local/regional technical and information standards will offer the best chance of later compatibility.

Patient access

This is too large a topic to be discussed here but suffice to say that most eHealth programmes in the developed world have adopted strategies that give patients access to their health records in some way. Numerous examples exist of allowing patients to disease-specific elements, e.g. diabetes, renal disease, etc., but these are almost always bespoke solutions that have not addressed the problem (that already besets clinical staff) of how the patient can get access to all of the appropriate information without having to memorise a host of usernames and passwords. What is required is a large-scale authentication and identification system to ensure that the patients see only what relates to them. Mechanisms must also be in place to make it impossible for the patients to directly change the information captured by the clinicians as part of their professional record – there should, however, be a process for reconciliation of errors. Too often also, no thought is given to supporting patients in understanding the meaning of what they have accessed. These are complex issues that will have to be addressed in the next few years. Increasingly, there is a perception that the medical record 'belongs' to the patient but experiments in letting patients be the custodian of their own records (outside of specific elements such as maternity records), e.g. with smartcards such as the European DiabCard (**B**) [7], have had very limited success.

Telemedicine

This is an area of diabetes care that has proved attractive, especially in remote and rural communities. The prospect of being able to maintain a therapeutic relationship with patients from afar has stimulated research into the feasibility and acceptability of using teleconferencing and remote monitoring. Smith *et al.* in Queensland (**B**) [8] successfully introduced teleconsultation for children with diabetes and other endocrine abnormalities. They delivered support for acute crises, education to patients and staff and routine clinical contact and emphasised the importance of this multimodality approach. Telemedicine must be used to solve identified problems rather than as an excuse to use new technology. The hardware is becoming more reliable and flexible in its mobility and use and so we are likely to see it being introduced more widely. It may have particular value in linking to small A&E departments without paediatric expertise so that the immediate care of children with diabetic ketoacidosis can be expedited.

Numerous schemes have been established with a view to encouraging patients (often adolescents) to monitor their blood glucose more effectively and to support them in using the results. These have ranged from downloading data from blood glucose meters integrated into mobile phones (Nokia, Finland) to emailing of results to the clinic. The 'Sweet Talk' programme in Dundee has introduced a system of patient-tailored text messages designed to improve adherence behaviour generally (**A**) [9].

In 2005, Farmer *et al.* published a meta-analysis of telemedicine interventions to support blood glucose monitoring in diabetes (**A**) [10]. Most of the studies they reviewed were of short duration and had small numbers of patients, so their conclusion, '*Telemedicine solutions for diabetes care are feasible and acceptable, but evidence for their effectiveness in improving HbA1c or reducing costs while maintaining HbA1c levels, or improving other aspects of diabetes management is not strong*', was perhaps unsurprising. There is a recurrent tendency to introduce such technology without consideration of proper evaluation.

Conclusion

Diabetes care is supported in numerous other ways by IT and doubtlessly many more will emerge in the coming years. We have yet to see the real impact of genomics and proteomics on medicine but when the genetics and phenotypes of diabetes are better understood, it will become even more critical to have technological support to ensure that individual patients receive best care. Early attempts better to organise research findings and literature to support care (see www.elib.scot.nhs.uk/portal/diabetes/Pages/) will become more tightly integrated with patient records.

Quite beyond the remit of this chapter but still a potent use of IT is the physical linkage of continuous blood glucose monitoring with insulin-pump algorithms which will, in the near future, close the loop so that patients can leave the technology to monitor and manage their blood glucose.

eHealth is a relatively new discipline and the application of the rigour which computers demand of record keeping will certainly be a challenge to a traditionally rather anarchic profession. Nonetheless, the potential benefits are huge for clinicians and their patients alike.

References

1 Morris AD, Boyle DI, MacAlpine R *et al.* The diabetes audit and research in Tayside Scotland (DARTS) study: electronic record linkage to create a diabetes register. DARTS/MEMO Collaboration. *BMJ* 1997; **315**: 524–8.

2 The Information Centre. *National Diabetes Audit Report for the Audit Period 2004/05: Key Findings about the Quality of Care for Children and Young People with Diabetes in England, Incorporating Registrations from Wales.* Available at: www.ic.nhs.uk

3 Grabert M, Schweiggert F, Holl RW. A framework for diabetes documentation and quality management in Germany: 10 years of experience with DPV. *Comput Methods Programs Biomed* 2002; **69**: 115–21.

4 Sequist TD, Gandhi TK, Karson AS *et al.* A randomized trial of electronic clinical reminders to improve quality of care for diabetes and coronary artery disease. *J Am Med Inform Assoc* 2005; **12**: 431–7.

5 *Directive 95/46/EC of the European Parliament and the Council of 24 October 1995 on the Protection of Individuals with Regard to the Processing of Personal Data and on the Free Movement of Such Data.* Available at: http://www.cdt.org/privacy/eurodirective/EU_Directive_.html

6 Corporate Author: Great Britain. *Data Protection Act (UK) 1998: Elizabeth II. Chapter 29: 8th Impression October 2003 (Incorporating Corrections).* Reprinted April 2003. Available at: http://www.opsi.gov.uk/ACTS/acts1998/19980029.htm

7 Engelbrecht R, Hildebrand C. *Diabcard: Improved Communication in Diabetes Care Based on Chip Card Technology.* Available at: http://www-mi.gsf.de/diabcard/nf_index.html

8 Smith AC, Batch J, Lang E *et al.* The use of online health techniques to assist with the delivery of specialist paediatric diabetes services in Queensland. *J Telemed Telecare* 2003; **9**(suppl 2): S54–7.

9 Franklin VL, Waller A, Pagliari C *et al.* A randomized controlled trial of Sweet Talk, a text-messaging system to support young people with diabetes. *Diabet Med* 2006; **23**: 1332–8.

10 Farmer A, Gibson OJ, Tarassenko L *et al.* A systematic review of telemedicine interventions to support blood glucose self-monitoring in diabetes. *Diabet Med* 2005; **22**: 1372–8.

Abbreviations

AAP	American Academy of Pediatrics
ACE	Angiotensin converting enzyme
ACR	Albumin creatinine ratio
ADA	American Diabetes Association
AER	Albumin excretion rate
AGREE	Appraisal of Guidelines, Research and Evaluation for Europe
AIRE	Autoimmune regulator
ALAD	La Asociación Latino Americana de Diabetes
APS I & II	Autoimmune polyendocrine syndromes 1 and 2
AUC	Area under the curve
BFST	Behavioural family systems therapy
BG	Blood glucose
BMI	Body mass index
BP	Blood pressure
BPA	British Paediatric Association
BSPED	British Society for Paediatric Endocrinology and Diabetes
CBT	Cognitive behavioural therapy
CD	Compact disk
CF	Cystic fibrosis
CFRD	Cystic-fibrosis-related diabetes
CGMS	Continuous glucose-monitoring system
CNS	Central nervous system
CRF	Chronic renal failure
CSII	Continuous subcutaneous insulin infusion
CTLA-4	Cytotoxic T lymphocyte antigen-4
CV	Cardiovascular
DAFNE	Diet adjustment for normal eating
DARTS	Diabetes Audit and Research in Tayside Study
DBP	Diastolic blood pressure
DCCT	Diabetes Control and Complications Trial
DESG	Diabetes Education Study Group
DH	Department of Health
DIDMOAD	Diabetes Insipidus, Diabetes Mellitus, Optic Atrophy and Deafness
DKA	Diabetic ketoacidosis
DNA	Deoxyribonucleic acid

DSME	Diabetes self-management education
DUK	Diabetes UK
EASD	European Association for the Study of Diabetes
ED	Eating disorder
EDIC	Epidemiology of Diabetes Interventions and Complications
ELISA	Enzyme-linked immunosorbent assay
EMA	Endomyseal antibodies
ENDIT	European Nicotinamide Diabetes Intervention Trial
ESPE	European Society for Pediatric Endocrinology
ESPGHAN	European Society of Paediatric Gastroenterology, Hepatology and Nutrition
FACTS	Families Adolescents and Children's Teamwork Study
FinnDiane	Finnish Diabetes Nephropathy Study
FPG	Fasting plasma glucose
fT_4	Free thyroxine
GAD-65/GADA	Glutamic acid dehydrogenase
GDG	Guideline development group
GFD	Gluten-free diet
GH	Growth hormone
GI	Glycaemic index
GL	Glycaemic load
GLP-1	Glucagon-like peptide 1
GRID	Genetic resource investigating diabetes
GWB2	Glucowatch Biographer 2
HbA1c	Glycated haemoglobin A1c
HBGM	Home blood glucose monitoring
HCP	Health care professional
HDL	High-density lipoprotein
HLA	Human leucocyte antigen
HMG-CoA	3-Hydroxy-3-methyl-glutaryl-CoA reductase
HNF	Hepatic nucleocyte factor
HSG	Hvidøre Study Group
HTA	Health technology assessment
IA-2	Tyrosine phosphatase-like molecule
IAA	Insulin autoantibodies
ICA	Islet cell antibodies
ICD	International classification of disease
IDDM1	Insulin-dependent diabetes mellitus susceptibility locus 1
IDDM2	Insulin-dependent diabetes mellitus susceptibility locus 2
IDDM12	Insulin-dependent diabetes mellitus susceptibility locus 12
IDF	International Diabetes Federation
IFG	Impaired fasting glucose

IFIH1	Interferon-induced helicase 1
IGF	Insulin-like growth factor
IGT	Impaired glucose tolerance
IPEX	Immune dysregulation, polyendocrinopathy, enteropathy X-linked syndrome
IPF	Insulin promoter factor
ISPAD	International Society for Pediatric and Adolescent Diabetes
IT	Information technology
KCNJ11	Potassium inwardly rectifying channel, subfamily J, member 11
LDL	Low-density lipoprotein
LJM	Limited joint mobility
LWPES	Lawson Wilkins Pediatric Endocrine Society
MDI	Multiple daily injections
MI	Motivational interviewing
MMR	Measles, mumps and rubella
MODY	Maturity-onset diabetes of the young
MUFA	Monounsaturated fatty acid
NAFL	Non-alcoholic fatty liver
NASH	Non-alcoholic steato-hepatitis
NDA	National Diabetes Audit
NH	Nocturnal hypoglycaemia
NHS	National Health Service
NPH	Neutral pH Hagedorn
NICE	National Institute for Clinical Excellence
NICE TA	NICE Technology Assessment
NSF	National Service Framework
OFSTED	Office for Standards in Education
OGTT	Oral glucose tolerance test
OMIM	Online Mendelian inheritance in man
OR	Odds ratio
PCOS	Polycystic ovarian syndrome
PCR	Polymerase chain reaction
PNDM	Permanent neonatal diabetes mellitus
PPARγ	Peroxisome proliferator-activated receptor gamma
PTPN22	Protein tyrosine phosphatase non-receptor type 22
P-WS	Prader–Willi syndrome
RCP	Royal College of Physicians
RCPCH	Royal College of Paediatrics and Child Health
RCT	Randomised controlled trial
RNA	Ribonucleic acid

SBP	Systolic blood pressure
SCI-DC	Scottish Care Information – Diabetes Collaboration
SDS	Standard deviation score
SH	Severe hypoglycaemia
SIGN	Scottish Intercollegiate Guideline Network
SNP	Single nucleotide polymorphism
SPE	Structured patient education
SSGCYD	Scottish Study Group for the Care of the Young with Diabetes
SUR	Sulphonyl urea receptor
T1DM	Type 1 diabetes mellitus
T2DM	Type 2 diabetes mellitus
T_3	Tri-iodothyronine
TCF	Transcription factor
TgA	Thyroglobulin antibodies
Th1	T helper 1
TNDM	Transient neonatal diabetes mellitus
TODAY	Treatment options for T2DM in adolescence and youth
TPO	Thyroid peroxidase
Treg	Regulatory T cells
TSH	Thyroid stimulating hormone
TTG	Tissue transglutaminase
UKPDS	United Kingdom Prospective Diabetes Study
VNTR	Variable number of tandem repeats
WHO	World Health Organization

Index

Page numbers in *italic* refer to figures; page numbers in **bold** refer to tables.

ABCC8 gene
  mutations in PNDM and TNDM, 203
  See also neonatal diabetes
acanthosis nigricans, 189
activity aspects, T1DM in very young children and, 66
acute management, polycystic ovarian syndrome (PCOS), 191
adolescence and diabetes, 76
  action research in, 83
  clinical perspectives
    adolescents with T1DM, 86
    anxiety and depression, 80
    associated diseases, 77
    behavioural problems, 79–80
    clinic non-attendance, 85
    eating disorders, 78
    emotional problems, 79–80
    glycaemic control deterioration aspects, 76
    insulin disorders, 78
    insulin omission, 77–8
    long-term consequences of diabetes, 79
    paediatric to adult service, transition of care from, 86
    physiological changes of puberty, 76
    psychological interventions, 80, **81**
    psychological issues, 77
    transfer-related aspects, 87
    transition of care, 87–90
    weight disorders, 78
    young adult clinics, effectiveness of, 86–7
  conceptualisations of, 82
  cultural perspectives, 80–3
  diagnostic criteria, 9
  insulin
    free mixing, 54
    management, 49, 54
  issues related to adolescence, 84
  management team structure, 17–18
  social perspectives, 80
  social support networks, 85
  study results, 83–4
  See also type 1 diabetes mellitus (T1DM); type 2 diabetes mellitus (T2DM)
aetiology, T1DM, 26
alcohol
  consumption and diabetes, 97–8, 108
  See also dietary management

algorithms, electronic reminders and, 224
alpha-glucosidase
  inhibitors, 184
  See also type 2 diabetes mellitus (T2DM) treatment
analogues, meglitinide, 184
antibody
  anti-CD3, 35
  antibody-negative child, 15
  autoantibodies, 15, 31
  islet cell, 31
antigen-presenting cells (APCs), 29
antioxidant
  nutrients, 108
  See also dietary management
anxiety
  adolescence considerations, 80
  psychological aspects, 148–9
autoantibody
  islet cell, 31
  markers, diabetes-associated, 15
autoimmune diseases
  screening for, 161
  T1DM, **30**

behavioural approaches
  adolescence and diabetes, 79–80
  in diabetes education, 117–18
  psychology and, 144, 146
  See also dietary management
bicarbonate
  therapy, 45
  See also diabetic ketoacidosis (DKA)
blood glucose
  monitoring, 69
  See also glucose monitoring; type 1 diabetes mellitus (T1DM) in very young children
body mass index (BMI), 162
British Society for Paediatric Endocrinology and Diabetes (BSPED) guidelines, 5

calpain-10, 177
  candidate genes for T2DM
    HNF1A, 178
    insulin gene, 178
    KCNJ11 gene, 179
    NEUROD1, 178
    PPARγ gene, 179

carbohydrate, 107
  assessment, 111
  counting, 111, 114
  counting (modern), 114
    carbohydrate to insulin ratios (level 3),
      114–15
    consistent carbohydrate intake (level 1), 114
    pattern management principles (level 2), 114
  See also dietary management
cardiovascular considerations
  diabetes and, 115–16
  See also dietary management
carer education, T1DM in very young children
      and, 67–8
carotenoids, 108
cataracts
  screening for associated conditions, 164
  See also ophthalmic complications
CD4 helper T cells, 32
CD8 T cells, 32
cerebellar hypoplasia, permanent neonatal
      diabetes with, 203
cerebral oedema, 46–8
  management, 47–8
  pathophysiology, 47
  See also diabetic ketoacidosis (DKA)
children and diabetes, 123
  continuous subcutaneous insulin infusion
      (CSII), 49, 50–53, 54
  diagnostic criteria, 9
  enterovirus infection in, 37
  insulin management
    free mixing, 54
    prepubertal, 49
    preschool, 49
  insulin regimens, 48, 50–53
  management team structure, 17–18
  rare forms of diabetes in
    cystic-fibrosis-related diabetes, 211, 213–14
    Prader–Willi syndrome (P-WS), 214–15
  See also dietary management; education in
      childhood diabetes; screening for
      associated conditions; type 1 diabetes
      mellitus (T1DM) in very young children
chromosome 6q
  anomalies, 200
  See also neonatal diabetes
chronic management, polycystic ovarian syndrome
      (PCOS), 191
chronic renal failure (CRF), 161
clinical
  assessment, diabetic ketoacidosis and, 44
  record, 222
  See also information technology
clinical perspectives (adolescence and diabetes)
  adolescents with T1DM, 86
  anxiety and depression, 80
  associated diseases, 77
  behavioural problems, 79–80
  clinic non-attendance aspects, 85
  eating disorders, 78
  emotional problems, 79–80

glycaemic control deterioration aspects, 76
  insulin
    disorders, 78
    omission, 77–8
  long-term consequences of diabetes, 79
  paediatric to adult service, transition of care
      from, 86
  physiological
    changes of puberty, 76
    interventions, 80, **81**
    issues, 77
  transfer-related aspects, 87
  transition of care, 87–90
  weight disorders, 78
  young adult clinics, effectiveness of, 86–7
Cochrane databases, 7
coeliac disease
  background and definition, 159
  complications, 159
  presentation and diagnosis, 159
  prevalence, 159
  screening, 160
    for autoimmune conditions, 161
    for associated conditions, 159
  treatment, 160
comorbidities treatment
  dyslipidaemia, 185–6
  hypertension, 186–7
  information technology and, 225
  See also type 2 diabetes mellitus (T2DM)
      treatment
complications, screening procedures performed for
  dental abnormalities, 167
  foot care, 165
  growth, 162
  hypertension, 163
  limited joint mobility, 166
  lipids profile, 165
  macrovascular disease, 165–6
  necrobiosis lipoidica, 167
  nephropathy, 162–3
  neuropathy, 166
  ophthalmic complications
    cataracts, 164
    retinopathy, 164
  skin changes, 166
  smoking, 166
confidentiality
  and consent, 225
  See also information technology
continuous glucose monitoring system (CGMS),
      56
  See also home blood glucose monitoring
      (HBGM); glucose monitoring
continuous subcutaneous insulin infusion (CSII)
  children and, 49, **50–3**
  special situations management and, 94
  See also insulin management
coordinated transfer process, 151
cow's milk
  proteins, 36
  See also trigger factors (T1DM)

C-peptide measurement, 15
CTLA-4 gene, 28, 29
cultural perspectives (adolescence and diabetes),
        80, 82–3
cystic-fibrosis-related diabetes (CFRD), 211
    diabetes and impaired glucose tolerance in
        impact of, 213
        treatment, 214
    insulin secretion defects in, 211

data
    sources, 6
    See also evidence-based health care
databases
    Cochrane, 7
    MEDLINE, 6
dental
    abnormalities, 167
    See also screening for associated conditions
depression
    adolescence and diabetes, 80
    eating disorders and, 116
    psychology, 148–9
    See also dietary management
diabetes
    antibody-negative child and, 15
    childhood. *See* children and diabetes
    classification, 9, 14
    C-peptide measurement, 15
    defined, 9
    diagnostic criteria, **10**
        adolescence, 9
        childhood, 9
    education. *See* education in childhood diabetes
    epidemiology, 9
    fasting insulin measurement, 15
    glycaemia, aetiological classification of, **11**
    impaired fasting glycaemia (IFG), 10
    impaired glucose tolerance (IGT), 10
    information technology and, 221, **223–4**
        clinical record, 222
        coding/terming, 222
        comorbidity, 225
        confidentiality and consent, 225
        data sharing, 222
        data standards, 222
        diabetes registers, 221
        electronic reminders and algorithms, 224
        patient access, 225–6
        telemedicine, 226
    long-term consequences in adolescents, 79
    management problems, 142
    management team structure, 17
        adolescence, 17–18
        childhood, 17–18
        glycaemic goals, 21
        multidisciplinary team approach, 18
        role of, **19**
        stabilisation in ambulatory versus in-hospital
            care, evidence for, **20**
    maturity-onset diabetes of the young (MODY),
        17

monogenic, 15, **16**
neonatal. *See* neonatal diabetes
oral glucose tolerance test (OGTT), 9–10
rare forms. *See* rare forms of diabetes
screening and, 161
special situations management in, 93
    alcohol consumption, 97–8
    exercise, 95–7
    fasting and feasting, 99–100
    illness, 93–4
    immunisation advice, 99
    recreational drug use, 98–9
    surgery, 97
    travel, 95
stress hyperglycaemia, 17
type 1 diabetes mellitus (T1DM), 9
    epidemiology, 12, **13**, 14
    prevention and cure, 34–5
    types
        T1DM, 14
        T2DM, 14
    See also adolescence and diabetes; dietary
        management; type 1 diabetes mellitus
        (T1DM); type 2 diabetes mellitus (T2DM)
Diabetes Education Study Group (DESG), 125
diabetes self management education (DSME),
        125–6
diabetes-associated autoantibody markers, 15
diabetic ketoacidosis (DKA), 5
    bicarbonate therapy, 45
    clinical assessment, 44
    fluid management
        fluid rate, 44
        fluid type, 44–5
    general issues-associated with, 44
    insulin therapy, 45
    management, 43
    monitoring, 46
    morbidity, 46
    mortality, 46
    pathophysiology, 42
    phosphate replacement, 45
    potassium replacement, 45
    prevention, 48
    resuscitation, 44
    subcutaneous insulin therapy and oral fluids,
        transition to, 46
    See also cerebral oedema; type 1 diabetes
        mellitus (T1DM)
diagnosis (psychological aspects)
    severity of presentation, 142
    treatment at home or in hospital, 142
dietary
    fat, 106–7
    See also carbohydrate
dietary management
    aims, 104–5
    alcohol intake, 108
    antioxidant nutrients intake, 108
    behavioural approaches in diabetes education,
        117–18
    carbohydrate

assessment, 111
  counting, 111, 114
  counting (modern), 114–15
  intake, 107
cardiovascular considerations, 115–16
development aspects, 105
dietary fat intake, 106–7
dietary guidelines, 116
eating disorders, 116–17
education and, 110
  education tools, 111
  structured patient education, 110–11
energy balance, 105
food
  plate, *113*
  pyramid, *112*
glycaemic control influence on, 109–10
glycaemic index (GI), 115
glycaemic load (GL), 115
growth potential, 105
non-starch polysaccharide (fibre) intake, 107
nutrients balance, 105
practical management, 109
protein intake, 106
psychological difficulties, 116–17
salt intake, 108
sucrose intake, 107
weight management, 108–9
dietitian role in diabetes management, **19**
disordered eating
  behaviour, 116–17
  See also dietary management
Dose Adjustment for Normal Eating (DAFNE), 126
drug use and diabetes, recreational, 98–9
dyslipidaemia, 185–6
  See also type 2 diabetes mellitus (T2DM)
    treatment

eating disorders
  adolescence and diabetes, 78
  dietary management and, 116–17
  psychology, 149–50
eating
  disordered, 116–17
  disturbance, 149–50
  See also psychology
education
  behavioural approaches in diabetes and, 117
  dietary management and
    education tools, 111
    structured patient education, 110–1
education in childhood diabetes, 123, 127–30
  barriers and consequences, 134–5
  defined, 124–5
  Diabetes Education Study Group (DESG), 125
  diabetes self management education (DSME),
    125–6
  Dose Adjustment for Normal Eating (DAFNE),
    126
  educational interventions, 125
  implementation aspects, 130–2, 135–6
  levels

level 1 (at diagnosis), 132, **133**
  level 2 (continuing education), 132, **133**, 134
  modes of education, 125
  principles and practice of, **131**
  structured patient education (SPE), 125–6
  T1DM and, 123
  T2DM and, 123
  therapeutic patient education, 125
electronic reminders and algorithms, 224
emotional
  problems, 79–80
  See also adolescence and diabetes
endomyseal antibodies (EMA), 160
energy balance, 105
energy intake
  carbohydrate, 107
  dietary fat, 106–7
  non-starch polysaccharide (fibre), 107
  protein, 106
  sucrose, 107
  See also dietary management
enterovirus
  infection, 37
  See also mumps; rubella
environmental factors (T2DM), 175–6
epidemiology, T1DM, 12, **13**, 14
evidence-based health care, 1
  data sources
    Cochrane databases, 7
    MEDLINE, 6–7
  evidence grading aspects, 3
    good practice points (GPP), 3
    guideline development groups (GDG), 3
  Fermat's last theorem proof and, 2
  guidelines, 3
    British Society for Paediatric Endocrinology
      and Diabetes (BSPED) guidelines, 5
    International Society for Pediatric and
      Adolescent Diabetes (ISPAD) guidelines,
      4, 6
    Lawson Wilkins Pediatric Endocrine
      Society/British Society of Paediatric
      Endocrinology and Diabetes
      (LWPES/BSPED) guidelines, 5–6
    National Institute for Clinical Excellence
      (NICE), 4, 6
  mathematical proof behind, 2
  scientific proof behind, 2–3
exercise and diabetes, 95–7
experience and expectations, understanding, 151

family
  conflict, 147–8
  interventions, 144, 146
  See also psychology
fasting
  and diabetes, 99–100
  insulin measurement, 15
fat
  dietary, 106–7
  See also dietary management
feasting and diabetes, 99–100

Fermat's
  theorem, 2
  See also evidence-based health care
fibre
  non-starch polysaccharide, 107
  See also dietary management
flavanoids, 108
flitting insulitis, 31
fluid management
  diabetic ketoacidosis and, 44
    fluid rate, 44
    fluid type, 44–5
  oral, 46
food
  advice, T1DM in very young children and,
    65–6
  plate, *113*
  pyramid, *112*
  See also dietary management
foot
  care, 165
  See also screening for associated conditions
FOXP3 mutations, 201
free mixing
  insulin, 54
  See also insulin management
frequency, neonatal diabetes
  ABCC8 gene mutations in PNDM and TNDM,
    203
  chromosome 6q anomalies, 200
  glucokinase mutations, 202
  insulin promoter factor 1 (IPF-1), 197
  IPEX (FOXP3 mutations), 201
  KCNJ11 permanent neonatal diabetes, 202
  permanent neonatal diabetes with cerebellar
    hypoplasia, 203
  Wolcott–Rallison syndrome, 201

GADA, 31
gene mutations
  ABCC8, 203
  glucokinase, 206
genetics
  HLA haplotypes and genotypes, 27
  maturity-onset diabetes of the young (MODY),
    204–6
    glucokinase gene mutations, 206–8
    transcription factors mutations, 208
  neonatal diabetes, 197
  type 1 diabetes mellitus (T1DM), 26, **27**
  type 2 diabetes mellitus (T2DM), 175–6
    calpain-10, 177
    candidate genes investigations, 178
    genome-wide scanning, 176
    HNF1A, 178
    HNF4A promoter variants, 177
    insulin gene, 178
    KCNJ11 gene, 179
    NEUROD1, 178
    PPARγ gene, 179
    TCF7L2, 177
genome-wide scanning

calpain-10, 177
HNF4A promoter variants, 177
TCF7L2, 177
See also type 2 diabetes mellitus (T2DM)
genotypes, HLA, 27
glucokinase mutations
  MODY and, 206
  neonatal diabetes and, 202
glucose monitoring
  continuous glucose monitoring system
    (CGMS), 56
  Glucowatch biographer (GWB2), 56–7
  glycaemic control and, 55
  T1DM in very young children and blood
    glucose, 69
glucose tolerance in cystic-fibrosis (CF), impaired
  impact of, 213
  treatment of, 214
Glucowatch biographer (GWB2), 56–7
  See also glucose monitoring
gluten-free diet (GFD), 160
glycaemia, aetiological classification of, **11**
glycaemic
  control
    deterioration aspects in adolescents, 76
    dietary management and, 109–10
    glucose monitoring and, 55
    T1DM in very young children and, 71
    targeting of, 144
  goals, 21
  index (GI), 115
  load (GL), 115
  See also diabetes management
glycated haemoglobin, 70–1
good practice points (GPP), 3
growth
  complications, screening procedures and, 162
  potential, 105
  See also dietary management
guideline development groups (GDG), 3
guidelines
  dietary, 116
  evidence-based health care, 3
    British Society for Paediatric Endocrinology
      and Diabetes (BSPED) guidelines, 5
    International Society for Pediatric and
      Adolescent Diabetes (ISPAD) guidelines,
      4, 6
    Lawson Wilkins Pediatric Endocrine
      Society/British Society of Paediatric
      Endocrinology and Diabetes
      (LWPES/BSPED) guidelines, 5
    National Institute for Clinical Excellence
      (NICE), 4, 6
    type 2 diabetes mellitus (T2DM) treatment, 180
  See also dietary management

haemoglobin, glycated, 70–1
haplotypes, HLA, 27
HbA1c
  diabetes management and, 143–4
  levels, 18

health care
  evidence-based. *See* evidence-based helath care
  providers, T1DM in very young children and,
    66–7
  See also education in childhood diabetes
heterozygous mutation of HNF-1$_\beta$, 204
HNF1A
  gene, 178
  See also type 2 diabetes mellitus (T2DM)
HNF-1γ, heterozygous mutation of, 204
HNF4A promoter variants, 177
home blood glucose monitoring (HBGM), 55
  See also continuous glucose monitoring system
    (CGMS); insulin management
human leucocyte antigen (HLA)
  haplotypes and genotypes, 27
  See also type 1 diabetes mellitus (T1DM)
hyperglycaemia, stress, 17
hypertension
  complications, screening procedures and, 163
  type 2 diabetes mellitus (T2DM) treatment and,
    186–7
hyperthyroidism, 158
  See also screening for associated conditions
hypoglycaemia
  avoidance, 58
  insulin regimen and, 54–5
  prevalence, 57
  risk factors, 57
  T1DM in very young children and, 69–70
    glycated haemoglobin and, 70–1
    monitoring goals, 70
  treatment, 57–8
  See also insulin management
hypoplasia
  cerebellar, 203
  See also neonatal diabetes

IDDM1 susceptibility locus for T1DM, 28
IDDM12, 28
IDDM2, 28
illness and diabetes, 93–4
immunisation advice and diabetes, 99
immunology, T1DM, 29, 31–34
impaired fasting glycaemia (IFG), 10
impaired glucose
  tolerance (IGT), 10
  tolerance in cystic-fibrosis (CF)
    impact of, 213
    treatment, 214
infective factors (T1DM)
  virus infections
    enterovirus infection, 37
    mumps, 36
    rubella, 36
  See also trigger factors (T1DM)
information technology, 221–2, **223–4**, 225–6
  clinical record, 222
  coding/terming, 222
  comorbidity, 225
  confidentiality and consent, 225
  data

    sharing, 222
    standards, 222
  diabetes registers, 221
  electronic reminders and algorithms, 224
  patient access, 225–6
  telemedicine, 226
inhibitors
  alpha-glucosidase, 184
  See also type 2 diabetes mellitus (T2DM)
    treatment
insulin
  carbohydrate and insulin ratios, 114
  disorders, 78
  gene, 178
  hypoglycaemia and, 54–5
  management. *See* insulin management
  omission, 77–8
  regimen, 54–5
  secretion defects in cystic-fibrosis (diabetes and
    impaired glucose tolerance in CF), 211
    impact of, 213
    treatment of, 214
  therapy
    diabetic ketoacidosis, 45–6
    T1DM in very young children and, 64–5
    T2DM treatment, 184–5
  See also adolescence and diabetes; type 2
    diabetes mellitus (T2DM)
insulin autoantibodies (IAA), 27
insulin management, 48
  adolescents, 49, 54
  children
    continuous subcutaneous insulin infusion
     (CSII), 49, **50–3**, 54
  continuous glucose monitoring
    continuous glucose monitoring system
     (CGMS), 56
    Glucowatch biographer (GWB2), 56–7
  continuous subcutaneous insulin infusion, 54
  free mixing aspects, 54
  glucose monitoring and glycaemic control, 55
  home blood glucose monitoring (HBGM), 55
  hypoglycaemia and insulin regimen, 54–5
  insulin regimens, 48–9, **50–3**
  prepubertal children, 49
  preschool children, 49
  T1DM, 48–9
  See also diabetic ketoacidosis
insulin promoter factor 1 (IPF-1) deficiency
  neonatal diabetes and, 197
  treatment, 200
International Society for Pediatric and Adolescent
  Diabetes (ISPAD) guidelines, 4, 6
IPEX (FOXP3 mutations), 201
  See also neonatal diabetes
islet in T1DM, pathology of, 29

joint mobility, limited, 166

KCNJ11 gene
  neonatal diabetes and, 202
  T2DM and, 179

ketone monitoring, 69
  See also type 1 diabetes mellitus (T1DM) in very
    young children

Lawson Wilkins Pediatric Endocrine
    Society/British Society of Paediatric
    Endocrinology and Diabetes
    (LWPES/BSPED) guidelines, 5–6
lifestyle changes, T2DM treatment and, 181
limited joint
  mobility, 166
  See also screening for associated conditions
lipids profile, 165
lipoidica, necrobiosis, 167
low-density lipoprotein (LDL), 165

macrovascular
  disease, 165–6
  See also screening for associated conditions
management
  cerebral oedema, 47–8
  diabetic ketoacidosis, 43–4
  neonatal diabetes, 197
mathematical proof, evidence-based health care's, 2
maturity-onset diabetes of the young (MODY), 17,
    204
  genetics, 204–6
  glucokinase gene mutations, 206–8
  management, 209–10
  T2DM and, 17, 177
  transcription factors mutations, 208
  See also neonatal diabetes
medicine, evidence-based. *See* evidence-based
    health care
MEDLINE database, 6, 7
meglitinide
  analogues, 184
  See also type 2 diabetes mellitus (T2DM)
    treatment
microalbuminuria, 163
mixing, insulin, 54
  See also insulin management
mobility, limited joint, 166
monitoring
  diabetic ketoacidosis, 46
  glucose, 55
    continuous glucose monitoring system
      (CGMS), 56
    Glucowatch biographer (GWB2), 56–7
    glycaemic control and, 55
    home blood glucose monitoring (HBGM), 55
  hypoglycaemia, 70
  T1DM in very young children and, 69–70
    blood glucose, 69
    ketone, 69
monogenic diabetes, 15, **16**
morbidity, diabetic ketoacidosis and, 46
multidisciplinary team approach, 18
mumps, 36
  See also enterovirus infection; rubella
mutations
  FOXP3, 201

glucokinase, 202
transcription factors, 208

National Institute for Clinical Excellence (NICE),
    3, 4, 6
necrobiosis lipoidica, 161, 167
  See also screening for associated conditions
neonatal diabetes
  ABCC8 gene mutations in PNDM and TNDM
    treatment, 203
  chromosome 6q anomalies treatment, 200
  genetics, 197
  glucokinase mutations treatment, 202
  insulin promoter factor 1 (IPF-1), 197, 200
  IPEX (FOXP3 mutations) treatment, 201
  KCNJ11 permanent neonatal diabetes
    treatment, 203
  management, 197
  permanent neonatal diabetes with cerebellar
    hypoplasia, 203
  very rare forms of, 203–4
  Wolcott–Rallison syndrome treatment, 201
  See also maturity-onset diabetes of the young
    (MODY)
nephropathy complications, screening procedures
    and, 162–3
NEUROD1
  gene, 178
  See also type 2 diabetes mellitus (T2DM)
neuropathy, 166
  autonomic, 167
  See also screening for associated conditions
non-alcoholic fatty liver disease (NAFLD), 187
  See also type 2 diabetes mellitus (T2DM)
    treatment
nutrients
  balance, 105
  antioxidant, 108
  See also dietary management
nutritional factors, type 1 diabetes mellitus
    (T1DM), 36

oedema, cerebral, 46–8
  management, 47–8
  pathophysiology, 47
  See also diabetic ketoacidosis (DKA)
ophthalmic complications, screening procedures
    and
  cataracts, 164
  retinopathy, 164
oral
  fluids, 46
  therapy
    with one agent, 182–3
    with two agents, 183
    See also diabetic ketoacidosis (DKA); type 2
      diabetes mellitus (T2DM) treatment
oral glucose tolerance test (OGTT), 9, 10

paediatric to adult service, transition of care from,
    86
  organisation of transition, 151

psychosocial aspects of, 150
See also adolescence and diabetes; psychology
parent and carer education, T1DM in very young
children and, 67–8
pathophysiology
cerebral oedema, 47
diabetic ketoacidosis, 42
polycystic ovarian syndrome, 189–90
T1DM management, 42
patient
access, 225–6
See also information technology
peer
relationships, 148
See also psychology
permanent neonatal diabetes with cerebellar
hypoplasia, 203
phosphate replacement, diabetic ketoacidosis and,
45
physiological changes of puberty in adolescents, 76
PNDM, ABCC8 gene mutations in, 203
polycystic ovarian syndrome (PCOS), 188–9
defined, 190
pathophysiology, 189–90
treatment
acute management, 191
chronic management, 191
See also type 2 diabetes mellitus (T2DM)
treatment
polysaccharide (fibre)
non-starch, 107
See also dietary management
potassium replacement, diabetic ketoacidosis and,
45
PPARγ
gene, 179
See also type 2 diabetes mellitus (T2DM)
practitioner–patient relationship, 150
Prader–Willi syndrome (P-WS), 214–15
pre-diabetes, 10
prepubertal children, insulin management in, 49
preschool children, insulin management in, 49
primary care involvement, transition and, 151
protein
intake, 106
See also dietary management
psychiatric
disorders, 148
See also psychology
psychoeducational interventions
psychology, 142
See also education
psychologist role in diabetes management, **19**
psychology
adolescence and diabetes, 77, 80, **81**
anxiety, 148–9
behavioural interventions, 144, 146
depression, 148–9
diabetes management, problems with, 142
diagnosis aspects
severity of presentation, 142
treatment at home or in hospital, 142

dietary, 116–17
eating
disorders, 149–50
disturbance, 149–50
everyday life problems, 147
family
conflict, 147–8
interventions, 144, 146
glycaemic control, targeting of, 144
HbA1c, improvement in, 143–4
independence, emergence of, 147
paediatric to adult services, transition from
organisation of transition, 151
psychosocial aspects of transition, 150
peer relationships, 148
psychiatric disorders and, 148
psychoeducational interventions, 142
psychosocial interventions, 144
T1DM, 141
See also adolescence and diabetes; dietary
management
puberty
physiological changes in adolescents of, 76
See also adolescence and diabetes

rare forms of diabetes, 197
in children
cystic-fibrosis-related diabetes (CFRD), 211,
213–14
Prader–Willi syndrome (P-WS), 214–15
maturity-onset diabetes of the young (MODY),
204
genetics, 204–6
glucokinase gene mutations, 206–8
management, 209–10
transcription factors mutations, 208
neonatal diabetes, 197
ABCC8 gene mutations in PNDM and
TNDM, 203
chromosome 6q anomalies, 200
glucokinase mutations, 202
insulin promoter factor 1 (IPF-1) deficiency,
200
insulin promoter factor 1 (IPF-1) treatment,
197
IPEX (FOXP3 mutations), 201
KCNJ11 permanent neonatal diabetes, 202
permanent neonatal diabetes with cerebellar
hypoplasia, 203
very rare forms of, 203–4
Wolcott–Rallison syndrome, 201
recreational drug use and diabetes, 98–9
resuscitation, diabetic ketoacidosis and, 44
retinopathy
screening for associated conditions, 164
See also ophthalmic complications
rubella, 36
See also enterovirus infection; mumps

salt, 108
See also dietary management
scientific proof, evidence-based health care's, 2, 3

screening, T2DM, 16, **17**
screening for associated conditions
  coeliac disease, 159
    background and definition, 159
    complications, 159
    presentation and diagnosis, 159
    prevalence, 159
    screening for autoimmune conditions, 161
    treatment, 160
  complications and, 162–167, **168**
    dental abnormalities, 167
    foot care, 165
    growth, 162
    hypertension, 163
    limited joint mobility, 166
    lipids profile, 165
    macrovascular disease, 165–6
    necrobiosis lipoidica, 167
    nephropathy, 162–3
    neuropathy, 166
    ophthalmic complications, 164
    skin changes, 166
    smoking, 166
  diabetes complications, screening for, 161
  hyperthyroidism, 158
  thyroid disease, 157–8
severity
  of presentation, 142
  See also psychology
skin
  changes, 166
  See also screening for associated conditions
smoking, 166
social
  perspectives (adolescence and diabetes), 80
  support networks, 85
  worker role in diabetes management, **19**
special situations management, 93
  alcohol consumption, 97–8
  exercise, 95–7
  fasting and feasting, 99–100
  illness, 93–4
  immunisation advice, 99
  recreational drug use, 98–9
  surgery, 97
  travel, 95
storm-and-stress conceptualisation, 82
stress hyperglycaemia, 17
structured patient education (SPE), education in
    childhood diabetes and, 125–6
subcutaneous
  insulin therapy, 46
  See also diabetic ketoacidosis (DKA)
sucrose, 107
  See also dietary management
sulphonylureas, 183
  See also type 2 diabetes mellitus (T2DM)
    treatment
surgery and diabetes, 97
susceptibility locus for type 1 diabetes mellitus
    (T1DM), 27
  IDDM1, 28

IDDM12, 28–9
IDDM2, 28–9

T cells
  CD4 helper, 32
  CD8, 32
  responses, 32
telemedicine, 226
  See also information technology
therapeutic patient education, 125
thyroglobulin (TgA), 157
thyroid disease
  T1DM and, 157–8
  TPO antibodies, 158
  See also screening for associated conditions
thyroid peroxidase (TPO), 157
tissue transglutaminase (TTG), 160
TNDM, ABCC8 gene mutations in, 203
tocopherols, 108
toxic factors, T1DM, 35
TPO antibodies, 158
transcription factors mutations, MODY and, 208
transition from paediatric to adult services
  organisation of transition, 151
  psychosocial aspects of transition, 150
  See also psychology
transition of care aspects in adolescents
  how to transfer, 88
  post transition aspects, 89–90
  recommendations for transition, 88–9
  transition service formation, 89
  where and when to transfer, 87
  See also adolescence and diabetes
travel and diabetes, 95
treatment
  at home/hospital, **142**
  See also psychology
trigger factors (T1DM), 35
  infective
    enterovirus infection, 37
    mumps infections, 36
    rubella infections, 36
    virus infections, 36
  nutritional
    cow's milk proteins, 36
  toxic, 35
  See also infective factors (T1DM)
type 1 diabetes mellitus (T1DM), 9
  adolescents and, 86–7
  aetiology, 26
  alcohol consumption and, 98
  autoimmune disease, **30**
  cardiovascular considerations and, 116
  in children. See type 1 diabetes mellitus (T1DM)
    in very young children
  clinical characteristics of, **16**
  dietary management and, 104
  education in childhood diabetes, 123, 126,
    128–30
  epidemiology, 12, **13**, 14
  exercise and, 96
  genetics, 26–7

HLA haplotypes and genotypes, 27
hyperthyroidism and, 158
IDDM1 susceptibility locus for, 28
IDDM2 susceptibility locus for, 28
immune pathogenesis in, 28
immunology
   diabetes prevention and cure, 34–5
   immune pathogenesis of, 31–4
   islet cell autoantibodies, 31
   pathology of the islet in, 29
management. *See* type 1 diabetes mellitus
   (T1DM) management
psychological aspects, 141
screening for associated conditions and, 157–8
susceptibility loci
   IDDM1, 28
   IDDM12, 28–9
   IDDM2, 28–9
   with LOD scores, **30**
thyroid disease and, 157–8
trigger factors, 35
   cow's milk proteins, 36
   enterovirus infection, 37
   infective, 36
   mumps infections, 36
   nutritional, 36
   rubella infections, 36
   toxic, 35
   virus infections, 36
See also adolescence and diabetes; type 2
   diabetes mellitus (T2DM)
type 1 diabetes mellitus (T1DM) in very young
   children, 63
activity aspects and, 66
food advice for, 65–6
glycaemic control, 71
glycated haemoglobin, 70–1
health-care providers for, 66–7
hypoglycaemia, 69–70
insulin therapy, 64–5
monitoring of
   blood glucose, 69
   goals, 70
   ketone, 69
parent and carer education, 67–8
treatment goals, 64
type 1 diabetes mellitus (T1DM) management, 42
cerebral oedema, 47
   management, 47, 48
   pathophysiology, 47
diabetic ketoacidosis
   bicarbonate therapy, 45
   cerebral oedema, 46
   clinical assessment, 44
   fluid management, 44
   fluid rate, 44
   fluid type, 44, 45
   general issues-associated with, 44
   insulin therapy, 45
   management, 43
   monitoring, 46
   morbidity, 46

mortality, 46
pathophysiology, 42
phosphate replacement, 45
potassium replacement, 45
prevention, 48
resuscitation, 44
subcutaneous insulin therapy and oral fluids,
   transition to, 46
hypoglycaemia
   avoidance, 58
   prevalence, 57
   risk factors, 57
   treatment, 57–8
insulin management, 48
   adolescents, 49, 54
   continuous glucose monitoring system
      (CGMS), 56
   continuous subcutaneous insulin infusion, 54
   free mixing aspects, 54
   glucose monitoring and glycaemic control, 55
   Glucowatch biographer (GWB2), 56, 57
   home blood glucose monitoring (HBGM), 55
   hypoglycaemia and insulin regimen, 54–5
   insulin regimens, 48–9, **50–3**
   prepubertal children, 49
   preschool children, 49
type 2 diabetes mellitus (T2DM), 175
alcohol consumption and, 98
clinical characteristics of, **16**
education in childhood diabetes, 123, 128–30
environmental factors in, 175–6
fasting and feasting aspects, 100
genetics, 175–6
   calpain-10, 177
   candidate genes investigations, 178
   genome-wide scanning, 176
   goals, 181
   HNF1A, 178
   HNF4A promoter variants, 177
   importance of, 175
   insulin gene, 178
   investigations, 176
   KCNJ11 gene, 179
   NEUROD1, 178
   PPARγ gene, 179
   TCF7L2, 177
guidelines, 180
management. *See* type 2 diabetes mellitus
   (T2DM) treatment
MODY and, 17
screening for, 16, **17**
type 2 diabetes mellitus (T2DM) treatment, 180
alpha-glucosidase inhibitors, 184
comorbidities treatment
   dyslipidaemia, 185–6
   hypertension, 186–7
insulin therapy, 184–5
lifestyle changes and, 181
management algorithm, 187–8
meglitinide analogues, 184
non-alcoholic fatty liver disease (NAFLD),
   187

type 2 diabetes mellitus (T2DM) treatment (*cont.*)
  oral therapy with one agent, 182–3
  oral therapy with two agents, 183
  polycystic ovarian syndrome, 188–9
    acute management, 191
    chronic management, 191
    defined, 190
    pathophysiology, 189–90
    treatment, 191
  sulphonylureas, 183

variable number of tandem repeats (VNTR),
    28
virus infections
  enterovirus infection, 37
  mumps, 36

rubella, 36
  See also trigger factors (T1DM)
vitamins, 108
  See also dietary management

weight
  disorders, 78
  management, 108–9
  See also adolescence and diabetes; dietary
    management
Wolcott–Rallison syndrome, neonatal diabetes
    and, 201

young adult clinics
  effectiveness of, 86–7
  See also adolescence and diabetes